Recent Advances in Pharmaceutical Science

Recent Advances in Pharmaceutical Science

Editor: Ralph Hahn

AMERICAN
MEDICAL PUBLISHERS
www.americanmedicalpublishers.com

AMERICAN
MEDICAL PUBLISHERS
www.americanmedicalpublishers.com

Cataloging-in-Publication Data

Recent advances in pharmaceutical science / edited by Ralph Hahn.
p. cm.
Includes bibliographical references and index.
ISBN 978-1-63927-551-9
1. Pharmacy. 2. Drugs. 3. Pharmacology. 4. Pharmaceutical industry. I. Hahn, Ralph.
RS92 .R43 2022
615.1--dc23

American Medical Publishers,
41 Flatbush Avenue,
1st Floor, New York,
NY 11217, USA

ISBN 978-1-63927-551-9 (Hardback)

Contents

Preface

Pharmaceutical sciences are a group of interdisciplinary fields of study that are concerned with the delivery, design, action and disposition of drugs. They use tools like physical, inorganic, analytical, and biochemical chemistry, epidemiology, statistics, chemical engineering, physics, chemometrics, etc. The pharmaceutical sciences are categorized into four main branches, namely, pharmacology, pharmaceutical chemistry, pharmaceutics, and pharmacognosy. Pharmacology studies the biochemical and physiological effects of drugs on human beings and pharmaceutical chemistry is the study of drug design. Pharmaceutics focuses on the study and design of drug formulation for best delivery, stability and patient acceptance. Pharmacognosy refers to the study of medicines that are derived from natural sources. This book discusses the fundamentals as well as modern approaches to pharmaceutical science. It traces the progress of this field and highlights some of its key concepts and applications. It aims to equip students and experts with the advanced topics and upcoming concepts in this area.

After months of intensive research and writing, this book is the end result of all who devoted their time and efforts in the initiation and progress of this book. It will surely be a source of reference in enhancing the required knowledge of the new developments in the area. During the course of developing this book, certain measures such as accuracy, authenticity and research focused analytical studies were given preference in order to produce a comprehensive book in the area of study.

This book would not have been possible without the efforts of the authors and the publisher. I extend my sincere thanks to them. Secondly, I express my gratitude to my family and well-wishers. And most importantly, I thank my students for constantly expressing their willingness and curiosity in enhancing their knowledge in the field, which encourages me to take up further research projects for the advancement of the area.

Editor

Hollow microspheres for gastroretentive floating- pulsatile drug delivery: preparation and in vitro evaluation

Maryam Maghsoodi[1*], Elham Hemati[2], Bahram Qadermazi[2], Zahra Yari[2]

[1] *Drug applied Research Center and Faculty of Pharmacy, Tabriz University of Medical Sciences, Tabriz, Iran*

[2] *Student Research Committee, Tabriz University of Medical Sciences, Tabriz, Iran*

ARTICLE INFO

Keywords:
Piroxicam
Floating microparticles
pulsatile systems

ABSTRACT

Purpose: A multiparticular floating-pulsatile drug delivery system was developed for time and site specific drug release of piroxicam. A blend of floating and pulsatile principles of drug delivery system would have the advantage that a drug can be released in the upper GI tract after a definite time period. ***Methods:*** Hollow microspheres were prepared by the emulsion solvent diffusion method using Eudragit S as an enteric acrylic polymer with piroxicam at various polymer/drug ratios in a mixture of dichloromethane and ethanol. Developed formulations were evaluated for yield, encapsulation efficiency, particle size, shape, apparent density, buoyancy studies and dissolution studies. ***Results:*** The obtained microballoons were spherical with no major surface irregularity and mean particle size ranging from 250 to 380 for different batches. Formulations show a slight amount of relaese ranging from 0.7 to 11% in acidic medium (SGF) with complete release of drug in simulated intestinal fluid (SIF) in less than 3 h. Encapsulation efficiency of different formulations varied from 90 to 98%. The optimum loading amount of drug in the particles was found to impart suitable floatable properties to the microballoons. With increasing polymer/drug ratio, buancy of the microballoons increases accompanied by simultaneous reduction of apparent particle density. ***Conclusion:*** A pulsatile release of piroxicam was demonstrated by a simple drug delivery system which could be useful in chronopharmacotherapy of rheumatoid arthritis.

Introduction

Pulsatile drug delivery system (PDDS) is based on principle of rapid release of a certain amount of drug within short time period after a predetermined off-release period, lag time.[1] Such novel drug delivery has been attempted for: (i) chronopharmacotherapy of diseases which show circadian rhythms in their pathophysiology[2]; (ii) avoiding degradation of active ingredients in upper GI tract, e.g. proteins and peptides[3]; (iii) for time programmed administration of hormones and many drugs such as isosorbidedinitrate, respectively to avoid suppression of normal secretion of hormones in body that can be hampered by constant release of hormone from administered dosage form and development of resistance[4,5]; (iv) to avoid pharmacokinetic drug–drug interactions between concomitantly administered drugs[6], etc. Chronopharmacotherapy for rheumatoid arthritis has been recommended to ensure that the highest blood levels of the drug coincide with peak pain and stiffness.[7] Morning stiffness associated with pain at the time of awakening is a diagnostic criterion of the rheumatoid arthritis and these clinical circadian symptoms are supposed to be outcome of altered functioning of hypothalamic–pituitary–adrenocortical axis.[8,9] A pulsatile drug delivery system that can be administered at night (before sleep) but that release drug in early morning would be a promising chronopharmaceutic system.

Oral pulsatile drug delivery systems that release drug after a lag period of 6–7 h usually release drug in large intestine [10] however, the viscous contents of lower part of GI tract cause hindrance to the drug diffusion and also enzymatic degradation of some drugs makes it an unfavorable site for drug release.[11] Moreover, the majority of drugs are preferentially absorbed from the upper part of the small intestine [12] hence, drug release at site of better absorption can improve therapeutic efficacy of drug. This is of more concern for drug delivery that is meant for pulse drug release after a lag period of 5–6 h following oral administration of dosage

***Corresponding author:** Maryam Maghsoodi (PhD), E-mail: maghsoodim@tbzmed.ac.ir

form. A blend of floating and pulsatile principles of drug delivery system would have the advantage that a drug can be released in the upper GI tract after a definite time period of no drug release (lag period). The major objectives of the present study were to develop a simple, multiparticulate, floating-pulsatile drug delivery system for obtaining no drug release during floating time followed by pulse drug release in small intestine. Additionally, multiple unit dosage forms provide many relative advantages over single unit dosage forms such as predictable GI transit time, greater product safety, etc..[13]

The essential features of this conceptual delivery system exhibit as a (a) multiparticulate system, (b) combination of gastroretentive and pulsatile principles in same dosage form, (c) single-step formulation process (d) idealistic drug release profile that is effective at morning time intended for a particular pathological condition based on chronotherapy, and (e) having low drug release in stomach suited for non-steroidal anti-inflammatory drug (NSAID) class of drug. Piroxicam, for symptomatic relief in rheumatoid arthritis, exhibits better toleration than indomethacin, naproxen, and enteric- coated acetylsalicylic acid hence; piroxicam was used as a model drug in this study.[14]

Materials and methods

Materials

Piroxicam, PX (Shasun Chemicals & Drugs, India), Eudragit S100, Eu S100 (MW ~ 135 KDa, Rohm GmbH, Germany), polyvinyl alcohol, PVA, (MW ~ 70 KDa, 88% hydrolyzed, Sigma, Germany), and ethanol and dichloromethane (Merck, Germany) were used. The Solvents were of analytical grade.

Preparation of the microballoons

PX (0.1- 0.6g) was dissolved with Eu S100 (0.6 g) in a mixed solution of ethanol (good solvent, 5 ml), and dichloromethane (bridging liquid, 5 ml). The microballoons were prepared by slowly adding the resultant solution (during 10 min) to 200 ml 0.1 N HCl containing 0.75 % of PVA (at 25 °C) placed in a cylindrical vessel (500 ml) equipped with three baffles under agitation (400 rpm) using a propeller type stirrer with four blades. After agitating the system for 20 min the solidified microballoons were recovered by filtration. The resultant products were dried in an oven at 50 °C for 6 h.

Determination of production yield and encapsulation efficiency of microballoons

All microballoon formulations were prepared in triplicate. Microballoons dried at 50 °C were then weighed and the yield of microballoon preparation was calculated using the formula (Eq. (1)):

$$\text{Production yield (\%)} = \frac{\text{Practical mass (microballoons)}}{\text{Theoretical mass (polymer + drug)} \times 100} \quad \text{Eq. (1)}$$

Microballoons were crushed and powdered by using a mortar. Accurately weighed of this powder was extracted in ethanol. The solution was then filtered, a sample of 2ml was withdrawn from this solution and assayed spectrophotometrically to determine the PX content of the microballoons. A calibration curve based on standard solutions of PX in ethanol was used to calculate the PX concentration.

The encapsulation efficiency (%) was calculated by using following Equation (Eq. (2)).

$$\text{Encapsulation efficiency (\%)} = \left(\frac{M_{actual}}{M_{theoretical}}\right) \times 100 \quad \text{Eq. (2)}$$

Where M_{actual} is the actual PX content in weighed quantity of powder of microballoons and $M_{theoretical}$ is the theoretical amount of PX in microballoons calculated from the quantity added in the fabrication process. The means of three assays were reported.

Measurement of micromeritic properties

Size distribution and mean diameter were determined by the sieving method. A total of 25 g of material was sieved using an Erweka vibration sieve (Erweka, Germany) through a nest of sieves. The vibration rate was set at 200 strokes/min and the sieving time was 10 min. The powder fractions retained by the individual sieves were determined and expressed as mass percentages. The morphology of the microballoonss was observed by optical microscopy (Nikon Labophot, Tokyo, Japan). Apparent particle density and roundness was determined by the projective image method as follows. Microballoons were placed on a glass plate and Heywood diameter, microballoon number, circumference of a projective image and area of a projective image were measured by an Image analyzing software (scion image analyzer). Subsequently, the apparent particle density and roundness were calculated according to Eq. (3) and Eq. (4), respectively.

$$\text{Apparent particle density } w/v = w/\sum(\pi d^3 n/6) \quad \text{Eq. (3)}$$

where W = weight of microballoons, V = volume of microballoons, d = Heywood diameter, and n = number of microballoons.

$$\text{Roundness of microballoons} = L^2/4\pi s \quad \text{Eq. (4)}$$

where L = circumference of a projective image and S = area of a projective image. When the roundness of microballoons was close to 1, the microballoons closely resembled spherical particles.

Flowability of the crystals was assessed by determining the angle of repose and the compressibility index (Carr index). The angle of repose was measured by a fixed funnel method.[15] The Carr index [16,17] is a measure of the propensity of a powder to consolidate. Changes occurring in packing arrangement during the taping procedure are expressed as the Carr index (CI).

CI= [(tapped density – bulk density) / tapped density] × 100
Eq. (5)

The Carr index reflects the packability of the powders, and there is also a correlation between the Carr index and the flowability of the crystals. The results presented are mean value of six determinations.

Differential scanning calorimetery (DSC)

The thermal characteristics of the microballoons and pure drug were determined using a differential scanning calorimeter (DSC60, Shimadzu, Japan). After calibration with indium and lead standards, samples of the crystals (3–5 mg) were heated (range 25-300°C) at 10 °C/min in hermetically sealed aluminum pans.

X-ray powder diffraction (XRPD)

In order to investigate polymorphism X-ray was used. The cavity of the metal sample holder of the X-ray diffractometer was filled with the ground sample powder and then smoothed with a spatula. X-ray diffraction pattern of PX samples was obtained using the X-ray diffractometer (Siemens, Model D5000, Germany) at 40 kV, 30 mA and a scanning rate of 0.06°/min over the range 2θ=5–40, using CuKα1 radiation of wavelength 1.5405A°.

Buoyancy percentage

Microballoons (100 mg) were spread over the surface of a USP XXIV dissolution apparatus (type II) filled with 900 mL 0.1 mol L^{-1}HCl containing 0.02% Tween 20.[18] The medium was agitated with a paddle rotating at 100 rpm for 8 h. The floating and the settled portions of microballoons were recovered separately. The microballoons were dried and weighed. Buoyancy percentage was calculated as the ratio of the mass of the microballoons that remained floating and the total mass of the microballoons.

In vitro release studies

The in vitro dissolution of microballoons was determined with a USP rotating paddle method (900 ml 0.1 N HCl or pH 7.4 phosphate buffer; 100 rpm; 37°C; n =3). At preset time intervals aliquots were withdrawn and replaced by an equal volume of dissolution medium to maintain constant volume. After suitable dilution, the samples were analyzed spectrophotometrically at 333.2 and 349.2 nm for the 0.1 N HCl and pH 7.4 phosphate buffer, respectively.

Results and discussion

The microballoons prepared in this study, as observed in Figure 1, were near spherical in shape with a central hollow core surrounded by a shell as shown in the photograph of a broken half of a microballoon. The cavity was supposedly formed as follows according to the previous reports.[19-21] As soon as the polymer solution was added to the aqueous medium, the ethanol diffused rapidly from the droplets of the polymer solution because of higher solubility of ethanol in water than dichloromethane. As ethanol diffuses through the aqueous solution, accompanied by simultaneous diffusion of water inside the sphere, the solubility of the polymer in the droplet is drastically reduced and reduces the coprecipitation of drug and polymer at the interface of the emulsion droplet, forming a solid shell covering the droplet. Dichloromethane evaporation appeared to be especially related to cavity formation in microballoons and properties of formed solid shell. Dichloromethane remaining as the central core diffused slowly due to its low water solubility. Therefore, the diffusion of dichloromethane began late, after the initial solidification, and formed a central hollow structure. As shown in photomicrographs the shape and shell thickness of the microballoons were different among the formulations. Preparation at higher polymer/drug ratio provided microballoons with a thin shell as to crumble upon touching and roundness close to 1 while the microballoons prepared at lower polymer/drug ratio showed thicker shell, probably arising as a trace of solvent evaporation.

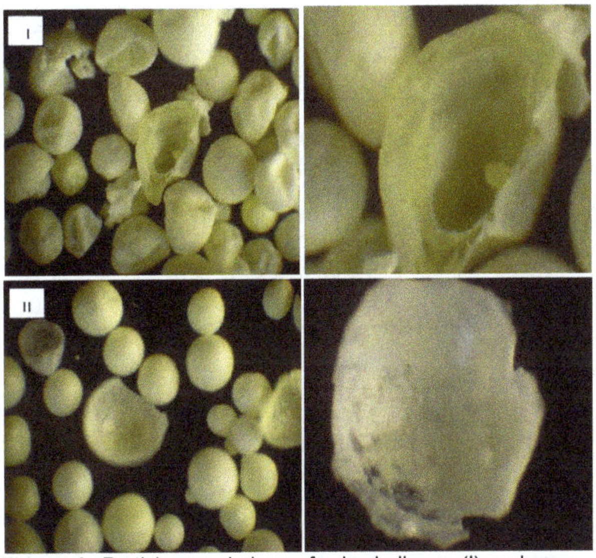

Figure 1. Particle morphology of microballoons (I): polymer: drug (1:1) and (II) polymer: drug (:1), right photographs (×100) left photographs (×500).

These results could be explained by considering the mechanism of formation of microballons as previously noted. Microballoons shells were conveniently formed by coprecipitation of drug and polymers, as well as successive evaporation of the inner solvent.

It is assumable that any factor which could modify the time needed to reach the physical state-transition boundaries of the polymeric solution (solution-gel-glass) during the hardening process will be effective in the polymer precipitation and consequently in solvent evaporation rate.[22]The polymer -to- drug ratio can be a critical factor during microballoon formation. The increase in polymer/drug ratio leads to a shorter time for the composition of the polymer solution to reach the viscous (gelation) boundary, resulting in a rapid film-like membrane formation on the droplets periphery. If the film-like polymeric membrane is quickly solidified, the microballoon structure is more fixed and thus solvent evaporation is delayed.[22] As previously explained a slow rate of evaporation of dichloromethane led to formation of porous microballoons as dichloromethane remained in the pockets preventing formation of a hard polymer shell. Thus it can be concluded that thin and porous structure of the microballoons shell prepared at higher polymer /drug ratio was attributed to slower rate of evaporation of dichloromethan as a consequence of rapid polymer shell formation.

On the other hand, the slower solidification of the polymeric shell at the droplet periphery due to decreasing polymer/drug ratio, delays creation of shell barrier to mass transfer, increases solvent evaporation rate and consequently increases the rigidity of the polymer shell.

Microballoons displaying diameters of between 250 and 380 µm (Table 1). Theparticle size increased with increasing the polymer / drug ratio. This is due to the increase in viscosity of the solution and the decrease in stirring efficiency. Also with increasing polymer/drug ratio, the hardening time of the microballoons was shortened. Consequently, a shorter time was provided for the breakup of droplets and larger microballoons were formed. Flowability results are shown in Table 1 as expressed in term of angle of repose and the compressibility index. All formulations showed high flowability as angle of repose ranged between 17.5 to 23 ° and the compressibility index ranged between7% to 11%. The excellent flow property indicates that the floating microballoons produced are non-aggregated (Table 1).

Table 1. Mean diameter, angle of repose, Carr's Index, yield and encapsulation efficiency of samples

samples		Mean diameter ± σ (µm)	sphericity	Angle of repose (°)	Carr's Index (%)	Yield (%)	Encapsulation efficiency (%)	Buancy 8h (%)	Apparent particle density (g/cm³)
Untreated PX		10.75±0.36	-	35.8±1.3	32.3±0.6	-	-	-	-
Eu:PX	1:1	250±110	0.98±0.02	17.5±0.9	7.0± 0.2	73.8±0.8	90.8±0.5	62.5±1.0	0.5±0.03
	2:1	290±80	0.96±0.03	20.7±1.0	10.8±0.3	70.6±1.0	92.5±0.6	77.7±0.9	0.29±0.03
	4:1	310±260	0.93±0.03	19.1±1.5	9.1±0.1	68.8±0.9	95.4±0.4	80.2±0.8	0.22±0.04
	6:1	380±220	0.92±0.02	23.0±0.6	11.0±0.3	65.5±1.1	98.3±0.4	85.4±1.1	0.19±0.04

Yield and encapsulation efficiency

The percentage yield of floating microballoons determined by weighing after drying was73, 70, 68 and 65% for microballoons prepare at 1:1, 2:1, 4:1 and 6:1 polymer/drug ratios, respectively. Decreasing yield of microballoons by increasing polymer/drug ratio ($p< 0.05$) may be due to higher viscosity of polymer which resulted in agglomeration of droplets and adhering to the vessel wall and propeller. As can be seen in Table 1, the encapsulation efficiencies were high in all formulations (>90%).The high encapsulation efficiencies probably result from the poor water solubility of the drug in the external aqueous phase. Slight loss of drug may be due to some dissolution prior to drop formation or during the hardening process in polyvinyl alcohol solution mixed with diffused ethanol.[23] The ratio 'polymer / drug' affected the resulting encapsulation efficiency. With more polymer/drug ratios, higher encapsulation efficiencies were produced. For instance, PX encapsulation efficiency was increased from 90.8% to 98.3 % as polymer:drug ratio was increased from 1:1 to 6:1.

This can either be attributed to the increased probability for the drug to be entrapped within the microballoons with increasing ratio of polymer to drug, and/or to the decreasing drug loss into the external water phase under these conditions. These results can be also related to hardening process of microballoons. Increasing polymer/drug ratio leads to a more viscous droplets and consequently faster solidification rate of microballoons. Therefore, the microballoon structure is more fixed and thus solvent and nonsolvent counter- diffusion is delayed. As a result, less water may be allowed to diffuse into the droplets and consequently less amount of drug will be carried by the solvent into the aqueous phase.[22]

DSC and X-ray diffraction results

The DSC curves and X-ray diffraction pattern of the microballoons are shown in Figure 2 and Figure 3, respectively. As shown in Figure 2, the melting peak of the drug in the microballoons disappeared with increasing the ratio of polymer/drug from 1:1 to 2:1, although the melting peak was observed in the physical mixtures of the drug and polymer with the same ratio. These indicated that PX had been disordered in the microballoons at 2:1 polymer/ drug ratio, suggesting that PX had been highly dispersed at this ratio, so as amorphous state.

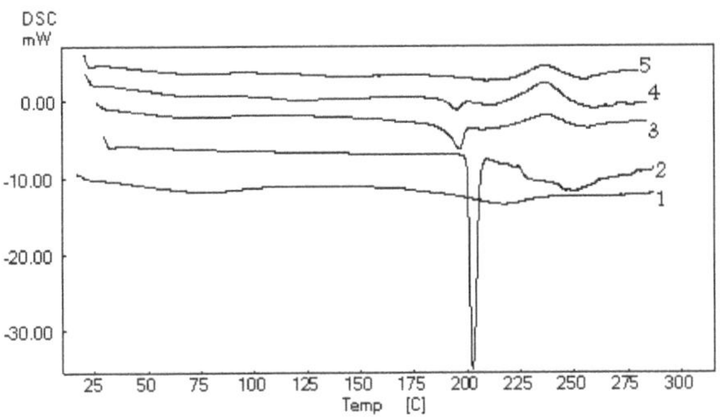

Figure 2. DSC scans of 1) polymer 2) untreated drug 3) polymer:drug (1:1), 4) physical .

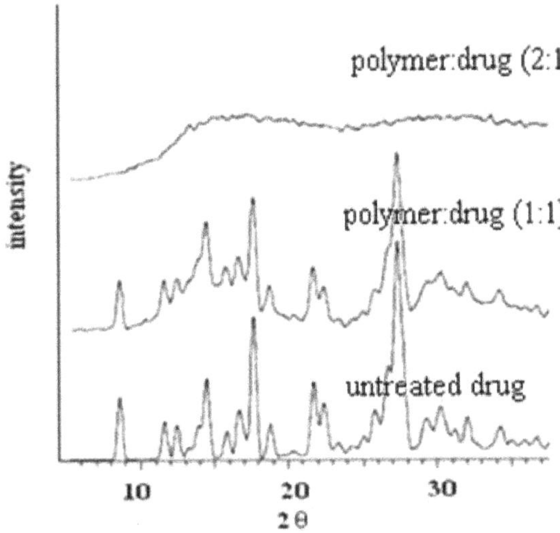

Figure 3. The X-ray diffraction patterns of untreated drug and microballoons prepared at polymer: drug ratios of 1:1 and 2:1.

This was further supported by the X-ray analysis data given in Figure 3, which shows the representative diffraction patterns for the pure drug, the microballoons prepared at 1:1 and 2:1 polymer/drug ratios. Characteristic peaks of piroxicam appeared at a diffraction angle of 2θ, at 8.99, 15.76, 23.02 and 25.85°. These values were comparable to those reported for form I of PX.[24] Crystalline peaks were observed in the 1:1polymer/drug ratio but no crystalline peaks of PX were found in the microballoons at 2:1 polymer /drug ratio. The scans and XRPD patterns of microballoons produced at 4:1 and 6:1 polymer/drug ratios are similar to 2:1 ratio and hence not all of them are shown. In summary, the DSC and XRPD data indicated no sign of interaction between the drug and the polymer and also showed that the PX inside the microballoons was changed only in its crystallinity.

Floating properties

To assess the floating properties, microballoons were placed in 0.1 HCl containing 0.02% polysorbate, in order to simulate surface tension of human gastric juice (35-50mN/m2).[18] Buoyancy of beads is directly related to performance of floating-pulsatile drug delivery system since lag time for beads is equivalent to their floating time.

Apparent particle density and buoyancy of microballoons prepared at various polymer/drug ratios were measured. It is noticeable that during the floating test, no swelling or gelation of the microballoons was found. In accordance with polymer/drug ratio (1:1, 2:1, 4:1 and 6:1), buoyancy and apparent particle density of the resulting microballoons varied distinctly as presented in Table 1. According to results, by increasing the polymer/drug ratio, the buoyancy of the microballoons largely increased, accompanied by decreased particle density. For instance, the microballoons prepared at 6:1 polymer/drug showed highest buoyancy as a consequence of lowest particle density. Therefore, it was concluded that the buoyancy of the microballoons appeared to be more greatly affected by the apparent particle density. Decreasing apparent particle density with increasing polymer /drug ratio could be explained by considering the mechanism of formation of microballons as previously noted. As can be seen in Figure 1, preparation at higher polymer/drug ratio provided larger microballoons with thinner shell. As previously described, this was attributed to slow rate of evaporation of dichloromethane as a consequence of rapid polymer shell formation.

Moreover, in other researches, it was observed that the microballoons of larger size, showed the longer floating time. Therefore, increasing buoyancy of microballons by increasing the polymer/drug ratio may also be attributed to larger particle size by increasing polymer/drug ratio (Table 1).[25,26]

In vitro drug release

Release of the drug from Eu S100 based microballoons was evaluated in pH 1.2 and 7.4. Release studies in SGF for 6 h showed only 0.7–11% cumulative drug release from beads of different batches (Figure 4).

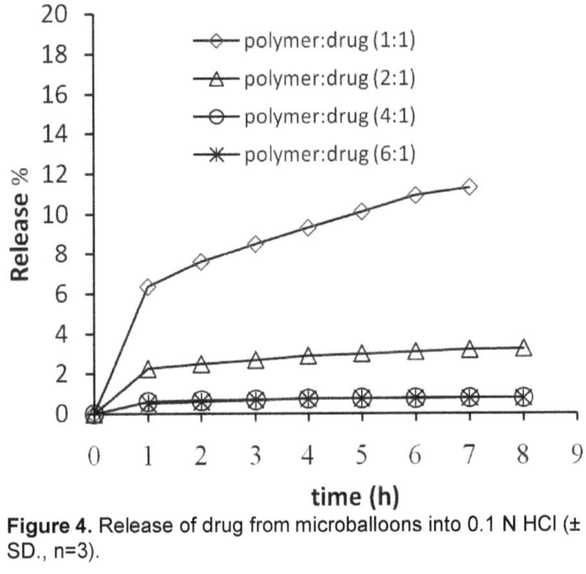

Figure 4. Release of drug from microballoons into 0.1 N HCl (± SD., n=3).

Since the acrylic polymer used is not soluble in acidic pH and starts to dissolve above pH 7[27], no marked amount of drug was released from the microballoons in SGF. Drug release from Eu S100 in SGF took place only through diffusion and drug release in SIF (pH 7.4) might have involved both mechanisms i.e. diffusion and erosion.

All the batches of beads showed fast disintegration and drug release in SIF due to pH dependent dissolving of Eudragit S. Complete drug dissolution from beads of each batch occurred during 3h in SIF, which would be useful in in vivo drug absorption from large surface area of small intestine. Small intestinal transit time for a drug formulation or for a meal is known to be almost constant at about 3 h.[28] As shown in Figure 5, although the drug release from beads of all batches was sufficiently rapid in SIF, the composition of bead showed significant effect on drug release rate and the drug release was inversely related to polymer/drug ratio. For example, batches prepared by using 6:1or 4:1 polymer/drug ratios showed marked slower drug release than beads prepared by using 2:1or 1:1 polymer/drug ratios. This significant effect of polymer/drug ratio on drug release in SIF may be attributed to formation of stronger and thicker gel formation with increase in polymer/drug that restrict the drug diffusion through the beads.

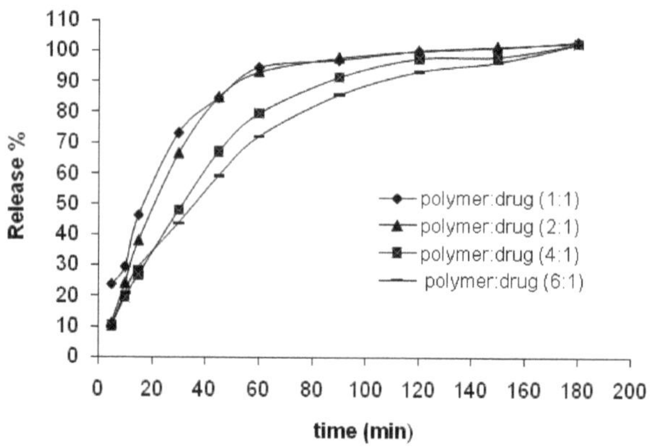

Figure 5. Release of drug from microballoons into pH 7.4 phosphate buffer (± SD., n=3).

Conclusion

As results showed, properties (buoyancy, apparent particle density, size and sphericity) of microballoons varied according to the polymer/drug ratio. Microballoons prepared at polymer/drug ratio higher than 2:1 were so brittle as to crumble upon touching and the buoyancy was higher probably due to lower apparent particle densities of these microballoons. The floating test revealed that approximately 85% of the microballoons with 6:1 polymer/drug ratio were still floating after 8h. During the floating test, no swelling or gelation of the microballoons was found, which suggested that they were dispersed individually in the stomach without adhesion to the mucosa. This property should avoid local irritation due to a localized overdose, which frequently occurs with the bioadhesion system. The beads showed fast drug release in SIF after sufficient floating time in SGF where no noticeable drug released. In conclusion, the piroxicam-loaded Eu S100 microballoons, prepared using a solvent diffusion method, have the qualities suitable for their successful use as pulsatile drug delivery system.

Acknowledgment

The financial support from the Drug applied Research Center of Tabriz University of Medical Sciences is greatly acknowledged.

Conflict of interest

The authors report no conflicts of interest. The authors alone are responsible for the content and writing of the paper.

References

1. Kikuchi A, Okano T. Pulsatile drug release control using hydrogels. *Adv Drug Deliv Rev* 2002; 54:53–77.
2. Sawada T, Kondo H, Nakashima H, Sako K, Hayashi M. Time-release compression-coated core tablet containing nifedipine for chronopharmacotherapy. *Int J Pharm* 2004; 280:103–111.
3. Rubinstein A, Tirosh B, Baluom M, Nassar T, David A, Radai R, Gliko-Kabir I, Friedman M. The rationale for peptide drug delivery to the colon and the potential of polymeric carriers as effective tools. *J Control Release* 1997; 46:59–73.
4. Terasawa E, Keen KL, Mogi K, Claude P. Pulsatile release of luteinizing hormone-release (LHRH) in cultured LHRH neurons derived from the embryolic olfactory placode of the rhesus monkey. *Endocrinology* 1999; 140:1432–1441.
5. Charloux A, Gronfier C, Lonsdorfer-Wolf E, Piquard F, Brandenberger G. Aldosterone release during the sleep-wake cycle in humans. *Am J Physiol* 1999; 276: E43–E49.
6. Sawada T, Sako K, Yoshihara K, Nakamura K, Yokohama S, Hayashi M. Timed-release formulation to avoid drug–drug interaction between diltiazem and midazolam. *J Pharm Sci* 2003; 92: 790–797.
7. Stehlin I. A time to heal: chronotherapy tunes in to body's rhythms. *FDA Consumer* 1997; 31:16.
8. Crofford LJ, Kalogeras KT, Mastorakos G, Magiakou MA, Kanik KS, Gold PW, Chrousos GP, Wilder RL. Circadian relationships between interleukin (IL)-6 and hypothalamic-pitutary-adrenal axis hormones: failure of IL-6 to cause sustained hypercortisolism in patients with early untreated rheumatoid arthritis. *J Clin Endocr Metab* 1997; 82: 1279–1283.
9. Cutolo M, Seriolo B, Craviotto C, Pizzorni C, Sulli A. Circadian rhythms in RA. *Ann Rheum Dis* 2003; 62: 593–596.

10. Niwa K, Takaya T, Morimoto T, Takada K. Preparation and evaluation of a time-controlled release capsule made of ethylcellulose for colon delivery of drugs. *J Drug Target* 1995; 3: 83–89.
11. Hoffman A, Stepensky D, Lavy E, Eyal S, Klausner E, Friedman M. Pharmacokinetic and pharmacodynamic aspects of gastroretentive dosage forms. *Int J Pharm* 2004; 277: 141–153.
12. Rouge N, Buri P, Doelker E. Drug absorption sites in the gastrointestinal tract and dosage forms for site-specific delivery. *Int J Pharm* 1996; 136: 117–139.
13. Ritschel WA. Targeting in the gastrointestinal tract: new approaches. *Methods Find Exp Clin Pharmacol* 1991; 13: 313–336.
14. Heynen G. Toleration and safety of piroxicam. *Eur J Rheumatol Inflamm* 1987; 8:86–93.
15. Pilpel N. The flow properties of magnesia. *J Pharm Pharmacol* 1964; 16: 705–16.
16. Carr RL. Evaluation flow properties of solids. *Chem Eng* 1965; 72:163–8.
17. Carr RL. Classify flow properties of solids. *Chem Eng* 1965; 72:69–72.
18. El-Gibaly I. Development and in vitro evaluation of novel floating chitosan microcapsules for oral use: comparison with non floating chitosan microballoons. *Int J Pharm* 2002; 249: 7–21.
19. Sato Y, Kawashima Y, Takeuchi H, Yamamoto H. Physicochemical properties to determine the buoyancy of hollow microballoons (microballoons) prepared by the emulsion solvent diffusion method. *Eur J Pharm Biopharm* 2003; 55:297–304.
20. Kawashima Y, Niwa T, Takeuchi H, Hino T, Itoh Y. Preparation of multiple unit hollow microballoons (microballoons) with acrylic resin containing tranilast and their drug release characteristics (in vitro) and floating behavior (in vivo). *J Control Release* 1991; 16:279–290.
21. Kawashima Y, Niwa T, Takeuchi H, Hino T, Itoh Y. Hollow microballoons for use as a floating controlled drug delivery system in the stomach. *J Pharm Sci* 1992; 81:135–140.
22. Re MI, Biscans B. Preparation of microballoons of Ketoprofen with acrylic polymers by a quasi-emulsion solvent diffusion method. *Powder technology* 1999; 101: 120-133.
23. Zaniboni HC, Fell JT, Collett JH. Production and characterization of enteric beads. *Int J Pharm* 1995; 125:151-155.
24. Vrecer F, Vrbinc M, Meden A. Characterization of piroxicam crystal modifications. *Int J Pharm* 2003; 256: 3-15.
25. Jain SK, Awasthi AM, Jain NK, Agrawal GP. Calcium silicate based microballoons of repaglinide for gastroretentive floating drug delivery: Preparation and in vitro characterization. *J Control Release* 2005; 107: 300-309.
26. Singh AN, Pathak K. Development and evaluation of dual controlled release microballoons containing riboflavin and citric acid: in vitro and in vivo evaluation. *J Microencapsul* 2011; 28: 442-54.
27. Yoo JW, Giri N, Lee CH. pH-sensitive Eudragit nanoparticles for mucosal drug delivery. *Int J Pharm* 2011; 403: 262-267.
28. Davis SS, Hardy JG, Fara JW. Transit of pharmaceutical dosage forms through the small intestine. *Gut* 1986; 27: 886–892.

2

Protective effect of NAC against malathion-induced oxidative stress in freshly isolated rat hepatocytes

Sara Mostafalou[1,2,4], Mohammad Abdollahi[3], Mohammad Ali Eghbal[1,2]*, Nazli Saeedi Kouzehkonani[1]

[1] *Drug Applied Research Center, Tabriz University of Medical Sciences, Tabriz, Iran.*

[2] *Department of Pharmacology and Toxicology, Faculty of Pharmacy, Tabriz University of Medical Sciences, Tabriz, Iran.*

[3] *Faculty of Pharmacy, and Pharmaceutical Sciences Research Center, Tehran University of Medical Sciences, Tehran, Iran.*

[4] *Students Research Committee, Tabriz University of Medical Sciences, Tabriz, Iran.*

ARTICLE INFO

Keywords:
Organophosphate Pesticides
Cytotoxicity
Oxidative Stress
Mitochondria
N-actylcycteine
Hepatocytes

ABSTRACT

Purpose: Induction of oxidative stress by Organophosphate compounds (OPs) has been previously reported. In the present work, the mechanism of protective effects of N-acetylcysteine as a glutathion (GSH) prodrug against malathion–induced cell toxicity was investigated. In this work, freshly isolated rat hepatocytes were used to determine the effect of NAC on malathion-induced cytotoxicity, formation of reactive oxygen species (ROS) and mitochondrial dysfunction. ***Methods:*** Rat hepatocytes were isolated using collagenase perfusion and then cell viability, mitchondrial membrane potential (MMP) and ROS formation were determined using trypan blue exclusion, Rhodamine 123 fluorescence and fluorogenic probe, 2', 7' -dichlorofluorescin diacetate (DCFH-DA), respectively. ***Results:*** Despite the protective effect of NAC on malathion-induced cell toxicity and MMP dysfunction, its efficacy against ROS formation was not adequate to completely protect the cells. ***Conclusion:*** Cytotoxic effects of malathion regardless of its cholinergic feature, is started with gradual free radical production but, the main factor that causes cell death, is mitochondrial dysfunction, so that reduction of ROS formation alone is not sufficient for cell survival, and the maintenance of mitochondrial integrity through different mechanisms is the most ameliorative factor specially at high levels of cell damage, as NAC seemed to protect cells with various fashions apart from ROS scavenging in concentrations higher than malathion's LC50.

Introduction

Malathion is one of the most widely used organophosphate compounds (OPs) applied in different fields like agriculture (as a pesticide), veterinary practice (as an ectoparasiticide), treatment of body lice on humans, food preparation and processing areas.[1] OPs are cholinesterase inhibiting chemicals and the main cause of pesticide poisonings.[2] Besides inhibiting cholinesterase (ChE), oxidative stress has been recently proposed as a main toxicity mechanism for OPs both in acute and chronic poisoning cases.[3-5] Increased lipid peroxidation and diminished antioxidant defense capacity particularly glutathione are important findings accounted for OPs toxicity.[6] Generation of oxidative intermediates induced by various agents has been predicated in cell death processes mainly mediated by the intracellular organelle mitochondriaMitochondria.[7] are important intracellular source of ROS because of being the oxidative phosphorylation station in the cells and a susceptive target for damaging effects of ROS under certain phathological situations owing to abundance of tetraacyl phospholipid cardiolipin in their membrane.[8-10] Mitochodrial membrane integrity is important for efficient oxidative phosphorylation.[11] While increased ROS production is a harmful outcome of mitochondrial dysfunction[12], there is lots of evidence underlining the responsibility of mitochondrial impairment for ROS signaling via apoptotic pathways.[13-14] Despite this, mitochondria have some antioxidant defense systems that help protect it against deleterious effects of ROS. The most important agents for mitochondrial antioxidant protection are the tripeptide glutathione (GSH) and multiple GSH-linked antioxidant enzymes.[15]

Considering oxidative stress induction by OPs pesticides, several studies proposed that a drug that could act as a multiplier of GSH content and a reductant would improve the cell tolerance towards OP-toxicity. In this regard, N-acetyl-L-cysteine (NAC) as a cell-permeable GSH prodrug that acts through direct scavenging of free radicals and revival of glutathione and cysteine can be a good candidate. Recently, our team reported that NAC can prevent toxicity of OPs in rats.[16]

***Corresponding author:** Mohammad Ali Eghbal (PHD), Drug Applied Research Center, and Faculty of Pharmacy, Tabriz University of Medical Sciences, Tabriz, Iran. E-mail: m.eghbal@utoronto.ca

The liver that is of extraordinary importance in detoxification of toxic metabolites acts as a potential site for OPs- induced damages.[17, 18] Since bio-transformation of thiono-OP as an imperative mechanism of their activation is mostly occurred in the liver, this organ is considered as one of the preliminary targets for malathion- induced toxicities.[19]

In this study, the role of mitochondrial dysfunction and enhanced ROS formation in malathion- induced cytotoxicity as well as the protective effect of NAC against it has been examined.

Materials and Methods

Chemicals

Bovine serum albumin, collagenase A from clostridium histolyticum and HEPES from Roche Diagnostics (Indianapolis, IN), 2',7'-dichlorofluorescin diacetate (DCFH-DA) and rhodamine 123 from Fluka (Italy), N-acetyl-cysteine (NAC) and 1-bromoheptane from Acros Pharmaceuticals, heparin sodium salt grade 1-A, trypan blue, methanol, and malathion 90% from Merck (Germany) were used in this study.

Animals

Male Sprague–Dawley rats (200–250 g) were obtained from the Laboratory of Animal Research Center of Tabriz University (Medical Sciences). The rats were housed in an air-conditioned room, under controlled temperature of 23 ± 1°C, relative humidity of 36 ± 6% and 12 h light/12 h dark conditions for 1 week before starting the experiments. They were allowed to feed with standard laboratory chaw and tap water *ad libitum*. Procedures involving animals and their care were conducted in conformity with the NIH guidelines for the care and use of laboratory animals.

Preparation of hepatocytes

Hepatocytes were isolated from adult male Sprague–Dawley rats (220–250 g), by a two-step collagenase perfusion of the liver as described previously.[20] After isolation, the cells were suspended (10^6cells/ml) in Krebs-Henseleit buffer (NaCl 118 mM; KCl 4.7 mM; KH_2PO_4 1.17 mM; $MgSO_4.7H_2O$ 1.19 mM; $CaCl_2.2H_2O$ 2.58 mM; $NaHCO_3$ 25mM) containing 12.5 mM HEPES (4-(2-hydroxyethyl)-1-piperazineethanesulfonic acid) and incubated under a stream of 95% O2 and 5% CO2 in continuously rotating round-bottomed 50 ml flasks at 37 °C for 30 minutes before the addition of chemicals. Stock solutions of chemicals were made either in incubation buffer or in methanol and added to the hepatocyte suspensions at the indicated time points. Cell viability was measured by Trypan blue exclusion method.[20] The hepatocytes used in this study were at least 85-90% viable immediately after isolation.

Exposure of hepatocytes to malathion and NAC

According to a previous report on the toxicity and metabolism of malathion in isolated rat hepatocytes [21] as well as our pilot studies, concentrations in the range of 0.5-1.5 mM were chosen to be used in this experimental set up. malathion was dissolved in methanol and NAC was dissolved in deionized double distilled water and added to the flasks containing the hepatocytes (10^6 cells /ml) at mentioned time intervals. 1- bromoheptane was dissolved in methanol and was added to the flasks 30 minutes before adding malathion. The utilized concentration of both NAC and 1- bromoheptane was 200 μM in cell suspensions.

Measurement of ROS formation

ROS formation was measured according to Eghbal et al., 2004b.[22] Briefly, DCFH-DA was dissolved in methanol. The final concentration of DCFH-DA in cell suspensions (10^6 cells per ml) was 1 μM. DCFH-DA was added to the cell suspensions at the same time as malathion and a 100 μl aliquot was taken and diluted in 2ml of the incubation buffer. The samples were taken and the fluorescence intensity was measured at the excitation wavelength 485 nm and the emission wavelength 530 nm.

Measurement of mitochondrial membrane potential

Mitochondrial membrane potential in hepatocytes was assessed by monitoring the uptake of the cationic dye, rhodamine 123 as described.[23-24] Isolated cells were extracted then resuspended in original media containing 1 μM rhodamine 123. After 10 minutes of incubation, the cells were centrifuged and the supernatant was measured with a Shimadzu RF-5000U spectrofluorimeter. The amount of dye remaining in the supernatant was inversely proportional to the membrane potential of the cells.

Statistical analysis

Statistical comparisons were carried out using a one-way analysis of variance (ANOVA) followed by the Bonferroni *t*-test (post-hoc) for multiple comparisons to determine statistical significance ($P < 0.05$) between treatments and control groups.

Results

Cytotoxic effect of malathion on freshly isolated rat hepatocytes

Figure 1 indicates the absolute toxicity of malathion in concentrations above 0.5 mM whereas the 1 and/or 1.5 mM caused significant cell death. Malathion at 2 mM caused 100% mortality 3 hours after incubation.

Effect of malathion on MMP in freshly isolated rat hepatocytes

Figure 2 illustrates the relative percentages of MMP in test groups in comparison with the control, where the 100 percent of Rhodamine 123 trapping occurred in the intact mitochondria. As shown, there was a significant difference in MMP of the malathion-treated cells (1 &1.5 mM) in comparison with the control.

Effect of malathion on ROS formation in freshly isolated rat hepatocytes

As shown in figure 3, ROS formation was significantly increased in 1 and 1.5 mM of malathion-treated cells in comparison with the control while 0.5 mM did not show a significant effect.

Effect of 1-bromoheptane on malathion toxicity

Table 1 compares the different rates of malathion-induced cytotoxicity in the cells pre-incubated with 1-bromoheptane to that in the cells treated with different concentrations of malathion only. In the presence of 1-bromoheptane, the cytotoxicity of malathion was intensified and the rate of cell mortality was increased even with nontoxic concentrations of malathion (0.25, 0.5 mM).

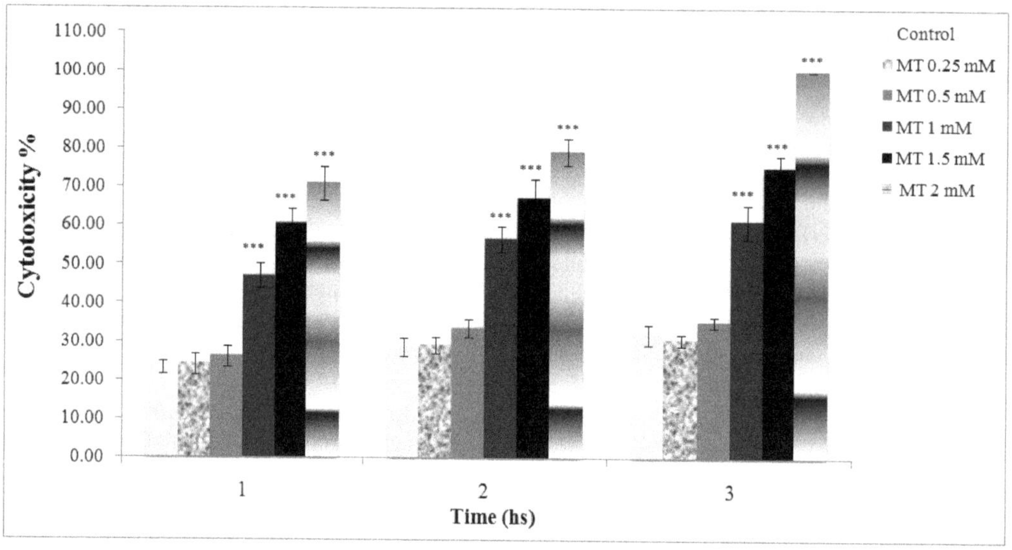

Figure 1. Cytotoxic effect of malathion on freshly isolated rat hepatocytes

Malathion was added to the flasks containing the hepatocytes to make the concentrations (1 and 1.5 mM) and cell viability was measured with uptake of trypane blue. All results were shown in mean ±S.E.M and are at least from 3 independent experiments. MT (malathion)

***Shows significant difference ($p<0.001$) with control

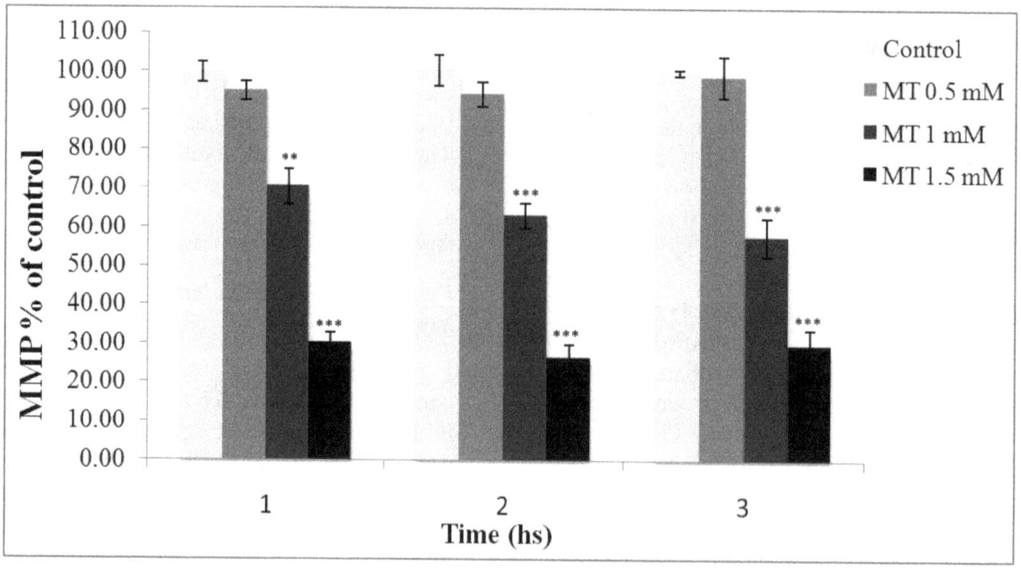

Figure 2. Effect of malathion on mitochondrial membrane potential in freshly isolated rat hepatocytes

Rhodamine was added to the aliquots of cell suspensions and the fluorescence amounts of the samples were measured with a Shimadzu RF-5000U spectrofluorimeter. The amount of dye remaining in the supernatant was inversely proportional to the membrane potential of the cells. All results were shown in mean ±S.E.M and are at least from 3 independent experiments. MT (malathion), MMP (mitochondrial membrane potential)

**Shows significant difference ($p<0.01$) with control

***Shows significant difference ($p<0.001$) with control

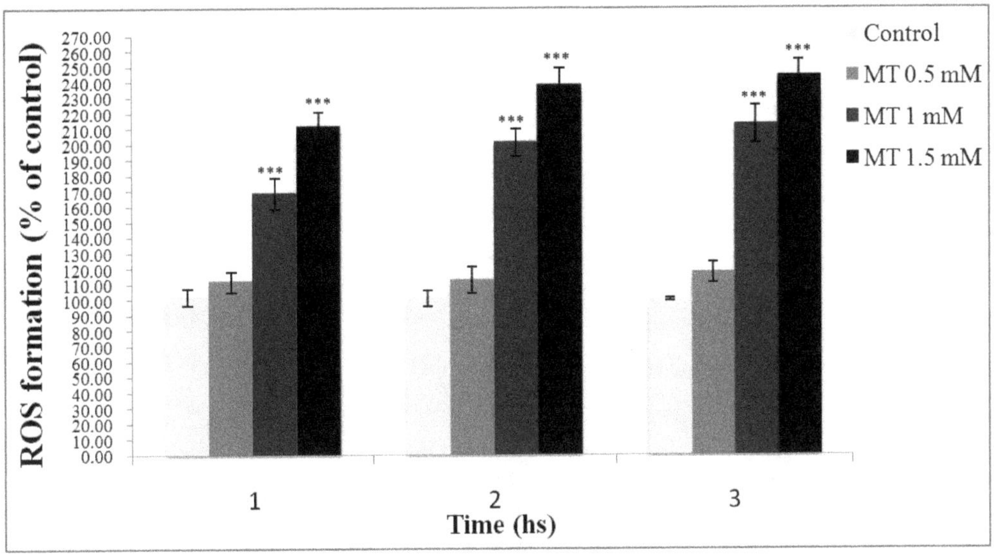

Figure 3. Effect of malathion on ROS formation in freshly isolated rat hepatocytes
DCF was added to the flasks containing hepatocytes at the same time as malathion and the fluorescence intensity was measured at the excitation wavelength 485 nm and the emission wavelength at 530 nm. All results were shown in mean ±S.E.M and are at least from 3 independent experiments. MT (malathion), ROS (reactive oxygen species)
***Shows significant difference ($p<0.001$) with control

Table 1. Effect of 1-bromoheptane on malathion cytotoxicity

Treatments \ Time Intervals	Cytotoxicity (%)		
	1 Hs	2 Hs	3Hs
Normal Cells (without treatment)	23.±1.7	28±2.3	32±2.7
" + MT 0.25mM	24±2.7	29±2.1	30±1.4
" + MT 0.5mM	26±2.6	33±2.3	35±1.4
" + MT 1mM	47±3.2 [c]	56±3.3 [c]	61±4.4 [c]
" + MT 1. 5mM	60±3.8 [c]	67±5.2 [c]	75±3.1 [c]
1-BH 200µM treated Cells	24±3.1	31±3.4	32±2.3
" + MT 0.25mM	43±2.8 [b]	46±3.4 [a]	49±3.5 [a]
" + MT 0. 5mM	48±4.1 [b]	55±2.9 [b]	57±4.3 [b]
" + MT 1mM	54±2.3 [c]	81±2.6 [c]	83±4.6 [c]
" + MT 1. 5mM	72±3.4 [c]	86±3.2 [c]	100±0.0 [c]

Hepatocytes were incubated in Krebs–Henseleit solution, pH 7.4 at 37 °C under the atmosphere of 95%O2/5%CO2.The samples were taken at mentioned time intervals and cell death was assessed by trypan blue exclusion method. All data were shown in mean ±S.E.M and are at least from 3 independent experiments.
a: Significant difference ($p<0.05$) with control
b: Significant difference ($p<0.01$) with control
c: Significant difference ($p<0.001$) with control

Protective effect of NAC against malathion-induced cytotoxicity
Figure 4 shows that NAC protected hepatocytes against malathion-induced cytotoxicity at different time intervals.

Protection by NAC of MMP against malathion toxicity
As shown in figure 5, NAC was able to prevent the reduction of MMP in malathion-treated cells in all 3 time intervals.

Effect of NAC on malathion-induced ROS formation
As shown in figure 6, NAC was able to prevent malathion- induced ROS formation only in the cells treated with 1 mM malathion.

Discussion
This study evaluated the cytotoxic effects of malathion as well as the protective effect of NAC against it in freshly isolated rat hepatocytes. The results indicate that NAC has beneficial effects on some parameters of malathion- induced cytotoxicity so that the decrease in

cell mortality, modification of altered MMP and reduction of ROS formation are obvious. The results of the present study indicate that hepatocytes were able to tolerate malathion in concentrations less than 0.5 mM, while the cell viability was significantly decreased at higher concentrations so that 100% cell mortality was seen in the group receiving 2 mM malathion after 3 hours incubation and the LC50 was estimated to be around 1mM in this experimental set-up.

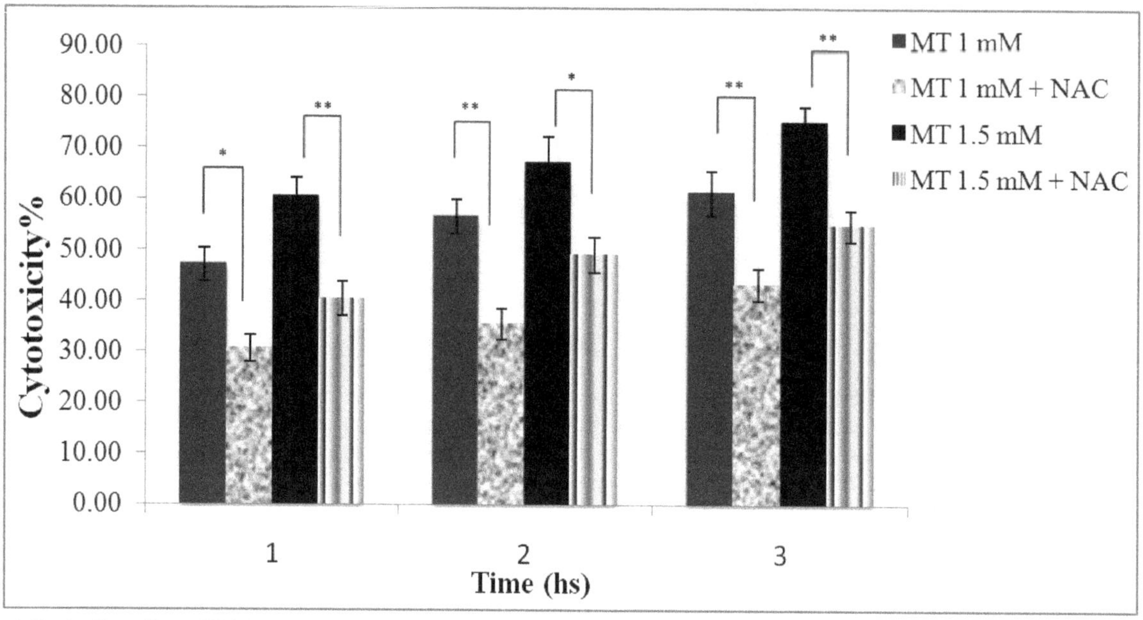

Figure 4. Protective effect of NAC against malathion toxicity in freshly isolated rat hapatocytes
Malathion (1 and 1.5 mM) and NAC (200μM) were added to the flasks containing the hepatocytes and cell viability was measured with uptake of trypane blue. All results were shown in mean ±S.E.M and are at least from 3 independent experiments. MT (malathion), NAC (N-acetylcysteine)
* Shows significant difference (p<0.05)
**Shows significant difference (p<0.01)

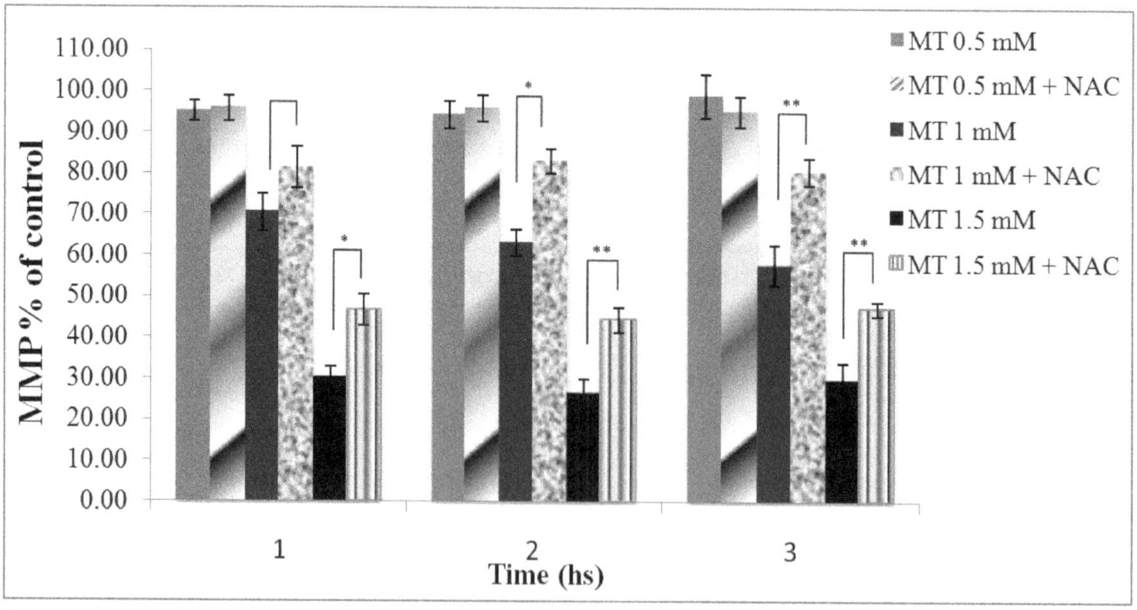

Figure 5. Protection of mitochondrial membrane potential against malathion toxicity by NAC
Rhodamine was added to the aliquots of cell suspensions and the fluorescence amounts of the samples were measured with a Shimadzu RF-5000U spectrofluorimeter. The amount of dye remaining in the supernatant was inversely proportional to the membrane potential of the cells. All results were shown in mean ±S.E.M and are at least from 3 independent experiments. MT (malathion), NAC (N-acetylcysteine), MMP (mitochondrial membrane potential)
* Shows significant difference (p<0.05)
**Shows significant difference (p<0.01)

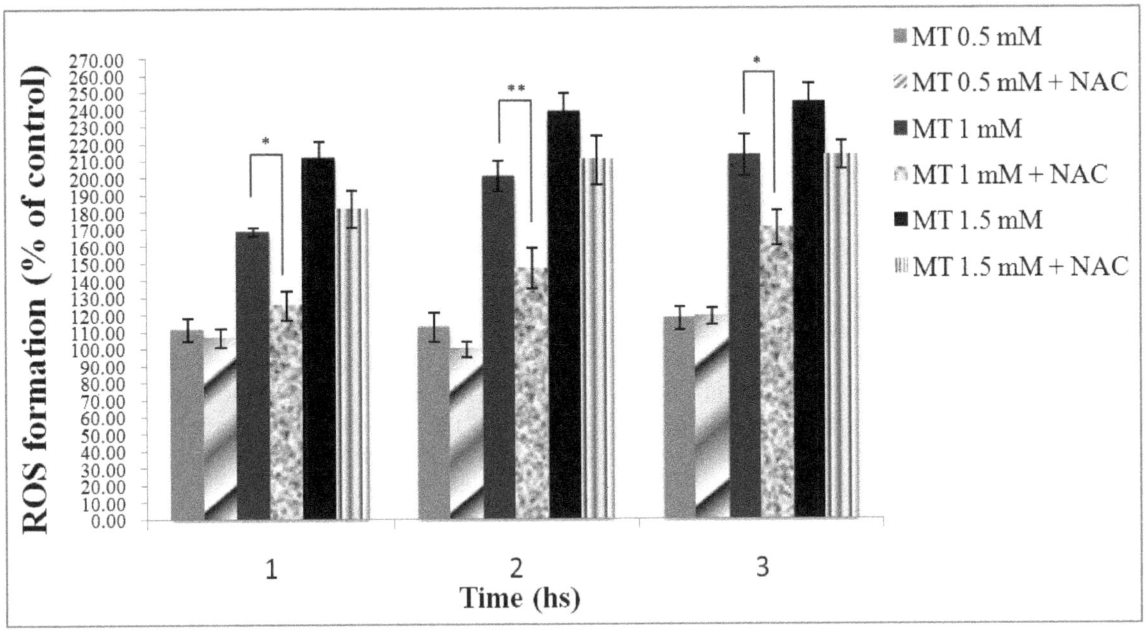

Figure 6. Effect of NAC on malathion – induced ROS formation in freshly isolated rat hepatocytes
DCF was added to the flasks containing hepatocytes at the same time as Malathion and the fluorescence intensity was measured at the excitation wavelength 485 nm and the emission wavelength at 530 nm. All results were shown in mean ±S.E.M and are at least from 3 independent experiments. MT (malathion), NAC (N-acetylcysteine), ROS (reactive oxygen species)
* Shows significant difference ($p<0.05$)
**Shows significant difference ($p<0.01$)

Malathion in its toxic concentrations in isolated rat hepatocytes (1, 1.5 mM) significantly increased ROS formation which is in parallel with the result of the previous studies showing the oxidative effects of various OPs in vitro [24], and also in vivo.[26-28]

The basis of OP toxicity in induction of oxidative stress has been speculated in two prospects; (a) redox-cycling activity recounted as the ability to accept an electron and produce free radicals that is subsequently followed by superoxide anions and hydrogen peroxide formation through transmission of an electron to oxygen and dismutation reactions, respectively; and (b) antioxidant depletion because of disruption of antioxidant homeostasis that results in increased ROS formation. [29-32]

This study not only confirmed the previous reports on the proxidative activity of OPs, but also examined if the toxicity of malathion could be an outcome of mitochondrial permeability transition (MPT). According to the results obtained from the rhodamine 123 uptake experiment, the loss of MMP significantly occurred in isolated rat hepatocytes incubated with 1 and/or 1.5 mM malathion. MPT is an important mechanism in various hepatotoxicities and defined as an abrupt increase in the inner mitochondrial membrane permeability to solutes of size less than 1500 Da. As a lethal event for the cells, MPT occurs with uncontrolled proton influx into matrix and is accompanied with dissipation of MMP, syncope of ATP synthesis, efflux of intramitochondrial ions specially calcium as well as mitochondrial swelling because of osmotic influx of water. It can be mediated by oxidative stress and causes increased oxidative stress.[24,33]

Two main functions of mitochondria are maintenance of cellular energy metabolism and regulation of cell death showing the unrivaled capacity of this organelle in ROS production. Indeed, mitochondrial respiratory chain is not only the main source of ROS production but also a sensitive target for the harmful effects of ROS. Ranjbar et al (2010)[34] have previously reported that malathion-induced mitochondrial dysfunction in rat brain is mostly mediated through oxidative stress. Since, release of cytochrom *c* toward triggering apoptosis can be largely mediated by mitochondria-generated ROS[35] as well as close correlation between apoptosis and collapse of MMP.[36] It can be ideated that hepatotoxic effect of malathion is mediated through occurrence of MPT toward programmed cell death. In addition, mitochondrial antioxidant defense system has a crucial role in the survival of cells.[37] But the most important factors for mitochondrial antioxidant protection are the tripeptide GSH and multiple GSH-linked antioxidant enzymes.[38,39] So we evaluated the effect of GSH-depleted condition induced by 1-bromoheptane on malathion cytotoxicity. 1-Bromoheptane and other 1-Halogenoalkanes are GSH-S-transferase substrates and produce a substantial depletion of cellular GSH with minimal effects on phase I biotransformation and minimal cytotoxicity. 1-bromoheptane is the most effective and least cytotoxic GSH-S-transferase substrate tested, and therefore has been used as a tool to modulate cellular GSH levels in isolated hepatocytes.[40] It is also clear that GSH depleted cells have adequate antioxidant and enzymatic systems to counteract physiological oxidative stress. It has been reported that treatment of cells with 1-bromoheptane depleted GSH by 87% within 30 min and the cells remained GSH-depleted for 4 hrs without significant cytotoxicity. A 30 fold higher concentration of 1-bromoheptane was required before cytotoxicity ensued. Therefore, 1-bromoheptane is particularly useful for studying the role of GSH in modulating xenobiotic cytotoxicity.[40,41] Paying attention to noticeable increase in mortality of hepatocytes incubated with 1-bromoheptane in this study, GSH depletion is considered as a main mechanism of malathion-induced toxicity. In other words, GSH plays a critical role in detoxification of malathion. As shown, in the presence of 1- bromoheptane, cytotoxicity of malathion was intensified and the rate of cell mortality was increased even with nontoxic concentrations of malathion (0.25, 0.5 mM)(table 1).

NAC, as a precursor of the sulfur amino acid, cysteine, exerts antioxidative effect by reacting directly with electrophiles or by facilitating generation of GSH, after incorporation into cells. It is a small molecule that passes freely through cell membranes into the intracellular compartments and is subsequently deacylated to deliver cysteine. As an antioxidant, NAC directly scavenges hydrogen peroxide, hydroxyl free radicals and hypochloric acid in vitro.[42-44] Furthermore, Saito et al[45] showed that administration of NAC or GSH results in a rapid and complete recovery of hepatic GSH level within 1 hour in mice and that the efficacy in supplying cysteine for recovery of GSH level and ROS scavenging in liver was similar between NAC and GSH treatment.

In this experimental set-up, NAC decreased malathion-induced cytotoxicity and ROS formation. Likewise, malathion-induced loss of MMP in freshly isolated rat hepatocytes was markedly terminated following NAC treatment. But the point is that NAC in malathion 1 mM-treated group declined cytotoxicity in parallel with both reduction of ROS formation and MMP obviation, whereas its cytoprotective effect in the next group (malathion 1.5 mM) is more similar to the pattern of MMP than the ROS one (Figures 5 & 6). Hence, it seems that maintenance of the cell survival is more related to the mitochondrial function integrity than the cellular ROS level, as the recent works on cell death mechanisms has focused on MPT. The mitochondrion has two redox-sensitive sites; one of them under the effect of mitochondrial GSH and the other influenced by NAD(P)H that can be modulated by ROS.[46] So, depletion of mitochondrial GSH may be considerably responsible for sensitization of cells to oxidative injury.[47] In hepatocytes, mitochondria include ~ 10-15 % of the total cellular GSH content. Lack of the enzymatic machinery for de novo GSH synthesis in mitochondria makes it dependent on GSH uptake from the cytosol by carrier-mediated transport systems located in the inner membrane. It means that inconvenience of the mitochondrial membrane can violate the function of these carriers towards the mitochondrial dysfunction.[48-50] NAC reduced toxicity in malathion 1.5 mM-treated hepatocytes in parallel with MMP upgrade but not distinctly ROS reduction. Thus, other mechanisms in addition to the ROS scavenging are responsible for the mitochondrial protective effects of NAC. In this regard, improvement of cellular energy supply is one of these proposed possible mechanisms, as the increasing effect of NAC on cytochrom c oxidase activity in mice synaptic mitochondria has been reported by Banaclocha & Martinez (1999).[51]Furthermore, Saito et al (2010)[45]explained that ameliorative effect of NAC on cellular ATP level in the liver may be the result of its capacity to supply substrates needed for Krebs cycle. Thereupon, improvement of energy supply to mitochondria may be responsible for the accelerated uptake of cytosolic GSH into mitochondria as was observed after GSH treatment previously.[45]

Conclusion

Based on the results of the current study, we cold conclude that the cytotoxic effects of malathion as a common OP, regardless of its cholinergic effect, is started with gradual free radical production but, the main factor that causes cell death, is mitochondrial dysfunction, so that reduction of ROS formation alone is not sufficient for cell survival, and the maintenance of mitochondrial integrity through different mechanisms is the most ameliorative factor specially at high levels of cell damage, as NAC seemed to protect cells with various fashions apart from ROS scavenging in concentrations higher than malathion's LC50.

Acknowledgments

This study was supported by a grant from Drug Applied Research Center, Tabriz University of Medical Sciences to M.A. Eghbal. This research received no specific grant from any other funding agency in the public, commercial, or not-for-profit sectors.

Conflict of interest

Authors declare no conflict of interest.

Abbreviations

OPs (Organophosphate Compounds), ROS (Reactive Oxygen Species), MMP (Mitochondrial Membrane Potential), GSH (Gluthatione), NAC (N-Acetylcysteine), DCFH-DA (2', 7' -Dichlorofluorescin Diacetate), LC50 (Lethal Concentration 50)

References

1. Gupta RC. Toxicology of Organophosphate and Carbamate Compounds. *Elsevier Academic Press*: 2006
2. Rahimi R, Nikfar S, Abdollahi M. Increased morbidity and mortality in acute human

organophosphate-poisoned patients treated by oximes: A meta-analysis of clinical trials. *Human and Experimental Toxicology*. 2006;25(3): 157-162.

3. Ranjbar A, Pasalar P, Abdollahi M. Induction of oxidative stress and acetylcholinesterase inhibition in organophosphorus pesticide manufacturing workers. *Human and Experimental Toxicology* 2002; 21(4): 179-182.
4. Ranjbar A, Solhi H, Mashayekhi FJ, Susanabdi A, Rezaie A, Abdollahi M. Oxidative stress in acute human poisoning with organophosphorus insecticides; A case control study. *Environ Toxicology and Pharmacology* 2005; 20 (1): 88-91.
5. Soltaninejad K, Abdollahi M. Current opinion on the science of organophosphate pesticides and toxic stress: A systematic review. *Medical Science Monitor* 2009;15(3): 75-90.
6. Abdollahi M, Mostafalou S, Pournourmohammadi S, Shadnia S. Oxidative stress and cholinesterase inhibition in saliva and plasma of rats following subchronic exposure to malathion. *Comparative Biochemistry and Physiology Part C Toxicology & Pharmacology* 2004; 137(1): 29-34.
7. Syng-Ai C, Kumari AL, Khar A. Effect of curcumin on normal and tumor cells: role of glutathione and bcl-2. *Molecular Cancer Therapy* 2004; 3: 1101–1108.
8. Kirkland RA, Franklin JL. Bax, reactive oxygen, and cytochrome *c* release in neuronal apoptosis. *Antioxidant & Redox Signaling* 2003; 5(5): 589-596.
9. Roue G, Bitton N, Yuste VJ, Montange T, Rubio M, Dessauge F, Delettre C, Merle-Beral H, Sarfati M, Susin SA. Mitochondrial dysfunction in CD47-mediated caspase-independent cell death: ROS production in the absence of cytochrome *c* and AIF release. *Biochimie* 2003; 85(8): 741-746.
10. Ahmed T, Tripathi AK, Suke SG, Kumar V, Ahmed RS, Das S, Banerjee BD. Role of HSP27 and reduced glutathione in modulating malathion-induced apoptosis of human peripheral blood mononuclear cells: Ameliorating effect of N-acetylcysteine and curcumin. *Toxicology in Vitro* 2009; 23: 1319-1325.
11. Shafiee H, Mohammadi H, Rezayat SM, Hosseini A, Baeeri M, Hassani S, Mohammadirad A, Bayrami Z, Abdollahi M. Prevention of malathion-induced depletion of cardiac cells mitochondrial energy and free radical damage by a magnetic magnesium-carrying nanoparticle. *Toxicology Mechanisms and Methods* 2010; 20(9): 538-543.
12. Eghbal MA, Pennefather PS, O'Brien PJ. H2S cytotoxicity mechanism involves reactive oxygen species formation and mitochondrial depolarisation.Toxicology 2004;203:69-76.
13. Lambert C, Apel K, Biesalski HK, Frank J. 2-Methoxyestradiol induces caspase-independent, mitochondria-centered apoptosis in DS-sarcoma cells. *International Journal of Cancer* 2004; 108(4): 493-501.
14. Karami-Mohajeri S, Abdollahi M. Toxic effects of organophosphate, carbamate, and organochlorine pesticides on cellular metabolism of lipids, proteins, and carbohydrates: A comprehensive review. *Hum Exp Toxicol* 2011; 30(9):1119-1140.
15. Czarna M, Jarmuszkiewicz W. Role of mitochondria in reactive oxygen species generation and removal, relevance to signaling and programmed cell death. *Postepy Biochemii* 2006; 52(2): 145-156.
16. Shadnia S, Dasgar M, Taghikhani S, Mohammadirad A, Khorasani R, Abdollahi M. Protective effects of α-tocopherol and N-acetyl-cysteine on diazinon-induced oxidative stress and acetylcholinesterase inhibition in rats. *Toxicology Mechanisms and Methods* 2007; 17 (2): 109-115.
17. Teimouri F, Amirkabirian N, Esmaily H, Mohammadirad A, Aliahmadi A, Abdollahi M. Alteration of hepatic cells glucose metabolism as a non-cholinergic detoxication mechanism in counteracting diazinon-induced oxidative stress. *Hum Exp Toxicol* 2006; 25(12): 697-703.
18. Amirkabirian N, Teimouri F, Esmaily H, Mohammadirad A, Aliahmadi A, Abdollahi M. Protection by pentoxifylline of diazinon-induced toxic stress in rat liver and muscle. *Toxicol Mech Methods* 2007; 17(4): 215-221.
19. Yang MC, McLean AJ, Rivory LP, Le Couteur DG. Hepatic disposition of neurotoxins and pesticides. *Pharmacoly Toxicology* 2000; 87: 286-291.
20. Moldeus P, Mogberg J, Orrenius S. Isolation and use of liver cells. *Methods in Enzymology*1978; 52: 60-71.
21. Malik JK and Summer HK. Toxicity and metabolism of malathion and its impurities in isolated rat hepatocytes: role of glutathione. *Toxicology and Applied Pharmacology* 1982; 66: 69-76.
22. Eghbal MA, Tafazoli S, Pennefather P, O'Brien PJ. Peroxidase catalysed formation of cytotoxic prooxidant phenothiazine free radicals at physiological pH. *Chemico-Biological Interactions* 2004; 151: 43–51.
23. Mingatto FE, Rodrigues T, Pigoso AA, Uyemura SA, Curti C, Santos AC. The critical role of mitochondrial energetic impairment in the toxicity of nimesulide to hepatocytes. *The Journal of Pharmacology and Experimental Therapeutics* 2002; 303(2): 601-607.
24. Anoush M, Eghbal MA, Fathiazad F, Hamzeiy H, Kouzehkonani NS. The protective effect of garlic extract against acetaminophen-induced loss of mitochondrial membrane potential in freshly isolated rat hepatocytes. *Iranian J. Pharm Sci* 2009; 5(3): 141-150.
25. Altuntas I, Kilinc I, Orhan H, Demirel R, Koylu H, Delibas N. The effects of diazinon on lipid

peroxidation and antioxidant enzymes in erythrocites in vitro. *Human and Experimental Toxicology* 2004; 23(1): 9-13.

26. John S, Kale M, Rathore N, Bhatnagar D. Protective effect ofVitamin E in dimethoate and malathion induced oxidative stress in rat erythrocytes. *The Journal of Nutritional Biochemistry* 2001; 12(9): 500-504.

27. Akhgari M, Abdollahi M, Kebryaeezadeh A, Hosseini R, Sabzevari, O. Biochemical evidence for free radicalinduced lipid peroxidation as a mechanism for subchronic toxicity of malathion in blood and liver of rats. *Human & Experimental Toxicology* 2003; 22: 205-211.

28. Shadnia S, Azizi E, Hosseini R, Khoei S, Fouladdel S, Pajoumand A, Jalali N, Abdollahi M. Evaluation of oxidative stress and genotoxicity in organophosphorus insecticide formulators. *Human and Experimental Toxicology* 2005; 24(9): 439-445.

29. Banerjee BD, Seth V, Bhattacharya A, Pasha ST, Chakraborty AK. Biochemical effects of some pesticides on lipid peroxidation and free-radical scavengers. *Toxicol Lett* 1999; 107(1-3):33-47.

30. Kovacic P. Mechanism of organophosphates (nerve gases and pesticides) and antidotes: electron transfer and oxidative stress. *Current Medicinal Chemistry* 2003; 10(24): 2705-2709.

31. Vidyasagar J, Karunakar N, Reddy MS, Rajnarayana K, Surender T, Krishna DR. Oxidative stress and antioxidant status in acute organophosphorous insecticide poisoning. *Indian J. Pharmacol* 2004; 36 (2): 76–79.

32. Possamai FP, Fortunato JJ, Feier G, Agostinho FR, Quevedo J, Wilhelm Filho D, Dal-Pizzol F. Oxidative stress after acute and sub-chronic malathion intoxication in Wistar rats. *Environ Toxicol Pharmacol* 2007; 23(2):198-204.

33. Reid AB, Kurten RC, McCullough SS, Brock RW, Hinson JA. Mechanisms of acetaminophen-induced hepatotoxicity: role of oxidative stress and mitochondrial permeability transition in freshly isolated mouse hepatocytes. *The Journal of Pharmacology and Experimental Therapeutics* 2005; 312(2): 509-516.

34. Ranjbar A, Ghahremani MH, Sharifzadeh M, Golestani A, Ghazi-Khansari M, Baeeri M, Abdollahi M. Protection by pentoxifylline of malathion-induced toxic stress and mitochondrial damage in rat brain. *Human and Experimental Toxicology.* 2010; 29 (10): 851-864.

35. Ott M, Gogvadze V, Orrenius S, Zhivotovsky B. Mitochondria, oxidative stress and cell death. *Apoptosis* 2007; 12(5): 913-922.

36. Yang J, Liu X, Bhalla K, Kim CN, Ibrado AM, Cai J, Peng TI, Jones DP, Wang X. Prevention of apoptosis by Bcl-2: release of cytochrome c from mitochondria blocked. *Science* 1997; 275: 1129-1132.

37. Han D, Antunes F, Canali R, Rettori D, Cadenas E. Voltage-dependent anion channels control the release of the superoxide anion from mitochondria to cytosol. *The journal of Biological Chemistry* 2003; 278(8): 5557-5563.

38. Soderdahl T, Enoksson M, Lundberg M et al. Visualization of the compartmentalization of glutathione and protein-glutathione mixed disulfides in cultured cells. *The FASEB Journal* 2003; 17(1): 124-126.

39. Marí M, Morales A, Colell A, García-Ruiz C, Fernández-Checa JC. Mitochondrial glutathione, a key survival antioxidant. *Antioxid Redox Signal* 2009; 11(11): 2685-2700.

40. Khan S and O'Brien P J. 1-bromoalkanes as new potent nontoxic glutathione depletors in isolated rat hepatocytes. *Biochemical and Biophysical Research Communications* 1991; 179 (1): 436-441.

41. Kanz M F, Dugas T R, Liu H and Cruz V S. Glutathione depletion exacerbates methylenedianiline toxicity to biliary epithelial cells and hepatocytes in rats. *Toxicological Sciences* 2003; 74: 447–456.

42. Custodio JBA, Cardoso CMP, Almeida LM. Thiol protecting agents and antioxidants inhibit the mitochondrial permeability transition promoted by etoposide: implications in the prevention of etoposide-induced apoptosis. *Chemico-Biological Interactions* 2002; 140(2): 169–184.

43. Soltan-Sharifi MS, Mojtahedzadeh M, Najafi A, Reza Khajavi M, Reza Rouini M, Moradi M, Mohammadirad A, Abdollahi M. Improvement by N-acetylcysteine of acute respiratory distress syndrome through increasing intracellular glutathione, and extracellular thiol molecules and anti-oxidant power: evidence for underlying toxicological mechanisms. *Human and Experimental Toxicology* 2007; 26 (9): 697-703.

44. Kamboj S S, Chopra K, Sandhir R. Neuroprotective effect of N-acetylcysteine in the development of diabetic encephalopathy in streptozotocin-induced diabetes. *Metab Brain Dis* 2008; 23(4): 427–443.

45. Saito C, Zwingmann C, Jaeschke H. Novel mechanisms of protection against acetaminophen hepatotoxicity in mice by glutathione and N-acetylcysteine. *Hepatology* 2010; 51(1): 246-254.

46. Constantini P, Chernyak BV, Petronilli V, Bernardi P. Modulation of the mitochondrial permeability transition pore by pyridine nucleotides and dithiol oxidation at two separate sites. *The Journal of Biological Chemistry* 1996; 271(12): 6746–6751.

47. Circu ML, Rodriguez C, Maloney R, Moyer MP, Aw TY. Contribution of mitochondrial GSH transport to matrix GSH status and colonic epithelial cell apoptosis. *Free Radical Biology & Medicine* 2008; 44: 768-778.

48. Meister A, Anderson M E. Glutathione. *Annual Review of Biochemistry* 1983; 52: 711–760.

49. Martensson J, Lai JC, Meister A. High-affinity transport of glutathione is part of a multi-component system essential for mitochondrial function. *Proceedings of the National Academy Sciences of the USA* 1990; 87(18): 7185-7189.
50. Han D, Canali R, Rettori D, Kaplowitz N. Effect of glutathione depletion on site and topology of superoxide and hydrogen peroxide production in mitochondria. *Molecular Pharmacology* 2003; 64(5): 1136-1144.
51. Banaclocha MM, Martinez N. *N*-Acetylcysteine elicited increase in cytochrome *c* oxidase activity in mice synaptic mitochondria. *Brain Research* 1999; 842: 249-251.

3

Evaluation and optimization of chitosan derivatives-based gene delivery system via kidney epithelial cells

S. Safari[1], M.H. Zarrintan[1*], M. Soleimani[2], F. A. Dorkoosh[3], H. Akbari[3], B. Larijani[4], M. Rafiee Tehrani[3]

[1] *Department of Pharmaceutics, Faculty of Pharmacy, Tabriz University of Medical Sciences, Tabriz, Iran.*

[2] *Department of Hematology, Faculty of Medical Science, Tarbiat Modares University, Tehran, Iran.*

[3] *Department of Pharmaceutics, Faculty of Pharmacy, Tehran University of Medical Sciences, Tehran, Iran.*

[4] *Endocrinology and Metabolism Research Center, Tehran University of Medical Sciences, Tehran, Iran.*

ARTICLE INFO

Keywords:
Chitosan derivatives
Gene delivery
Epithelial cells

ABSTRACT

Purpose: Non-viral vectors have been widely proposed as safer alternatives to viral vectors, and cationic polymers have gained increasing attention because they can form self-assembly with DNA. Chitosan is also considered to be a good candidate for gene delivery systems, since it is already known as a biocompatible, biodegradable, and low toxic material with high cationic potential. However, low solubility and transfection efficiency need to be overcome prior to clinical trial. In this work, we focus on alkyl modified chitosan which might be useful in DNA condensing and efficient gene delivery. ***Methods***: N, N- Diethyl N- Methyl (DEMC) and N- Triethyl Chitosan (TEC) were synthesized from chitosan polymer. In order to optimize the polymers for gene delivery, we used FITC-dextran (FD). Then the optimized polymer concentrations were used for gene delivery. Fluorescent microscope was used, in order to evaluate the polymers' efficiency for gene delivery to human embryonic kidney epithelial cells (HEK 293T). ***Results***: This modification increased chitosan's positive charge, thus these chitosan derivatives spontaneously formed complexes with FD, green fluorescence protein plasmid DNA (pEGFP), red fluorescence protein plasmid DNA (pJred) and fluorescent labeled miRNA .Results gained from fluorescent microscope showed that TEC and DEMC were able to transfer FD, DNA and miRNA (micro RNA) to HEK cell line. ***Conclusion***: We conclude that these chitosan derivatives present suitable characteristics to be used as non-viral gene delivery vectors to epithelial cells.

Introduction

In the past decade, Cationic polymers have been proposed as an alternative approach to the viral vectors. Generally, cationic polymers form efficient complexes with DNA and interact with cells. Polymer/DNA complexes are more stable than cationic lipids, and they protect DNA against nuclease degradation. [1] Examples include diethylaminoethyl dextran [2], poly(L-lysine) (PLL) [3], polyethylenimine (PEI) [4], gelatin [5], polyamidoamine dendrimers [6], and chitosan. [7] Both PEI and the dendrimers are effective gene carriers, but both are synthetic and not biodegradable, which means that their potential toxicity is a concern. Although biodegradable, PLL forms polyplexes with lower transfection efficiency than that of PEI and the dendrimers.

Among non-viral vectors, chitosan has been considered to be a good gene carrier candidate, since it is known as a biocompatible, biodegradable, and low toxic material with high cationic potential [8], and it has functional groups that allow simple coupling of extracellular and intracellular targeting ligands. [9] However, the low specificity and low transfection efficiency of chitosan must be overcome for its use in clinical trials. Up to now many chemical modifications have been done on chitosan. These chemical modifications include hydrophilic [10], hydrophobic [11], pH-sensitive [12], thermosensitive [13] and cell-specific ligand [14] groups for enhancement of cell specificity and transfection efficiency of chitosan in vitro. One of the subtypes of hydrophobic modification of chitosan is alkylated chitosan(ACSs).

Alkylated chitosans synthesized for gene deliveries are, N-dodecylated chitosan (NDC) [15], alkyl bromide [16] and trimethlyated chitosan oligomers [17]. Hydrophobic units in the polymeric carriers may assist dissociation of polymer/DNA complexes, to facilitate release of DNA which otherwise would be strongly bound through ionic interactions between cationic units and phosphates of DNA. [18] These favorable characteristics of the hydrophobic units lead to higher transfection

***Corresponding author:** Mohammad Hossein Zarrintan (PhD), E-mail: zarrintanmh@yahoo.com

efficiency of chitosan than polymer systems using only ionic interactions. In the hydrophilic modification of chitosan by alkylation, Kean et al. proposed that TMC, a quaternized form of the chitosan, makes the chitosan soluble over a wide pH range, increases gene –polymer intraction and increases its transfection efficiency with less toxicity. [19]

Human Embryonic Kidney Epithelial Cells (HEK 293 Line), are a specific cell line originally derived from human embryonic kidney cells grown in tissue culture. An important variant of this cell line is the 293T cell line that contains, in addition, the SV40 Large T-antigen, that allows for episomal replication of transfected plasmids containing the SV40 origin of replication. This allows for amplification of transfected plasmids and extended temporal expression of the desired gene products. [20]

The aim of the present work is to show the effect of another chemical modification of chitosan in gene delivery. DEMC and TEC were synthesized from chitosan polymer. In order to optimize the polymers for gene delivery, we used FITC-dextran (FD). Then the optimized polymer concentrations were used for gene delivery. Fluorescent microscope was used, in order to evaluate the polymers' efficiency for gene delivery to human embryonic kidney epithelial cells (HEK 293T).

Materials and Methods

Materials

Low molecular weight chitosan from Primex, Iceland. Ethyliodide, methyl iodide, and sodium borohydride were obtained from Sigma (Vienna, Austria). Sodium hydroxide, *N*-methyl pyrrolidone (NMP) and sodium iodide were purchased from Merck (Darmstadt, Germany). HEK 293T cell line was purchased from NCBI (Tehran, Iran). Flourescein isothiocyanate-dextran (sigma, USA), Plasmid extraction kit (Fermentas Miniprep Kit, Lithuania), RPMI 1640 (Gibco-BRL, UK), FBS (Fetal Bovine Serum, Gibco® In vitrogen Ltd, UK), Lipofectamine™ 2000 (in vitrogen, USA), Scramble-miRNA (Exiquon, USA), DMEM (Dulbecco's modified Eagle, Gibco-BRL, UK), all were obtained from stem cell technology institute (Tehran, Iran).

Synthesis and characterization of N-triethyl chitosan

TEC was prepared by a method reported by Avadi et al [21] At the beginning, we distributed chitosan. (DD=97%) in *N*-methyl pyrrolidone and it was mixed at room temperature. Then sodium hydroxide, sodium iodide and ethyl iodide was added to the mixture and it was heated at 60 °C for 6 hours under stirring. The product chitosan–N+(CH2CH3)3I– was precipitated with acetone and separated by centrifugation. In order to separate the N-methyl pyrrolidone between the TEC chains and get a better NMR, the precipitate was left for one week in acetone under gentle stirring. To exchange I– with Cl–, the polymer was dissolved in 10% aqueous sodium chloride solution and stirred for 3 h. The polymer was precipitated with acetone, centrifuged and dried to obtain a white water-soluble powder. The polymer structure, the degree of quaternization and zeta potential were characterized by H-NMR and Malvern zeta sizer.

Preparation and characterization of N-diethylmethyl chitosan

DEMC was prepared by a two-step method reported by Avadi et al. [22] In the first step chitosan was dissolved into 1% acetic acid solution and formaldehyde solution was added. After stirring for 1 h, NaBH4 was added and the stirring continued for 16 h. Then the solution pH was adjusted to 10 by adding 1 M NaOH solution and a white precipitant was yield. In the second step, methyl chitosan was dispersed in *N*-methyl pyrrolidone and after 4h of sttiring, sodium hydroxide; ethyl iodide and sodium iodide were added. Reaction was carried out with stirring for 6 h at 60 C. Finally acetone was added and the precipitant of chitosan derivative was collected. In order to separate the *N*-methyl pyrrolidone between the TEC chains and get a better NMR, the precipitate was left for one week in acetone under gentle stirring. For exchanging I- with Cl-, the polymer was dissolved in sodium chloride (10%) solution. The polymer was precipitated with acetone, centrifuged and dried to obtain a white water-soluble powder. The polymer structure, the degree of quaternization and zeta potential were characterized by H-NMR and Malvern zeta sizer.

Plasmid preparation

The EGFP and Jred plasmids were used to monitor gene transfer and transgene expression after transfection. The plasmid was transformed in Escherichia coli ($DH_{5\alpha}$). After thawing DH5α on ice for 15 minutes, it was aliquot (100 uL) into pre-chilled 1.5 mL microfuge tubes. 10 ng/uL of plasmid was added to 100 uL cells and mixed. DH5α / plasmid mix were incubated on ice for 20 minutes and heat shocked at 45°C for 42 seconds. 800 ul of LB (liquid broth) was added to the cells with shaking for 1h, and then centrifuged. Transformed cultures were plated on LB plates containing 100 μg/ml ampicillin and incubated for 12-16 h. 5 ul of the cells were mixed with 5 ml LB containing ampicillin and gently mixed at 37°C. After 16 h the transformed bacteria were centrifuged and the plasmid was isolated via Plasmid Miniprep Kit. The Plasmid concentration and purity were determined using BioPhotometer Eppendorf (Hamburg, Germany) and electrophoresis on 1.5% agarose gel. The gels were stained with ethidium bromide and photographed on a UV transilluminator (Uvidoc, Bridgeville, UK). The plasmid size and purity are shown in figure 1. Compared to 1kb DNA Ladder (GeneRuler™, Fermentase) the plasmid is pure and its size is approximately 7 kbp. The plasmid concentration was 1 μg/μl.

HEK293T cell line preparation

HEK293T cells were cultured in plates. The cells medium was Dulbecco's modified Eagle (DMEM) with 10% (V/V) fetal bovine serum (FBS), 100 u/ml penicillin and 100 u/ml streptomycine. They were cultured at 37C in a humidified atmosphere of 5% CO2 and 95% air. The cells were used for transfection at 70-80% confluency, 24 h post-seeding.

Fluorescein isothiocyanate-dextran transfection

In order to optimize the system for gene delivery, we used Flourescein isothiocyanate-dextran (FD) (Figure 2). HEK 293T cell line, which are the standard cells for transfection, were used for system optimization. In order to calculate the amount of TEC and DEMC for transfection we used different polymer/FD ratios. To obtain a complex between FD (20 ug/ml) and each quaternized derivative, we prepared different polymer concentrations. The polymer concentration (polymer/FD (w/w) ratio) that were used for TEC and DEMC on HEK cell line were: 0.0001% (0.05), 0.0004% (0.2), 0.002% (0.8), 0.003% (1.6), 0.006% (3.2), 0.01% (6.4), 0.03% (12.8), 0.05% (25.60), 0.1% (51.20), 0.25% (125), 0.5% (250) and 1% (500) and 2% (1000). Polymer/FD complexes were prepared by adding the polymer solution to FD solution (1:1) and incubating for 2h at room temperature under gentle stirring on incubator stirrer.

600000 cells/cm^2 HEK cells were cultured in 6 well plates as described above. Prior to transfection, culture medium was removed and culture medium without FBS was added. After 2h polymer/FD complexes were added to the cells. Then the cells were incubated at 37°C on low speed shaker for 15 min. The cells were seen with fluorescent microscope after 5h.

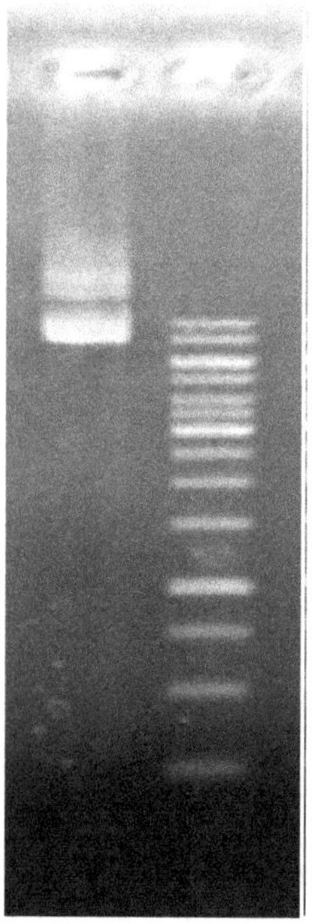

Figure 1. Plasmid size and purity compared to DNA ladder.

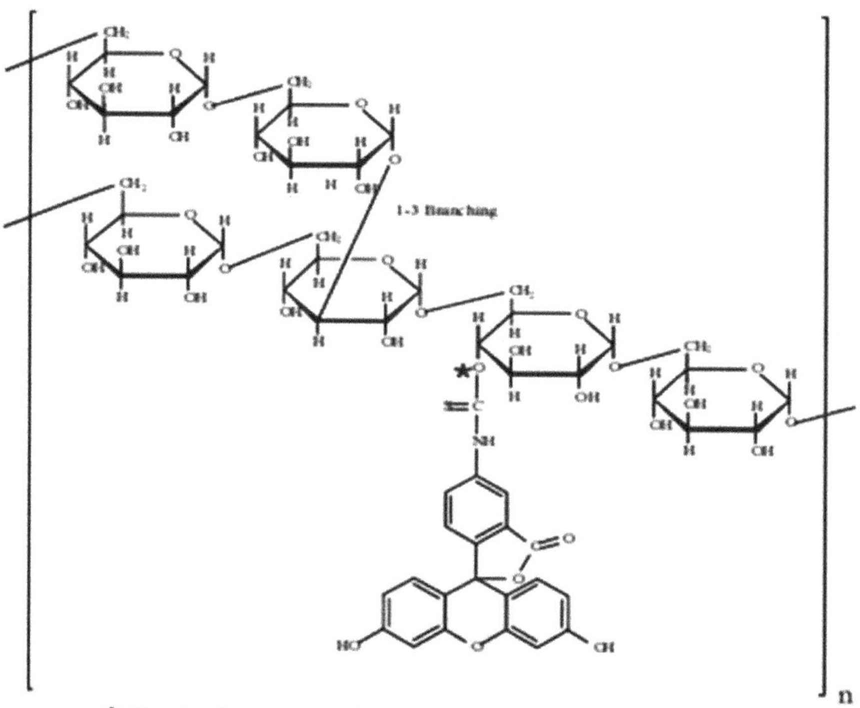

★ The site of attachment of FITC is assumed to be randomly associated with any free hydroxyl group

Figure 2. FITC-dextran structure

miRNA transfection

The miRNA was brought from Exiquon Company (Control, miRCURY knockdown probe, 5 nmol in 200 µL, 5`-fluorescein labeled) (Figure 3). The chitosan derivatives (TEC and DEMC) were dissolved separately in DMEM without serum. Polymer/miRNA complexes were prepared by adding polymer solution to miRNA solution (50 nM) at equal volume and quickly mixed before incubating them at room temperature for 30 min.

2.5×10^4 HEK293T cells were cultured in 96 well plates. Prior to transfection, culture medium was removed and the cells were rinsed with phosphate-buffered saline (PBS, pH 7.4). 100 µl/well of polymer–miRNA complexes, miRNA alone or Lipofectamine 2000–miRNA (prepared according to protocol) complexes were added to wells. The cells were incubated at 37C. The transfected cells were detected with fluorescence microscope after 5h.

GTGTAACACGTCTATACGCCCA

5`-fluorescein labeled

Figure 3. Scramble-miRNA

Plasmid (pEGFP and pLEX-JRed) transfection

Two kinds of plasmids (1 ug) were used for HEK cell transfection with TEC and DEMC: 1) pLEX-JRED (from stem cell technology institute (Tehran, Iran)) which produced red fluorescent protein and 2) pEGFP which produced green fluorescent protein after transfection. Thus these plasmids could easily be detected and used for transfection optimization. (Figure 4, 5)

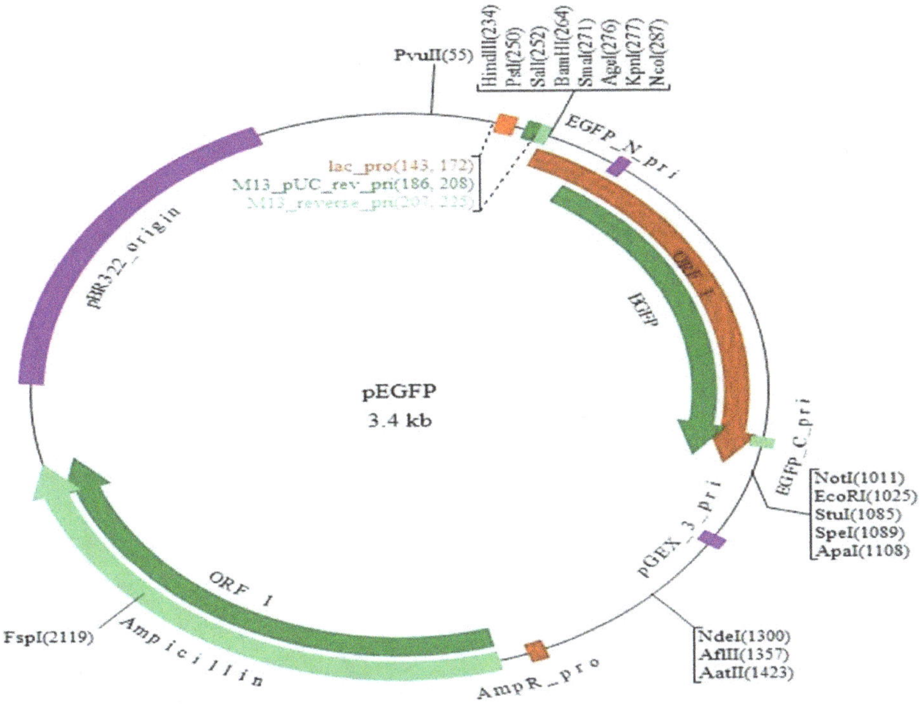

Figure 4. pEGFP (Enhanced green fluorescent protein plasmid)

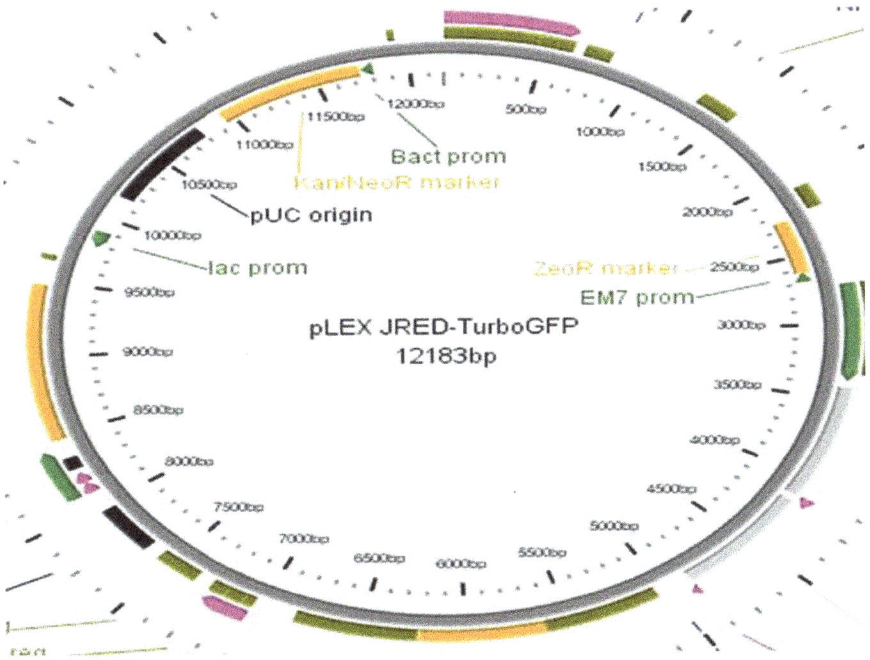

Figure 5. Jred (Red fluorescent protein plasmid)

HEK293T cells were cultured in 6 well plates. Prior to transfection, culture medium was removed and the cells were rinsed with phosphate-buffered saline (PBS, pH 7.4). The cells were incubated with plasmid alone, polymer/plasmid complexes with both chitosan derivatives and also Lipofectamine 2000-plasmid (prepared according to protocol) at 37°C. After 5 h the formulations were removed, the cells were rinsed with PBS and grown in culture medium for 24 h to allow for GFP expression and detected with fluorescent microscope.

Results and discussion

Polymer preparation

The H-NMR spectrum, data and polymer peaks for TEC and DEMC can be seen in the below figures. (Figure 6, 7)

For TEC, the triple signal at 1.2 ppm was attributed to the CH3 groups of the ethyl substituents, while the CH2 groups at the quaternized site are superimposed by the 2-H and 6-H protons of the polysaccharide backbone. The intense band at 4.8 ppm was due to HDO (solvent). The integral of CH3 of ethyl groups versus the other protons was used to calculate the degree of quaternization. According to the NMR peak, the percent of quaternization of TEC is 21%. Also TEC's zeta potential is +36.5 mV.

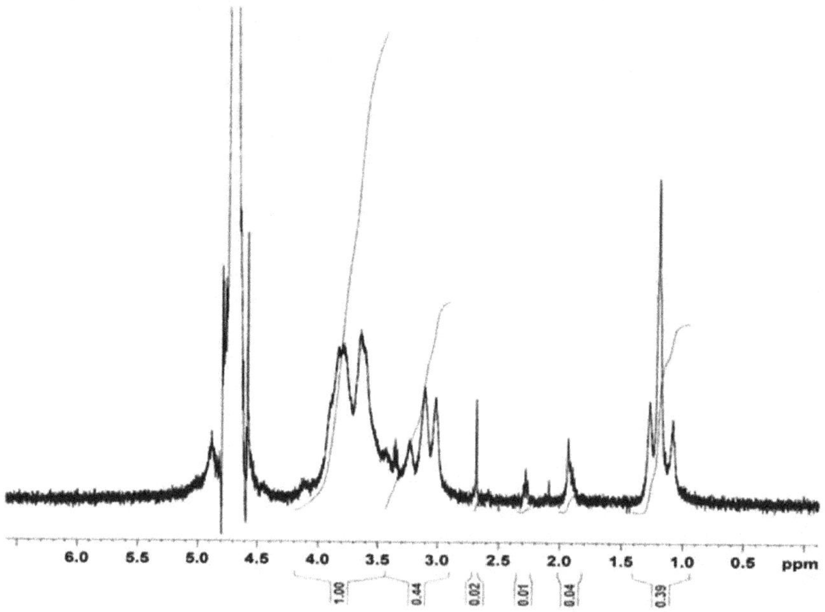

Figure 6. H-NMR of TEC

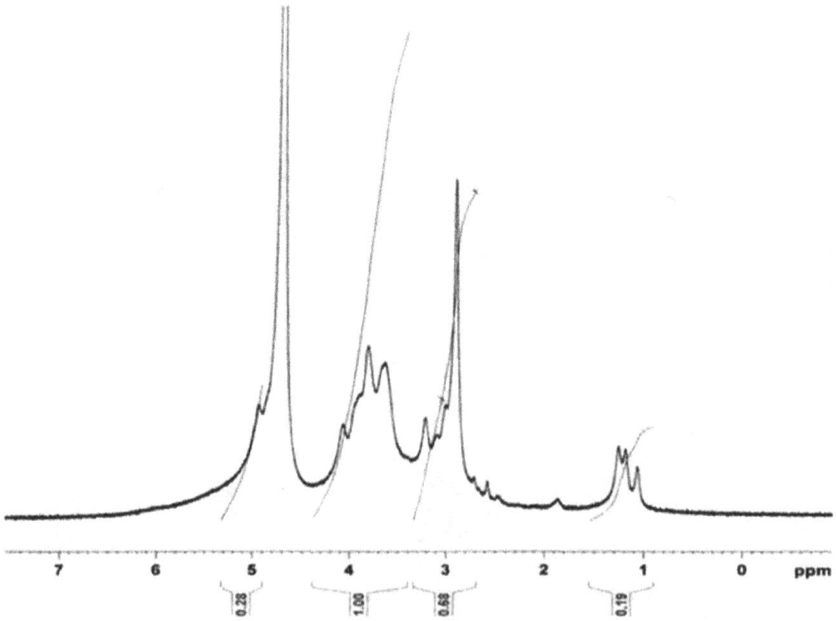

Figure 7. H-NMR of DEMC

According to DEMC H-NMR, the signal at 1.3 ppm was attributed to CH3 groups of the ethyl substituent and the signal at 3 ppm is related to the CH3 group of methyl. While H2-H6 protons of the polysaccharide backbone are superimposed by the CH2 groups. The intense band at 4.8 ppm was related to HDO. The integral of CH3 of ethyl groups versus the other protons was used to calculate the degree of

quaternization. According to the NMR peak, the percent of quaternization of DEMC is 21%. Its zeta potential is +58 mV.
According to results, because of their positive charge, both polymers are suitable for complex formation with negative charged Flourescein isothiocyanate-dextran and plasmids.

Cell transfection with FD/chitosan derivatives complexes

After research it was found that the best FD transfection with TEC and DEMC is at 2% (polymer/FD: 1000) polymer concentration. Transfection was completed after 5h. The transfected HEK cells with TEC/FD and DEMC/FD were seen with fluorescent microscope (Figure 8-10). As it can be seen in these figures the cells transfected with FD are green fluorescent.
FITC-dextran (FD) is primarily used for studying permeability and transport in cells and tissues. The advantages of FD are that just like nucleic acids. It has negative charge and because of its fluorescence part, it can easily be detected inside the cells. Also in a study done by Sushma et al. preparation of thiol-modified gelatin nanoparticles for intracellular DNA delivery was evaluated. [23] In this study the gelatin concentration used for gene delivery was 1% (w/v). Compared to our study, which 2% (w/v) of DEMC and TEC was used for FD transfection, lower concentration of gelatin is needed for FD transfection. Up to now no studies have been done on FD transfection with chitosan derivatives.

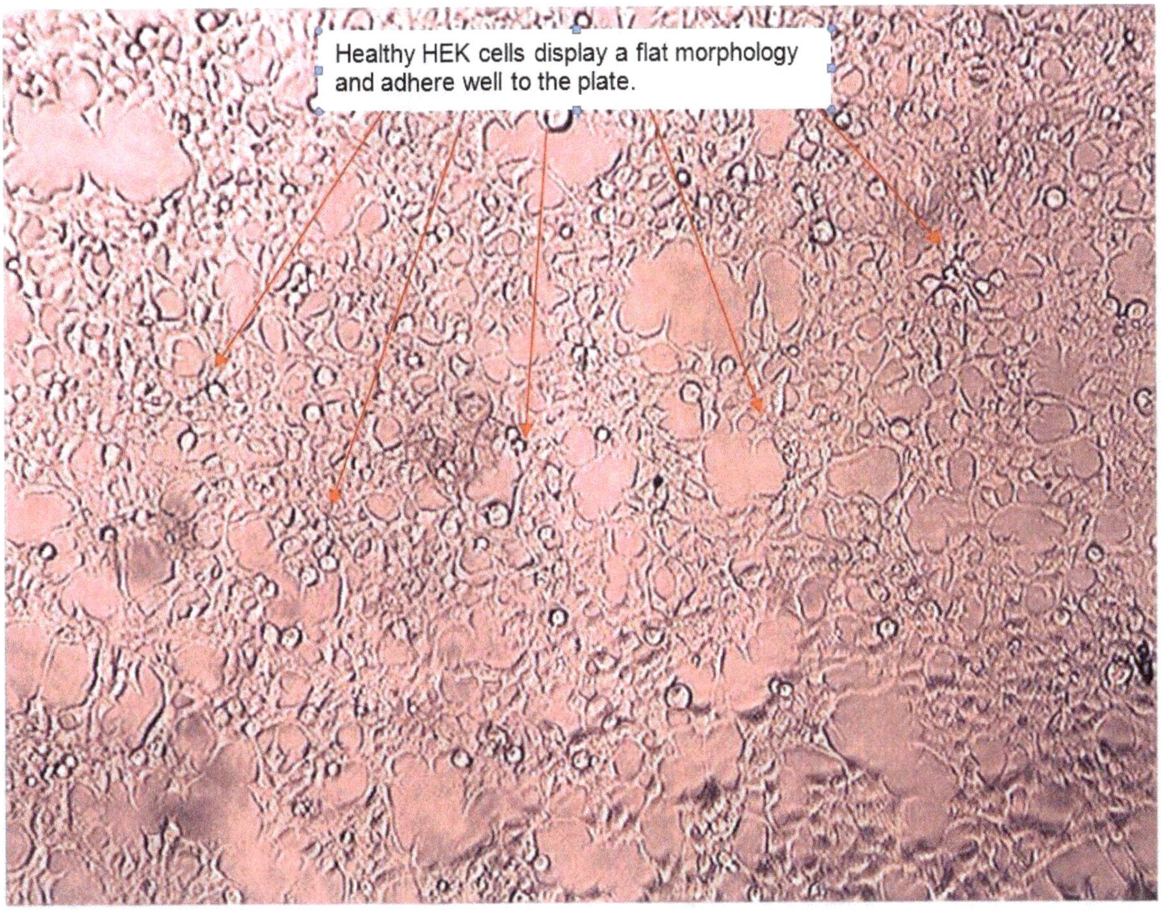

Figure 8. HEK 293T cells (Human Embryonic Kidney Epithelial Cells)

miRNA transfection

Since the miRNA was fluorescein labeled so, like fluorescence dextran (FD), it was detected after 5 hours in the cell cytoplasm. As it can be seen in the figures below (Figure 11, 12), the miRNA can be seen in the cells as green fluorescent dots. The transfected cells with lipofectamine are seen in figure 13. As it can be seen there was no obvious transfection for uncomplexed miRNA (Figure 14).
The positively charged head group of polymers makes electrostatic complexes with the negatively charged phosphate ions on the base backbone on miRNA. Thus, DEMC/miRNA and TEC/miRNA complexes are prepared by this mechanism. From the gained results, it is concluded that TEC and DEMC could be used for miRNA delivery to epithelial cell lines. In a study done by Katas et al. chitosan nanoparticles for siRNA delivery was developed by chitosan hydrochloride and chitosan glutamate and it was concluded that low concentration and low molecular weight of chitosan is needed for RNA delivery. [24]

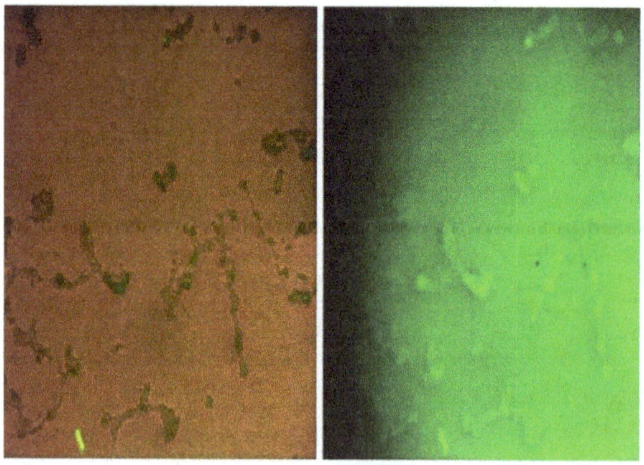

Figure 9. HEK 293T cell line transfected with TEC/ FD complexes.

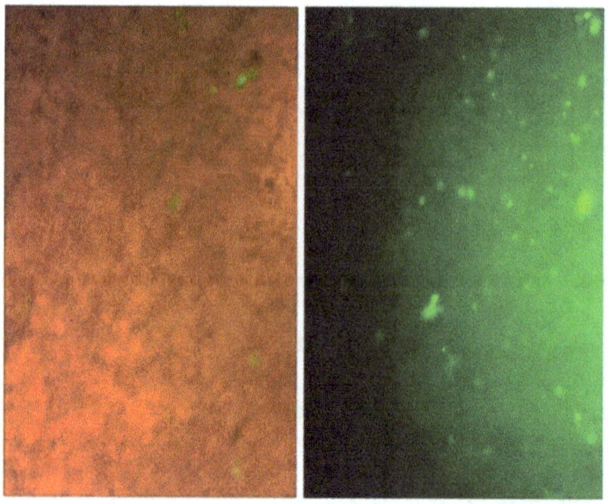

Figure 12. HEK 293T cell line transfected with DEMC/ miRNA complexes.

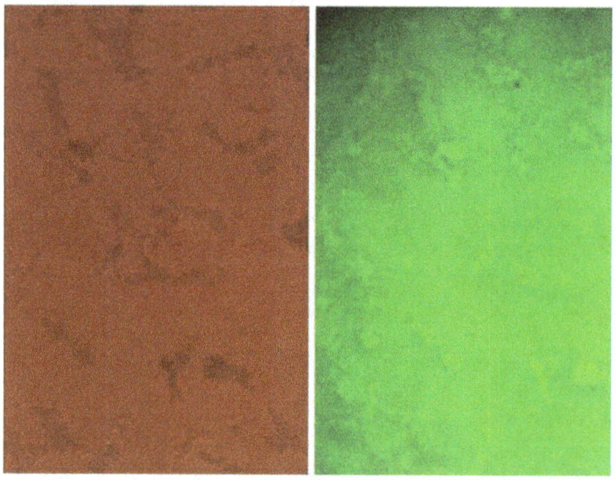

Figure 10. HEK 293T cell line transfected with DEMC/ FD complexes.

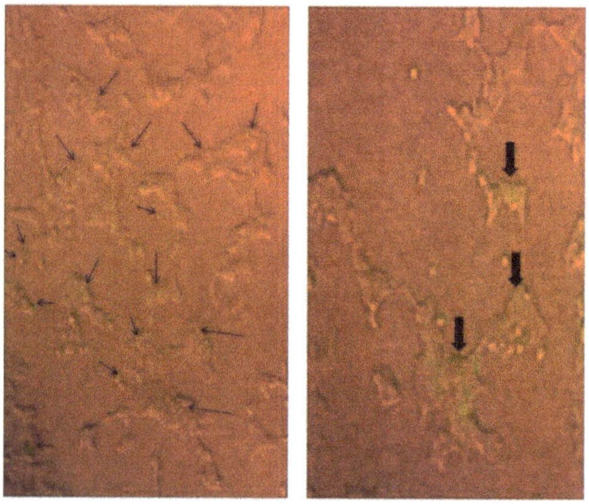

Figure 13. HEK 293T cell line transfected with lipofectamine/miRNA

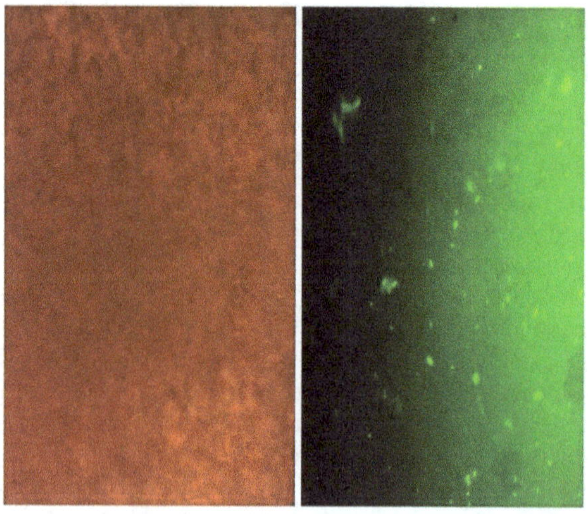

Figure11. HEK 293T cell line transfected with TEC/ miRNA complexes.

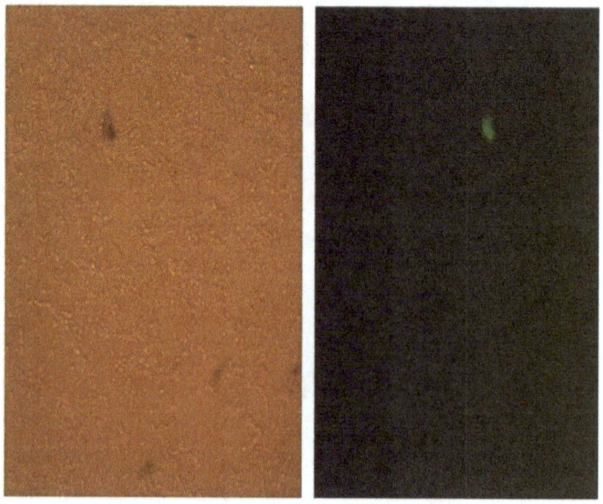

Figure 14. HEK 293T cell line transfected with miRNA

Plasmid transfection

As it can be seen in Figure 15-19, approximately 80-90% of the HEK cells are transfected with TEC and DEMC complexed with pEGFP and pJred. Compared with lipofectamine (positive control) and plasmid transfected (negative control), the results with pEGFP and pJred are seen as green flouresent protein and red flourecent protein.

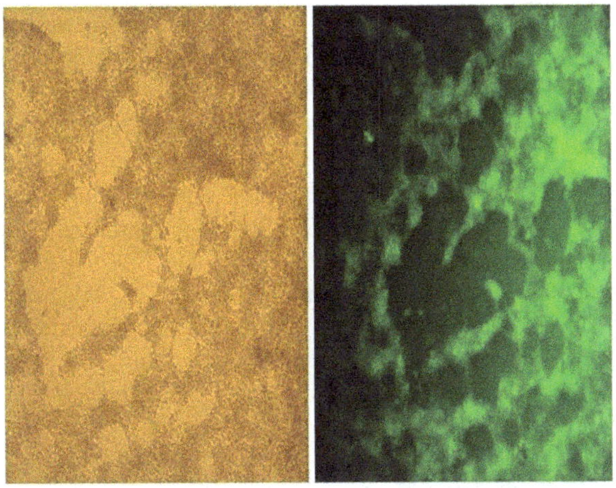

Figure 15. HEK 293T cell line transfected with TEC/pEGFP

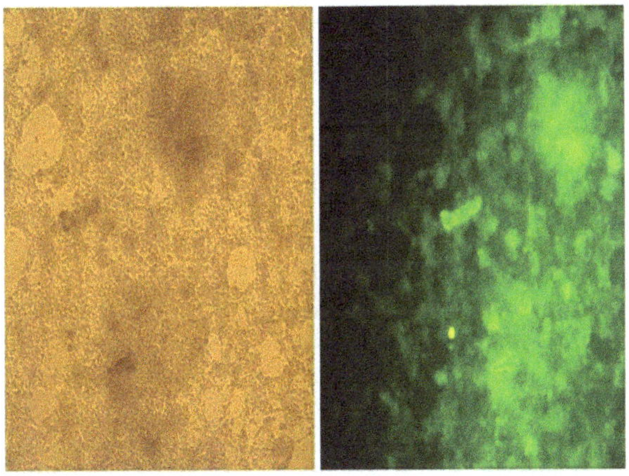

Figure 16. HEK 293T cell line transfected with DEMC/pEGFP

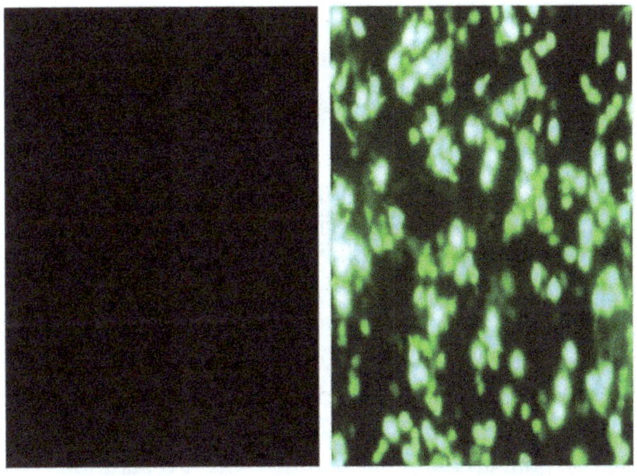

Figure 17. HEK 293T cell line transfected with lipofectamine/pEGFP (right) and pEGFP (left)

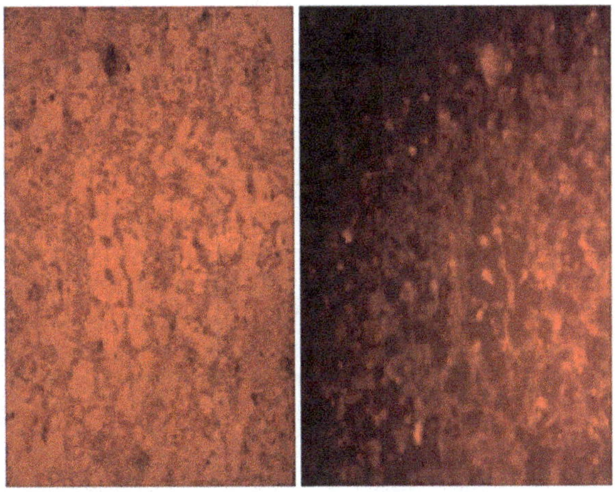

Figure 18. HEK 293T cell line transfected with TEC/Jred

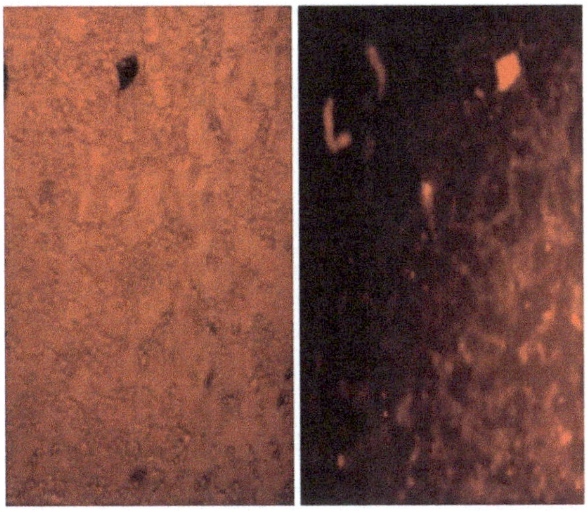

Figure 19. HEK 293T cell line transfected with DEMC/Jred

As stated in the introduction many studies have been done on chitosan derivatives for gene delivery. Among these studies Kiang et al. formulated chitosan-DNA nanoparticles with poly(propyl acrylic acid) which enhanced gene expression.[25] Also Mao et al. increased transfection to HEK cells by attaching transferrin to chitosan.[26]

So up to now, according to the transfection results, the polymer concentration required for cell transfection is 2%. With this polymer/concentration we had transfection in most of the HEK cells. Triethyl chitosan (TEC) and Diethylmethyl chitosan (DEMC) are quaternized and more hydrophobic then TMC so we could use the advantages of both hydrophobic and hydrophilic modification of chitosan in gene delivery. Quaternizing the polymer increases gene –polymer intraction and increases its transfection efficiency and hydrophobic modifications of chitosan increases transfection efficiency by modulating complex interactions with cells, such as adsorption on cell surfaces and cell uptake.

Conclusion

Based on the assumption that quaternization may increase the DNA condensing ability of chitosan, we have prepared quaternized derivatives of chitosan polymer, Triethyl chitosan (TEC) and Diethylmethyl chitosan (DEMC) .These derivatives proved to transfect HEK 293T cells to a high extent. Considering that HEK cells are the standard cell line for transfection evaluation the transfection results in this cell line could be used in order to transfect other epithelial cell lines including pancreatic cancer cells (the results will be published). Up to now these results indicate that these partially quaternized chitosan derivatives are promising agents to be used in gene and miRNA, which are used widely in cancer therapy [27,28], delivery.

Acknowledgements

The authors would like to acknowledge the stem cell technology institute (Tehran, Iran) for generous use of equipment.

Conflict of interest

The authors report no conflicts of interest.

References

1. Gao X, Huang L. Potentiation of cationic liposomemediated gene delivery by polycations. *Biochemistry* 1996;35:1027–1036.
2. Danna KJ, Sompayrac LM. Efficient infection of monkey cells with DNA of simian virus 40. *Proc Natl Acad Sci USA* 1981;78:7575–7578.
3. Wu GY, Wu CH. Receptor-mediated in vitro gene transformation by a soluble DNA carrier system. *J Biol Chem* 1987;262:4429–4432.
4. Boussif O, Lezoualc'h F, Zanta MA, Mergny MD, Scherman D, Demeneix B, et al. A versatile vector for gene and oligonucleotide transfer into cells in culture and in vivo: polyethylenimine. *Proc Natl Acad Sci USA* 1995;92:7297–7301.
5. Truong-Le VL, August JT, Leong KW. Controlled gene delivery by DNA-gelatin nanospheres. *Hum Gene Ther* 1998;9:1709–1717.
6. Haensler J, Szoka FC JR. Polyamidoamine cascade polymers mediate efficient transfection of cells in culture. *bioconjug Chem* 1993;4:372–379.
7. Rolland AP. From genes to gene medicines: recent advances in nonviral gene delivery. *Crit Rev Ther Drug Carrier Syst* 1998;15:143–198.
8. Lee KY, Kwon IC, Kim YH, Jo WH, Jeong SY. Preparation of chitosan self-aggregates as a gene delivery system. *J Control Release* 1998;51:213–220.
9. Dang JM, Leong KW. Natural polymers for gene delivery and tissue engineering. *Adv Drug Deliv Rev* 2006;58: 487–499.
10. Satoh T, Kano H, Nakatani M, Sakairi N, Shinkai S, Nagasaki T. 6-Amino-6-deoxy chitosan. Sequential chemical modifications at the C-6 positions of N-phthaloylchitosan and evaluation as a gene carrier. *Carbohydr Res* 2006;341:2406–2413.
11. Hu F, Zhao M, Yuan H, You J, Du Y, Zeng S. A novel chitosan oligosaccharide-stearic acid micelles for gene delivery: properties and in vitro transfection studies. *Int J Pharm* 2006;315:158–166.
12. Jones RA, Cheung CY, Black FE, Zia JK, Stayton PS, Hoffman AS, et al. Poly(2-alkylacrylic acid) polymers deliver molecules to the cytosol by pH-sensitive disruption of endosomal vesicles. *Biochem J* 2003;372:65–75.
13. Dang JM, Sun DD, Shin-Ya Y, Sieber AN, Kostuik JP, Leong KW. Temperature-responsive hydroxybutyl chitosan for the culture of mesenchymal stem cells and intervertebral disk cells. *Biomaterials* 2006;27:406–418.
14. Hashimoto M, Morimoto M, Saimoto H, Shigemasa Y, Yanagie H, Eriguchi M, et al. Gene transfer by DNA/ mannosylated chitosan complexes into mouse peritoneal macrophages. *Biotechnol Lett* 2006;28:815–821.
15. Liu WG, Yao KD, Liu QG. Formation of a DNA/ N-dodecylated chitosan complex and salt-induced gene delivery. *J Appl Polym Sci* 2001;82:3391–3395.
16. Liu WG, Zhang X, Sun SJ, Sun GJ, Yao KD, Liang DC, et al. N-alkylated chitosan as a potential nonviral vector for gene transfection. bioconjug *Chem* 2003;14:782–789.
17. Thanou M, Florea BI, Geldof M, Junginger HE, Borchard G. Quaternized chitosan oligomers as novel gene delivery vectors in epithelial cell lines. *Biomaterials* 2002;23: 153–159.
18. Kurisawa M, Yokoyama M, Okano T. Transfection efficiency increases by incorporating hydrophobic monomer units into polymeric gene carriers. *J Control Release* 2000;68:1–8.
19. Kean T, Roth S, Thanou M. Trimethylated chitosans as non-viral gene delivery vectors: cytotoxicity and transfection efficiency. *J Control Release* 2005;103:643–653.
20. Graham FL, Smiley J, Russell WC, Nairn R. Characteristics of a human cell line transformed by DNA from human adenovirus type 5. J Gen Virol 1977;36: 59–74.
21. Avadi M R, Zohourian-Mehr MJ, Younessi P, Amini M, Rafiee-Tehrani M, Shafiee A. Optimized synthesis and characterization of n-triethyl chitosan, *J Bioact Compt Polym* 2003;18: 469–480.
22. Avadi MR, Sadeghi AMM, Erfan M, Moezi L, Dehpour AR, Younessi P, Rafiee- Tehrani M, Shafiee A N,N-Diethyl N-methyl chitosan as an enhancing agent for colon drug delivery. *J Bioact Compat Polym* 2004;19: 421–433.
23. Kommareddy S, Amiji M. Preparation and evaluation of thiol-modified gelatin nanoparticles for intracellular DNA delivery in response to

glutathione. *Bioconjug Chem* 2005 16(6):1423-1432.

24. Katas H, Alpar HO. Development and characterization of chitosan nanoparticles for siRNA delivery. *J Control Release* 2006;115:216–225.
25. Kiang T, Bright C, Cheung CY, Stayton PS, Hoffman AS, Leong KW. Formulation of chitosan-DNA nanoparticles with poly(propyl acrylic acid) enhances gene expression. *J Biomater Sci Polymer Ed* 2004;15:1405–1421.
26. Mao HQ, Roy K, Troung-Le VL, Janes KA, Lin KY, Wang Y, et al. Chitosan-DNA nanoparticles as gene carriers: synthesis, characterization and transfection efficiency. *J Control Release* 2001;70:399–421.
27. Lundstrom K. Micro-RNA in disease and gene therapy. *Curr Drug Discov Technol* 2011 Jun 1;8(2):76-86.
28. Gardlik R, Celec P, Bernadic M. Targeting angiogenesis for cancer (gene) therapy. *Bratisl Lek Listy* 2011;112(8):428-34.

4

In vitro evaluation of tetrazoles as a novel class of Antimycobacterium tuberculosis agents

Mohite P.B.[1, 3*], **Bhaskar V.H.**[2]

[1] *Department of Pharmaceutical Chemistry, MES's College of Pharmacy, Sonai, Ahmednagar, Maharashtra, India.*

[2] *Department of Pharmaceutical Chemistry, MP Patel College of Pharmacy, Kapadwanj, Gujrat, India.*

[3] *Research Scholar, Department of Pharmacy, Vinayaka Missions University, Salem, Tamilnadu, India.*

ARTICLE INFO

Keywords:
Azatidinones
Tetrazole
Antimycobacterial activity
TAACF

ABSTRACT

Purpose: We report here the antimycobacterial activity of some already synthesized tetrazole derivatives containing tetrazole against Mycobacterium tuberculosis strain H37Rv. ***Methods***: In vitro evaluation of the antitubercular activity was carried out within the Tuberculosis Antimicrobial Acquisition & Coordinating Facility (TAACF) screening program for the discovery of novel drugs for the treatment of tuberculosis. Under the direction of the US National Institute of Allergy and Infectious Diseases (NIAID), Southern Research Institute that coordinates the overall program. The method of TAACF was followed for evaluation of activity. ***Results***: This new structural class of compounds showed high activity against the bacilli. The activity depends on the substituent's present in azatidinone core. Compounds having a 4-$MeOC_6H_4$ 4-$N(CH_3)_2C_6H_4$ group as the substituent on β-lactam ring were active. The highest activity was registered for compounds having 4-$MeOC_6H_4$ as substituent. ***Conclusion***: The new compounds showed high potency and promising antitubercular activity and should be regarded as new hits for further development as a novel class of Antimycobacterium tuberculosis agents.

Introduction

Infection with Mycobacterium tuberculosis affects much of the world population, despite the fact that drugs for treating tuberculosis (TB) were available for over half a century. Each year, it is estimated that 9.2 million new cases appear, of which many lead to death[1-4]. The World Health Organization (WHO) has estimated that approximately 2 billion people worldwide are latently infected with M. tuberculosis and approximately 10% will develop the active disease during their lifetime. In addition, tuberculosis is a frequent HIV co-infection and a major cause of death among people living with HIV-AIDS. In recent years, multidrug-resistant (MDR-TB) and extensively drug-resistant (XDR-TB) tuberculosis strains emerged and tuberculosis can be considered one of the most significant threats to global health. [5, 6] The current TB treatment takes 6e12 months and requires a combination of three or four drugs that were developed almost half a century ago: isoniazid, streptomycin, rifampin and pyrazinamide (Figure 1). The narrow choice of antibiotics, lengthy treatment regimens, and patient noncompliance has provided conditions for acquired antibiotic resistance that led to worldwide emergence of strains resistant to virtually all available drugs. [5-7]

Since mid-1985s a renewed interest in the discovery of new antitubercular drugs led to the appearance of new classes of compounds active against M. tuberculosis. [8-10] Nowadays several agents belonging to the fluoroquinolone, oxazolidinone, diarylquinoline, and nitroimidazo-oxazole/-oxazine classes are in various stages of development. [2-4, 11] However, new clusters of extensively drug resistant tuberculosis may always appear and, currently, there is still an urgent demand for new and more effective anti-TB drugs possessing new modes of action. According to the literature, tetrazole can be synthesized from the from benzonitrile and sodium azide in presence of ammonium chloride.[12, 13] They can also be synthesized from hydrazoic acid. During the last few years, our research group developed a simple and efficient method to synthesize 5-phenyl tetrazole and its different derivative. Similarly tetrazole are found to possess different pharmacological activities like antimicrobial[14], antibacterial[15], antifungal[16], analgesic[17], anti-inflammatory[18], Antinociceptive[19], antitubercular activity[20], anticancer.[21]

***Corresponding author:** Mohite P.B . Department of Pharmaceutical Chemistry,MES's College of Pharmacy, Sonai, University of Pune, Pune, Maharashtra, India. E-mail:mohitepb@gmail.com

To the best of our knowledge the tetrazole containing azatidinones were never evaluated as antitubercular agents, either as a core or incorporated as substituent's in other base structures. Herein we describe the in vitro activity against M. tuberculosis strain H37Rv of this novel structural class of azatidinones containing tetrazoles which were previously synthesized and reported. Thus, a single molecule containing more than one pharmacophore, each with different mechanism of action could be beneficial for the treatment of tuberculosis. Taking inspiration from the above, and as a part of our enduring research on the "chemistry-driven" approach of tetrazoles, we have struck a rich lode of novel bioactive agents and report herein the influence tetrazole containing azatidinone scaffold combination on the antimycobacterial effect.
These compounds showed high activity against the bacilli.

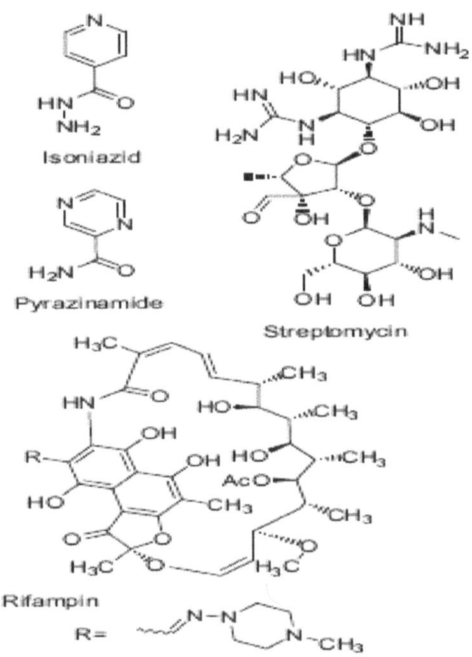

Figure 1. Drugs currently used for TB treatment

Materials and Methods

The scaffold analogues of tetrazole viz.A1-A7 were synthesized and characterized as reported earlier [22] by our research group (Figure 2).

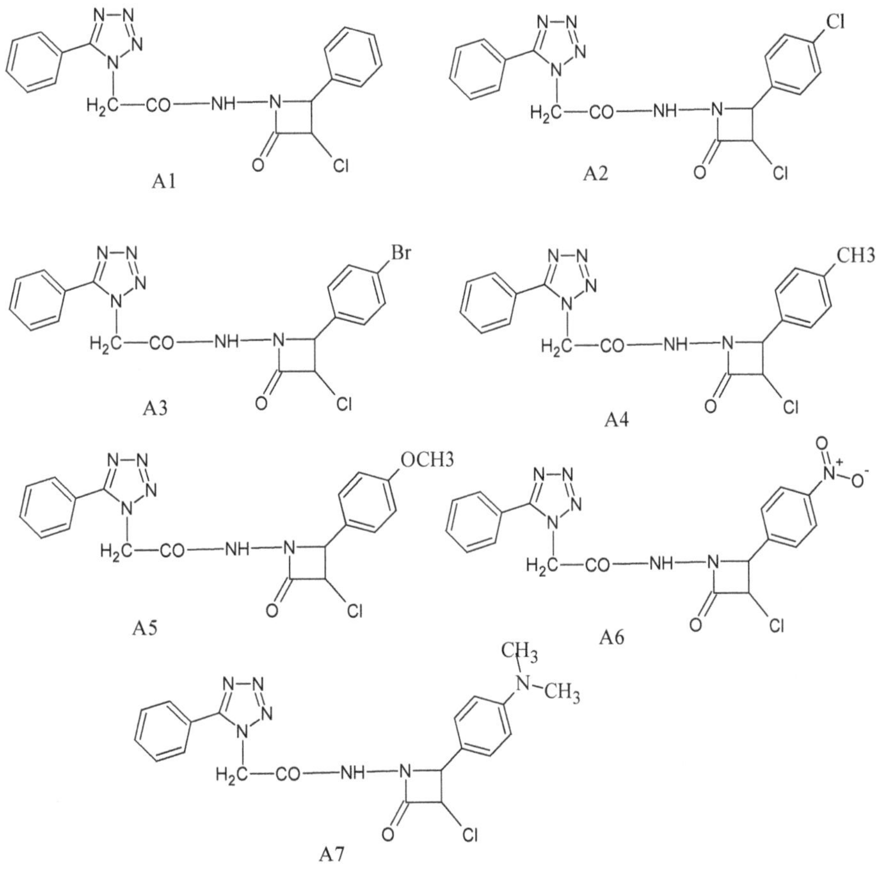

Figure 2. Structure of different tetrazole derivatives (A1-A7).

In vitro antitubercular activity

In vitro evaluation of the antitubercular activity was carried out within the Tuberculosis Antimicrobial Acquisition & Coordinating Facility (TAACF) screening program for the discovery of novel drugs for the treatment of tuberculosis. Under the direction of the US National Institute of Allergy and Infectious Diseases (NIAID), Southern Research Institute that coordinates the overall program. All the new tetrazole were screened for antimycobacterial activity on the M. tuberculosis strain H37Rv according to procedures previously published by the TAACF organization[23]. All the new tetrazole were screened for antimycobacterial According to the information on the TAACF webpage[24] and NIAID webpage[25] the IC90 of the compounds is determined as a primary screen. Any compound having an IC90 ≥10 mg/mL is considered active for antitubercular activity.

Procedure for the Resazurin MIC Assay

The resazurin MIC assay, developed by Collins and Franzblau (1997), is a colorimetric assay used to test compounds for antimycobacterial activity. A color change from blue to pink is observed when growth occurs. Compounds are initially tested at a single point concentration of 10 µg/ml against *Mycobacteruim tuberculosis* H37Rv (H37Rv), obtained from Colorado State University, Fort Collins, CO. If compounds are active at the 10 µg/ml level, they are further tested in an MIC assay at 8 concentrations in a dose range between 10 to 0.078 µg/ml.

Receipt and Preparation of Test Compounds

Upon receipt, test compounds [A1-A7] are logged into the inventory spreadsheet and placed in a -20°C freezer. The day of the experiment, one vial from each compound is reconstituted using the supplier's recommended solvent to achieve a stock concentration of 3.2 mg/ml.

Inoculum Preparation

H37Rv is grown in Middlebrook 7H9 broth medium (7H9 medium) supplemented with 0.2% (v/v) glycerol, 10% (v/v) ADC (albumin, dextrose, catalase), and 0.05% (v/v) Tween 80. The bacteria are inoculated in 50 ml of 7H9 medium in 1 liter roller bottles that are placed on a roller bottle apparatus in an ambient 37oC incubator. When the cells reach an OD600 of 0.150 (equivalent to ~1.5 x 107 CFU/ml), they are diluted 200-fold in 7H9 medium.

Single Point Concentration Procedure

The procedure is the same as that used for the MIC procedure described below, but only the first 2 fold dilution is made that reduces the stock solution to 1.6 mg/ml. An additional 1:10 dilution is made in water (see Step 3 below) which reduces the stock solution further to 0.16 mg/ml. Addition of 6.25 µl of the 1:10 dilution to the wells in a final volume of 100 µl will give rise to a concentration equivalent to 10 µg/ml (see Step 2 below).

MIC procedure

1. 20 µl of the 3.2.mg/ml of test was added to 96 -well microtitre plate.
2. Two fold dilutions were made by the addition of 20 µl of diluents.
3. Each dilution is further diluted 1:10 in sterile water (10 µl of dilution in 90ul of sterile water)
   Note: The additional 10-fold dilution in water is required when DMSO is used as solvent to minimize toxicity to the bacteria. For uniformity in the assay procedure, this dilution step is used even if water or other solvents are used.
4. 6.25 µl of each dilution is transferred to duplicate 96-well test plates.
5. 93.75 µl of the cell suspension (~ 104 bacteria) in 7H9 medium is added to the test plates.
6. Positive, negative, sterility and resazurin controls are tested.
   a. Positive controls include: rifampicin and isoniazid
   b. Negative controls include:
      i. cell culture with solvent and water
      ii. cell culture only
   c. Sterility controls include:
      i. media only
      ii. media with solvent and water
   d. Resazurin control includes one plate containing the diluted compounds with resazurin only. No bacterial suspension is added. This control plate is needed to verify whether the compound reacts with resazurin that could possibly elicit fluorescence.
7. The 96 well test plates are incubated in an ambient 37°C incubator for 6 days.
8. After the 6 day incubation, 5 µl of a 0.05% sterile resazurin solution is added to each well of the 96-well plate. The plates are placed in an ambient 37°C incubator for 2 days.
9. After the 2 day incubation, a visual evaluation and fluorimetric read-out is performed. The results are expressed as µg/ml (visual evaluation) and as IC50 and IC90 (fluoremetric readout)

Results and discussion

The results summarized in Table 1, shows that most of the tetrazole were active against Mycobacterium tuberculosis and the activity depends on substituents present in azatidinone core.

Different tetrazole derivatives of general structure A1-A7 having different aryl substituents on azatidinone core were efficiently synthesized. The activity of these compounds against M. tuberculosis strain H37Rv was assessed and most of the molecules proved to be active. Their activity depends on phenyl ring substituents. Compounds having a 4-methoxyphenyl and 4-dimethylamino phenyl unit, are highly active when compared with isoniazid and rifampin. The compound having 4-chlorophenyl,4-Bromophenyl on azatidinone core are also found to be moderately active. In case of methoxy and dimehtylamino, the IC90 varies from 0.18 (A5) to 0.14 mM (A7).The results of MIC was depicted in figure 3,4.These novel molecules are new promising antitubercular hit compounds.

Table 1. showing dilution of dose level of test compound

Expected final dose level In μg/ml	Test compound =3.2 μg/ml	Dilution
10	1st dilution of 8= 1.6 μg/ml	Dilute 1:2
5	2nd dilution of 8= 8 μg/ml	Dilute 1:2
2.5	3rd dilution of 8= 4 μg/ml	Dilute 1:2
1.25	4th dilution of 8= 2 μg/ml	Dilute 1:2
0.625	5th dilution of 8= 1 μg/ml	Dilute 1:2
0.312	6th dilution of 8= 0.05 μg/ml	Dilute 1:2
0.156	7th dilution of 8= 0.025 μg/ml	Dilute 1:2
0.078	8th dilution of 8= 0.0125 μg/ml	Dilute 1:2

Table 2. Antibacterial activity of compound A1-A7 against M. tuberculosis strain $H_{37}Rv$

Entry	Compound	R	MIC (μg/ml)	IC50 (μg/ml)	IC90 (μg/ml)
1	A1	C_6H_5	>10	NT	NT
2	A2	4-ClC_6H_4	>6.25	NT	NT
3	A3	4-BrC_6H_4	>6.25	NT	NT
4	A4	4-MeC_6H_4	>10	NT	NT
5	A5	4-MeOC_6H_4	0.156	0.11	0.18
6	A6	4-$NO_2C_6H_4$	>10	NT	NT
7	A7	4-$N(CH_3)_2C_6H_4$	0.156	0.12	0.14
8	Rifampin	-	0.006	-	-
9	Isoniazid	-	0.063	-	-
10	Control	Growth	-	-	-

*NT-not tested

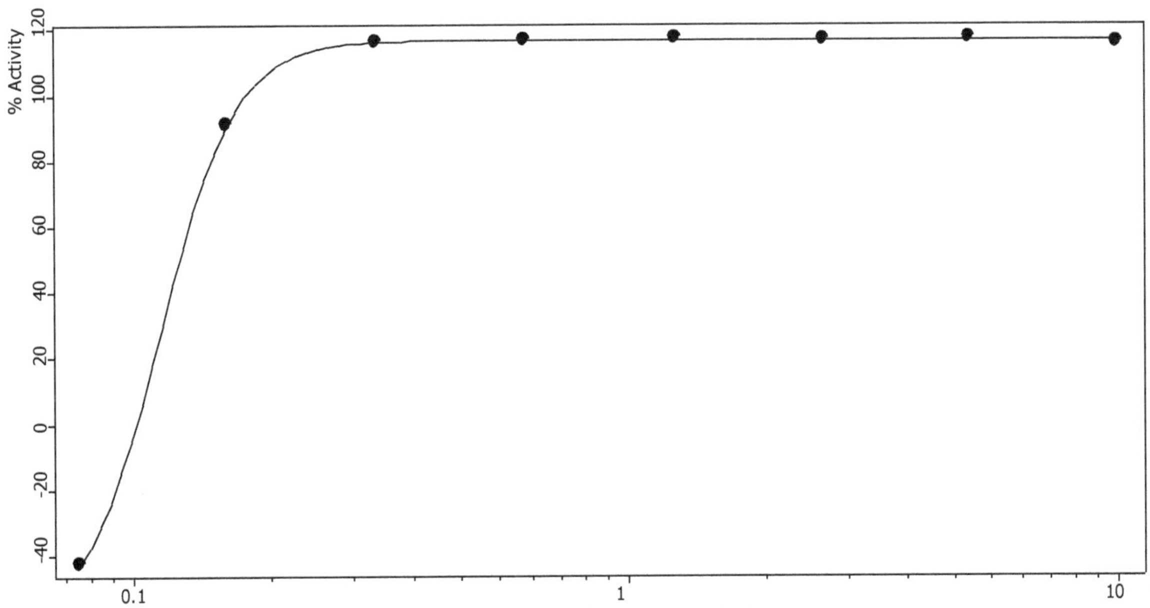

Figure 3. MIC graph of compound A5

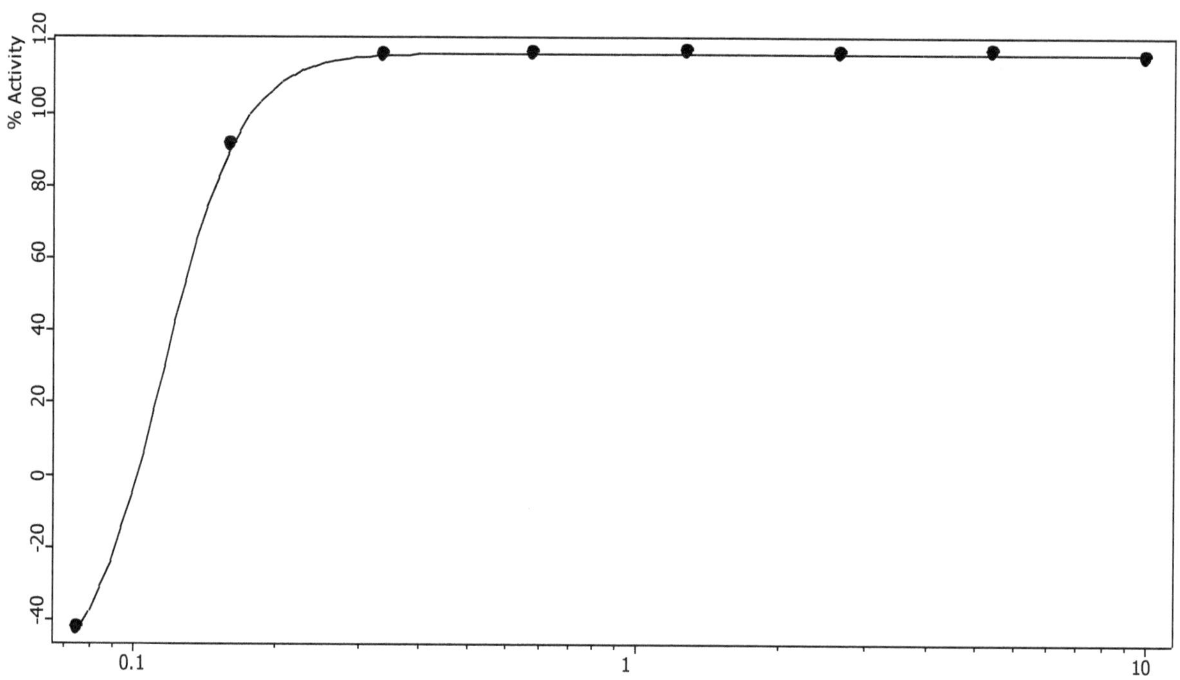

Figure 4. MIC graph of compound A7

Furthermore, as the compounds discussed herein have no structural similarity to any other compounds active against M. tuberculosis, this may indicate that they may act by a new mechanism of action.Further structural modifications of the identified hits are in progress in order to enhance the efficacy of this new structural class of compounds active against M. tuberculosis.

Conclusion

The different tetrazole derivatives containing azatidinone may serve as good antimycobacterial agents which may help the medicinal chemist in drug discovery and development. The obtained results prove the necessity for further investigations to clarify the features underlying the Antimycobacterial potential of tested compounds.

Acknowledgements

Antimycobacterial data were provided by the Tuberculosis Antimicrobial Acquisition and Coordinating Facility (TAACF) through a research and development contract with the US National Institute of Allergy and Infectious Diseases.

Conflict of interest

All the authors report no conflicts of interest.

References

1. Dye C. Doomsday postponed? Preventing and reversing epidemics of drug-resistant tuberculosis. *Nat Rev Microbiol* 2009;7:81-7.
2. Ginsberg AM. Emerging drugs for active tuberculosis. *Semin Respir Crit Care Med* 2008;29:552-9.
3. Showalter HD, Denny W. A roadmap for drug discovery and its translation to small molecule agents in clinical development for tuberculosis treatment of Tuberculosis. *Tuberculosis* 2008;88 (1):S3-17.
4. Tomioka H, Tatano Y, Yasumoto K, Shimizu T. Recent advances in antituberculous drug development and novel drug targets. *Expert Rev Respir Med* 2008;2:455-71.
5. Goldman RC, Laughon BE, Reynolds RC, et al. Programs to facilitate tuberculosis drug discovery: the tuberculosis antimicrobial acquisition and coordinating facility. *Infect Disord Drug Targets* 2007;7(2) :92-104.
6. Nguyen L, Thompson CJ. Foundations of antibiotic resistance in bacterial physiology: the mycobacterial paradigm. *Trends Microbiol* 2006;14(7):304-12.
7. Shi R, Itagaki N, Sugawara I. Overview of Anti-Tuberculosis (TB) Drugs and Their Resistance Mechanisms. *Mini Rev Med Chem* 2007;7(11):1177-85.
8. Ballell L, Field RA, Duncan K, Young RJ. New Small-Molecule Synthetic Antimycobacterials. *Antimicrob Agents Chemother* 2005;49(6):2153-63.
9. Nayyar A, Jain R. Recent advances in new structural classes of anti-tuberculosis agents. *Curr Med Chem* 2005;12(16): 1873-86.
10. Tangallapally RP, Sun D, Rakesh, Budha N, Lee RE, Lenaerts AJ, Meibohm B. Discovery of Novel Isoxazolines as Anti-tuberculosis Agents. *Bioorg Med Chem Lett* 2007;17(23):6638-42.
11. Laughon BE. New tuberculosis drugs in development. *Curr Top Med Chem* 2007;7(5):463-73.

12. Mohite PB, Pandhare RB, Khanage SG, Bhaskar VH. A novel approach for synthesis of substituted tetrazoles. *Digest journal of nanomaterials and biostructures* 2009;4(4):803-7.
13. Mohite PB, Pandhare RB, Khanage SG, Bhaskar VH. Synthesis and Anti-Inflammatory Activity of Some 5-Phenyl-1-(Acyl)-1, 2, 3, 4-Tetrazole. *Journal of Pharmacy Research* 2010;3(1):43.
14. Bhaskar VH, Mohite PB, Pandhare RB, Khanage SG. Synthesis and in vitro antimicrobial activity of some novel chalcones containing 5-phenyl tetrazole. *Acta pharm sci* 2010;52:505-10.
15. Mulwad VV, Pawar RB, Chaskar AC. Synthesis and Antibacterial Activity of New Tetrazole Derivatives. *J Korean Chem Soc* 2008;52(3): 249-56.
16. Upadhayaya RS, Jain S, Sinha N, Kishore N, Chandra R, Arora SK. Synthesis of novel substituted tetrazoles having antifungal activity. *Eur J Med Chem* 2004;39:579-92.
17. Bachar SC, Lahiri SC. Synthesis of chloro and bromo substituted 5-(indan-1′-yl) tetrazoles and 5-(indan-1′-yl) methyltetrazoles as possible analgesic agents. *Pharmazie* 2004;59:435-8.
18. Mohite PB, Bhaskar VH. Design, synthesis, characterization and biological evaluation of some novel 1, 5 disubstituted tetrazole as potential anti-inflammatory agents. *Journal of Optoelectronics and Biomedical Materials* 2010;2(4):231-7.
19. Rajasekaran A, Thampi PP. Synthesis and antinociceptive activity of some substituted-{5-[2-(1, 2, 3, 4-tetrahydrocarbazol- 9-yl)ethyl]tetrazol-1-yl}alkanones. *Eur J Med Chem* 2005;40:1359-64.
20. Adamec J, Waisser K, Kunes J, Kaustova J. A note on the antitubercular activities of 1 aryl-5-benzylsulfanyltetrazoles. *Arch Pharm*(weinheim) 2005; 338(8):385-9.
21. Mohite PB, Bhaskar VH. Synthesis, characterization and evaluation of anticancer activity of some tetrazole derivatives. *Journal of Optoelectronics and Biomedical Materials* 2010; 2(4):249-59.
22. Mohite PB, Bhaskar VH. Synthesis and biological activities of some 3-chloro-4-(substituted phenyl)-1-{[2-oxo-2-(5-phenyl-1H-tetrazol-1-yl) ethyl] amino} azetidin-2-one as potential antibacterial agents. *Orbital Elec J Chem* 2010;2(4):347-55.
23. Collins LA, Franzblau SG. Microplate alamar blue assay versus 460 system for high-throughput screening of compounds against Mycobacterium tuberculosis and Mycobacterium avium. Antimicrob *Agents Chemother* 1997;41:1004-9.
24. http:www.taacf.org (accessed 02.02.10).
25. www. niaid.nih.gov

5

Design of vancomycin RS-100 nanoparticles in order to increase the intestinal permeability

Badir Delf Loveymi[1,2], **Mitra Jelvehgari**[1,3*], **Parvin Zakeri-Milani**[1,4], **Hadi Valizadeh**[1,5]

[1] *Faculty of Pharmacy, Tabriz University of Medical Sciences, Tabriz, Iran.*

[2] *Biotechnology Research Center, Tabriz University of Medical Sciences, Tabriz, Iran.*

[3] *Drug Applied Research Center, Tabriz University of Medical Sciences, Tabriz, Iran.*

[4] *Liver and Gastrointestinal Diseases Research Center, Tabriz University of Medical Sciences, Tabriz, Iran.*

[5] *Research Center for Pharmaceutical Nanotechnology, Tabriz University of Medical Sciences, Tabriz, Iran.*

ARTICLE INFO

Keywords:
Vncomycin
Nanoparticles
Eudragit RS100
Physicochemical properties

ABSTRACT

Purpose: The purpose of this work was to preparation of vancomycin (VCM) biodegradable nanoparticles to improve the intestinal permeability, using water-in-oil-in-water (W/O/W) multiple emulsion method. ***Methods***: The vancomycin-loaded nanoparticles were created using double-emulsion solvent evaporation method. Using Eudragit RS100 as a coating material. The prepared nanoparticles were identifyed for their micromeritic and crystallographic properties, drug loading, particle size, drug release, Zeta potential, effective permeability (P_{eff}) and oral fractional absorption. Intestinal permeability of VCM nanoparticles was figured out, in different concentrations using SPIP technique in rats. ***Results***: Particle sizes were between 362 and 499 nm for different compositions of VCM-RS-100 nanoparticles. Entrapment efficiency expansed between 63%-94.76%. The highest entrapment efficiency 94.76% was obtained when the ratio of drug to polymer was 1:3. The in vitro release studies were accomplished in pH 7.4. The results showed that physicochemical properties were impressed by drug to polymer ratio. The FT-IR, XRPD and DSC results ruled out any chemical interaction betweenthe drug and RS-100. Effective intestinal permeability values of VCM nanoparticles in concentrations of 200, 300 and 400 μg/ml were higher than that of solutions at the same concentrations. Oral fractional absorption was achieved between 0.419-0.767. ***Conclusion***: Our findings suggest that RS-100 nanoparticles could provide a delivery system for VCM, with enhanced intestinal permeability.

Introduction

Vancomycin is a glycopeptide antibiotic that has been in clinical use for nearly 50 years to treat methicillin-resistant Staphylococcus aureus infections.[1] It is water soluble, having a high molecular weight, and poorly absorbed after oral administration. It is well known that VCM, is very poorly absorbed from the GI tract, usually generating serum concentrations that are minimal or undetectable.[2-5] VCM was very stable in the supernatant of intestinal mucosal homogenate and that its binding to gastric mucin. VCM exhibited a secretory-oriented manner in both the jejunum and ileum. known P-glycoprotein modulators, significantly enhanced the serosal -to- mucosal permeation of VCM. It was suggested that intestinal P-glycoprotein might be involved in the poor absorption of VCM from rat small intestine as a potent barrier.[6] Nanoparticulate polymeric delivery systems have been investigated as a possible accessibility to increase the oral drug availability. Biodegradable particulate carrier systems are of interest as potential means for oral delivery to enhance drug absorption, improve bioavailability and targeting of therapeutic agents to specific organ,[7-10] because it is nontoxic biodegradable polymer and well tolerated by the human body. Eudragit RS-100 is a polymer has been commonly employed for the preparation of controlled-release oral pharmaceutical dosage forms.[11] As Eudragit RS-100 is insoluble at physiological pH values, therefore it has been utilized as a good polymer for the preparation of pH-independent sustained-release formulations of drugs. Various non-biodegradable polymers with good biocompatibility such as Eudragit and ethyl cellulose were used in the preparation of nanospheres.[11] The presence of a polymeric wall supplies a protection from the gastrointestinal

***Corresponding author:** Mitra Jelvehgari (PHD), Department of Pharmaceutics, Faculty of Pharmacy, Tabriz University of Medical Sciences, Tabriz, Iran. E-mail: jelvehgri@tbzmed.ac.ir

environment and may lengthen contact of nanospheres with the epithelium that may be enough to increase the bioavailability of certain drugs.[12-16] In the present investigation, VCM was incorporated in Eudragit RS-100 nanoparticles, with the aim of ameliorating intestinal permeability. Loading of VCM, a hydrophilic antibiotic, into RS-100 microparticles can be problematic owing to its high hydrophilicity . The most used technique to encapsulate hydrophilic molecules is the double (water-in-oil-in-water, W/O/W) emulsification method, followed by solvent extraction/evaporation.[17] Aqueous solution of the hydrophilic compound is first emulsified in organic solution of the polymer. The primary emulsion is then poured into a large volume of water with or without surfactant. The double emulsion technique has fairly good encapsulation efficiency for hydrophilic compounds; however, particle size is usually larger than with single emulsion technique.[18] Multiple emulsions of the W/O/W type are excellent candidates for controlled and sustained release of hydrophilic drugs due to the existence of a middle oil layer that accomplishes as a liquid membrane.[19]

However, there have been no reports on preparing VCM nanoparticles using RS-100 and assessing their intestinal permeability. One of the most used classic techniques in the study of intestinal absorption of compounds has been the single-pass intestinal perfusion (SPIP) model, which provides experimental conditions nearer to what is encountered following oral administration.[12-16] SPIP is the most used classic technique employed in the study of intestinal absorption of compounds in which a non-absorbable marker such as phenol red is used to adjust the water flux.[20] SPIP proposes a simple and relevant method of permeability evaluation and coordinates very much with the true absorption properties in human beings.[21] The applicability of the method is assessed by testing the physiological function of the rat intestine during perfusions. This technique has lower delicacy to pH variations and it maintains an intact blood supply to the intestine.[12-16] The objective of this study was improving intestinal permeation. It sounds alternative formulations are needed to extend the time over which the VCM intestinal level remains high enough and therefore enhance the oral performance of this suitable antibiotic. Reversed-phase high performance liquid chromatography (HPLC) is the most credible approach to the assay.[22] In this study, we identified P_{eff} and oral fractional absorption (F_a) of VCM in the rat intestine.

Materials and Methods

Materials

Vanko® was obtained from Jaberebnehyan Pharmaceutical Company, Iran. Eudragit RS-100 was purchased from RÖhm Pharma GMBh, Weiterstadt, Germany. Poly vinyl alcohol (PVA) with molecular weight of 95000 Da was provided byAcros Organics, Geel, Belgium. Dichloromethane, methanol, glacial acetic acid, triethanolamine, hydrochloric acid, potassium chloride, acetone, sodium chloride, sodium hydrogen phosphate (dibasic), potassium dihydrogen phosphate were received from Merck, Darmstadt, Germany. Dialysis bag (10,000 Da) for invitro release studies was procured from Biogene (Mashhad, Iran). Male Wistar rats were purchased from the animal house of Tabriz University of Medical Sciences. All other reagents used were analytical grade.

Preparation of nanoparticles

VCM- Eudragit RS100 nanoparticles were prepared by the W1/O/W2 modified solvent evaporation method Using different ratios of drug to polymer (1:1, 1: 2 and 1: 3). Briefly, 5 ml of aqueous internal phase was emulsified for 120 s in 20 ml of methylene chloride (containing 100, 200 and 300 mg Eudragit RS-100) using homogenizer with 24000 rpm. This primary emulsion was added into 25 ml of a 0.2% PVA aqueous solution while stirring using a homogenizer for 3 min, immersed in an ice water bath, to create the water in oil-in-water emulsion. Approximately five ml of NP suspension was prepared after solvent evaporation under reduced pressure (Evaporator, Heidolph, USA). Nanoparticles were separated from the bulk suspension by centrifugation (Hettich universal 320R, USA) at 21,460×g for 20 min. The supernatant was kept for drug assay as described later and the precipitated nanoparticles were collected by filtration and washed with three portions of 30 ml of water and were redispersed in 5 ml of purified water before freeze-drying. After lyophilization, the dried nanoparticles were resuspended in 50 ml of Phosphate buffered saline (PBS)12hrs before perfusion. Blank nanoparticles (without drug) were prepared under the same conditions without drug.[23,24]

Nanoparticle size

A laser light scattering particle size analyzer (SALD-2101, Shimadzu, Japan) was used to determine the particle size of the drug, polymer and nanoparticulate formulations. Samples were suspended in distilled water (nanoparticles and polymer) or acetone (drug) in a 10 cm cuvette and stirred continuously during the particle size analysis.

Zeta potential measurement

The zeta potential of a nanoparticle is commonly used to characterise the surface charge property of nanoparticles. It shows the electrical potential of particles is influenced by the composition of the particle and the medium in which it is dispersed. Currently principal technique involved in zeta potential determination is laser doppler anemometry. Nanoparticles with a zeta potential above (+/-) 30 mV have been shown to be stable in suspension, as the surface charge prohibits aggregation of the particles.[25] These might result in stronger repulsive interactions among the particles, and hence, higher stability of the particles is achieved.[26] The zeta potential can also be used to determine whether a charged active material is encapsulated within the centre of the nanocapsule or adsorbed onto the surface.[25] Zeta potential was measured by Zetasizer (Malvern instruments, England). The samples were diluted with 0.1 mM NaCl solution at a series of pH values in order to maintain a constant ionic strength and measured in automatic mode. Each sample was repeated measured three times and the values reported were the mean value for two replicate samples. Zeta potential is an important consideration, since membranes often bear (negative) surface charge. Therefore, to enhance the particle cellular uptake, the surface of particles might be adjusted by positively charged surface functional groups.[25] Zeta potential measurement is made to optimize formulation parameters and to make predictions regarding the storage stability of the colloidal dispersion.[28]

Determination of drug loading (DL), encapsulation efficiency (EE) and production yields (PY)

DL can be done by two methods:

- Incorporating at the time of nanoparticles production (incorporation method)
- Absorbing the drug after formation of nanoparticles by incubating the carrier with a concentrated drug solution (adsorption /absorption technique).[29] For determinating of DL, freeze-dried nanoparticles was dissolved in a known volume of methanol.The amount of VCM was quantified by measuring the absorbance at 279.6nm . Another method for determining of DL is measuring the amount of non-entrapped VCM in the external aqueous solution. The results of these two methods were consistent. Ideally, a successful nanoparticulate system should have a high DL capacity thereby reduce the quantity of matrix materials for administration.[29] DL and EE very much depend on the solid-state drug solubility in matrix material or polymer (solid dissolution or dispersion), which is related to the polymer composition, the molecular weight, the drug polymer interaction and the presence of endfunctional groups (ester or carboxyl).[30-32] The EE of VCM in RS-100 nanoparticles was determined spectrophotometrically (UV-160, Shimadzu, Japan) at 280.2 nm by measuring the amount of non-entrapped VCM in the external aqueous solution (indirect method) before freeze-drying. The external aqueous solution was procured after centrifugation of the colloidal suspension for 20 min at 21,460×g at 25°C. A standard calibration curve was plotted with the VCM solution (aqueous solution of 0.2% PVA). The EE (%) was calculated according to the following equation:

$$\text{encapsulation efficiency (\%)} = (\text{actual drug content in nanoparticles/theoretical drug content}) \times 100.$$

Independently of the drug-to-polymer weight ratio, the PY % (expressed as practical mass *100/Theoretical mass(polymer+drug)) are relatively high.[33] All of the experiments were performed in triplicate.

X-ray diffraction, Infrared spectroscopy and differential scanning calorimetry (DSC) studies

Powder X-ray diffraction (XRD) patterns of the pure drug and polymer and also nanoparticles were obtained using an X-ray diffractometer (Siemens D5000, Munich, Germany) equipped with a graphite crystal monochromator (CuKα) (a voltage of 40 KV and a current of 20 mA) as X-ray source to observe the physical state of the drug in the microspheres. The scanning rate was 6°/min over the range of 5-70° and with an interval of 0.02°. FTIR spectra were recorded to assess the compatibility of the drug and polymer.[34] The infrared (IR) spectra of VCM powder, physical mixture of drug and polymer, and prepared nanoparticles were recorded on an IR-spectrophotometer(range 450-4000 cm^{-1}) (BomemHartmann & Brann, Canada) by the KBr pellet technique. Samples were prepared in KBr disks (2 mg sample in 20 mg KBr). Sample analysis were carried out by the E2 OMNIC software for analysis. With reasonable intensity, the spectrum was saved for further analysis at 1 cm^{-1} resolution. Differential scanning calorimetry (DSC) was employed to identify any changes in the thermal behavior of VCM nanoparticles compared to original materials. DSC was also used to study the thermal behavior of the granules of the raw material and the film of polymers.[35] DSC analysis was performed using a DSC-60 calorimeter (Shimadzu, Japan). The instrument was equipped with a TA-60WS thermal analyzer, FC-60A flow controller and TA-60 software. Samples of VCM, polymer, physical mixture and agglomerates were located in an aluminum crucible and were heated ranging 25-300 °C at a scanning rate of 10 °C/min under a nitrogen atmosphere. A similar pan contain indium was used as reference.

Dissolution study

The in vitro release of the drug from the polymeric nanoparticles was studied by the dialysis bag diffusion technique and under sink conditions for all nanoparticles formulations. The dialysis bag retained nanoparticles and allow the diffusion of the drug immediately into the recipient compartment.[36] A set amount of nanoparticles (20 mg drug) was added to 200 ml dissolution medium (PBS, pH 7.4), an in vitro dissolution medium imitates the pH and salt concentrations in the body, preheated and maintained at 37±1 °C in a water bath, then stirred at 100 rpm. Then 3 ml of the medium were withdrawn at preset times by an automatic sampling system (Erweka DT 70, Erweka GmbH, Heusenstamm, Germany), (0.5, 1, 2, 3, 4, 5, 6, 8, 12 and 24 hrs). Each sample was centrifuged at 21,460×g for 10 min. An equal volume of fresh medium was added after each sampling. The amount of

VCM in the release medium was determined by UV at 279.8 nm.[37] Each experiment was performed in triplicate.

Calibration curve

Accurately weighed quantities of VCM hydrochloride were dissolved in a PBS, pH 7.4 to acquire solutions with known concentrations in the range of 31.25–500μg/ml. The spectra of these solutions were registered against the same medium, and absorption was measured in the 279.8 nm by spectrophotometer. Each experiment was performed in triplicate, After that the calibration graph was plotted.

Perfusion solution

The perfusion solution was prepared by dissolving 7g NaCl, 0.2g KCl, 1.44 g Na2HPO4(anhydrous) and 0.24g KH_2PO_4 in one liter of distilled water. The pH of prepared PBS was 7.4. preparatory experiments showed that there was no considerable adsorption of the compounds on the tubing and syringe. Primary stock solution of drug, phenol red and nanoparticles was prepared in PBS.[15] Then it was diluted to 200-400μg/ml to make a working solution and standards for calibration curves and quality control samples were prepared using serial dilution of working solution in PBS. This range was selected based on the concentration that were going to used in animal studies. All standards were freshly prepared for every study.

In situ permeation studies

Adult male Wistar rats (200-250 g) were housed in air conditioned. Rats were maintained on 12 h light- dark cycle and fasted 12-18 h before experiment. However drinking water was accessible. Rats were divided into control and test groups. In each group three concentration levels of VCM (200, 300 and 400 μ g /ml) were used in separate experiments. Rats were anaesthetized using an intraperitoneal injection of pentobarbital (50 mg/kg) and placed on a heated pad to keep normal body temperature. A small midline cut was made in the abdomen and a 10 cm section of the small intestine was identified and cannulated. Care was taken to handle the small intestine gently and to minimize the surgery in order to maintain an intact blood reserve. The entire surgical area was then covered with Parafilm to reduce evaporation. Blank perfusion buffer was infused for 10 min by a syringe pump (Palmer, England) followed by perfusion of different concentrations (200, 300, 400 μ g/ml) of VCM (prepared from its powder or its nanoparticles) at a flow rate of 0.2 ml/min for 80 min. Outlet samples were collected at appropriate intervals (40, 50, 60, 70, 80 min with half hour lag time for balance) in microtubes. The volume of sample for each time interval was 2 ml. When the experiment was completed, the length of segment was measured and the animal was euthanatized with a cardiac injection of overdose of sodium pentobarbital. Samples were stored at -20 °C until analysis. Samples from perfusion study were filtered and directly injected onto HPLC column. Effective permeability coefficients (P_{eff}) were calculated from the steady-state concentrations of compounds in the collected perfusate, which is considered to be reached when the concentration level of phenol red was at the steady state level. It was reached about 30 min after the beginning of the perfusion, which is approved by plotting the ratio of the outlet to inlet concentrations (corrected for water transport) versus time. The intestinal net water flux (NWF, μ l/h/cm) was calculated according to following equation:

$$NWF= Qin(1-(Ph.redout/Ph.redin))/l$$

Where (Ph.red(in)) and (Ph.red(out)) are the inlet and outlet concentrations of phenol red. A negative net water flux showes loss of fluid from the lumen to the serosal side. A positive net water flux indicates secretion of fluid into the segment.[38] P_{eff} was calculated using the following equation according to the parallel tube model:

$$P_{eff} = -Qln(Cout/Cin)/2\pi r\ell$$

In which Cin is the inlet concentration and Cout is the outlet concentration of compound which is corrected for volume change in segment using phenol red concentration in inlet and outlet tubing. Q is the flow rate (0.2 ml/min), r is the rat intestinal radius (0.18 cm) and ℓ is the length of the segment. [39] In all animal studies "Guide to the care and use of experimental animals" by Canadian Council on Animal Care, was followed. [40] The P_{eff} for passively absorbed compounds is on average 3.6 times higher in humans compared to rats. Solutes with carrier-mediated absorption deviate from this relationship, which indicates that an absolute scaling of active processes from animal to man is difficult, and therefore needs further investigation. The oral fractional absorption of drugs after oral administration in humans (fa) can be estimated from this equation:

$$Fa=1-e^{-(2.P_{eff,man}.t_{res}/r.f)}$$

Where t_{res} and r are the average small intestinal transit time and radius in humans, and are assumed to be 3 hrs and 1.75cm, respectively. The relationship between our human P_{eff} and Fa (from in vivo pharmacokinetic studies), expressed as correction factor f was determined by non- linear regression. The f-value was then used for simulation and prediction of Fa in vivo in man. The f is approximately 2.8.[38]

Chromatographic conditions

Perfusion samples were analyzed using a modified reversed-phase high performance liquid chromatography (RP-HPLC) method. Reverse-phase

HPLC was achieved at room temperature. HPLC system containing an autosampler (Hewlett-Packard 1050 Series), quaternary pump thermostat, variable-wavelength UV–Vis spectrophotometer detector (all from Hewlett-Packard, Waldbronn, Germany). The analytical methodology was demonstrated for specificity, accuracy, precision and sensitivity. Wavelength ultraviolet spectrophotometric detector (Knauersmartline 2500) set at 430 nm and 254 nm for phenol red and VCM, respectively. EZChrom Elite version 2.1.7 was used for data attainment, data reporting and analysis. The mobile phase for VCM analysis consisted of 30% (v/v) methanol and 70% (v/v) of glacial acetic acid aqueous solution (0.75%) adjusted to pH 5.5. For phenol red analysis the mobile phase consisted of 45% (v/v) KH_2PO_4 0.05 M and 55% (v/v) methanol adjusted with triethanol amine to pH 2.6. The mobile phases were filtered with a 0.45 mm pore size cellulose membrane filter, and degassed before use. Analytical column used for chromatographic separations was packed with Adsorbosil ODS C18 (250 × 4.6 mm) 5 μm with precolumn. 20 μl of samples or calibration standards were injected directly onto the column and were eluted with a gradient consisting of phosphate buffer. Until termination of the run at 20 min, the flow rate was 1 ml/min. The system was equilibrated for 20 min under the starting conditions before injecting the next sample. Under the mentioned conditions the retention times for VCM and phenol red were 5 min and 13.8 min, respectively. Runs contained quality control samples (QC) at three concentrations levels. Calibration curves were acquired by plotting the phenol red and VCM peak area against their concentrations in standard solutions.[41,42] Each determination was carried out in triplicate (SD within 0.09).

Results

Micromeritics properties

Encapsulation efficiencies of VCM nanoparticles are reported in Table 1. It is evident from Table 1 that the encapsulation efficiency was affected by the ratio of drug:polymer. Mean particle diameter and production yield of the different nanoparticles are also shown in Table 1. The encapsulation efficiency of the drug depended on the solubility of the drug in the solvent and continuous phase. Youan & et al. have been reported Similar observation. VCM is insoluble in organic solvents used to dissolve the polymer and thus cannot migrate from the internal into the external aqueous phase via diffusion through the organic polymer solution. Entrapment efficiency of polypeptides was increased by enhancing the viscosity creators.[43] Despite the hydrosolubility of VCM, favoring the leakage of the drug into the external aqueous phase, entrapment efficiencies were rather high. It is assumed that VCM is localized at the interfaces (either internal water in oil or external oil in water). Therefore a considerable amount of drug is supposed to be adsorbed at the outer surface. In addition, the elimination of the organic solvent under reduced pressure favors its fast evaporation followed by the polymer precipitation, thus reducing the movement of the drug to the external phase. At the ratio of drug to polymer 1:3 the amount of drug entrapment was 23.69% which was very near to the theoretical value (25%).

The particle size data show that prepared nanoparticles were of submicron size and of small polydispersity, which indicated a relatively narrow particle size distribution. An increase in particle size from 362 nm to 499 nm with a decrease in the theoretical drug loading was also observed (Table 1). As it can be seen, the particles size are increased with increasing polymer amount.[44,45] When the dispersed phase with higher viscosity was poured into the dispersion medium, bigger droplets were formed with larger mean particle size. It has also been reported that the particle size increases with increasing the content in hydrophobic polymer. It can be assigned to that fact that with the higher diffusion rate of non-solvent to polymer solution the smaller size of nanocapsules is easily obtained.[46] A volume-based size distribution of drug, polymer, and drug-loaded nanoparticles indicated a log–probability distribution. The increase in drug content of the nanoparticles with increased theoretical drug loading has emerged in the decreased particle sizes displayed ($p<0.05$).

Table 1. Effect of drug: polymer ratio on drug loading efficiency, production yield, particle size zeta potential and polydispersity index of vancomycin nanoparticles

Formulation code	Drug: polymer ratios	Production yield (%±SD)	Theoretical drug Content (%)	Mean drug Entrapped (%±SD)	Drug loading efficiency (%±SD)	Mean particle Size (nm±SD)	Zeta Potential (mV±SD)	Polydispersity Index (PDI)
F_1	1:1	96.38 ±1.65	50	30.25 ±1.04	63 ± 2.19	362±29.26	18.1±8.82	0.0099
F_2	1:2	97.84 ±1.54	33.33	29.79 ±1.12	89.37±2.36	430±31.94	25.7±9.72	0.0055
F_3	1:3	98.35 ±1.87	25	23.69 ±1.02	94.76± 1.95	499 ± 110	24.1±7.17	0.0034

The average yield of 97% is in the normal range does not indicate any unexpected vanishment of products.
Zeta potential is the potential difference the dispersion medium and stationary layer of fluid attached to the dispersed particles. The significance of zeta potential is that its value can be pertained to the stability of colloidal dispersion.[28] The zeta potential indicates the degree of repulsion between near, similarly charged particles in dispersion. As to the zeta potential, the larger its absolute value is, the more likely the suspension is to be stable, since the charged particles repel one another and thus defeat their natural tendency to aggregate.[47] The zeta potential measurements showed posetively-charged particle surfaces, varying from 18.1 to 25.7mV. Drug-loaded nanoparticle indicated positive charge, because VCM is cationic drug and changed the charge of nanoparticles. All the gained values were then acceptable and favoring a good stability. The zeta potential of three nanosphere formulations is shown in Table 1. Blank nanoparticles like nanoparticles had a positive charge (15.7 mV).

DSC Analysis

DSC was employed to study the crystallinity of nanoparticles. DSC studies were carried out to confirm compatibility.[48] The thermal behavior of drugs, physical mixture of drug and polymer, and formulations was studied. Any sudden or forceful change in the thermal behavior of the drug or polymer may indicate a possible drug-polymer interaction.[49] The endothermic peak of the pure drug was observed at about 82.10°C (Figure 1) and Eudragit RS100 showed an amorphous state. The physical mixture of VCM and RS100 showed nearly the same thermal behavior as the individual components, indicating that there was no interaction between the drug and the polymer in the solid state. Indeed, in the thermogram of the nanoparticles containing Eudragit RS, there was endothermic peak at 219.92°C which accords to the melting point of drug in the nanoparticles. In the DSC curve of physical mixture of drug and polymer, and formulations F1, F2 and F3, the characteristic peaks of drug were observed. The results showed that there is no incompatibility between drug and polymers.

Powder X-ray diffractometry

XRPD is a powerful tool to identify any changes in crystallinity of drug (polymorphism).[50] Comparison of the X-ray diffraction patterns of VCM and nanoparticles prepared with RS-100 (Figure 2) showed no remarkable reduction in the peak intensities, suggesting that the expanse of VCM crystallinity was not reduced by the polymer. The X-ray diffraction patterns of pure drug and Eudragit RS showed that the pure drug is crystalline in nature (Figure 2). As shown in Figure 2, Eudragit RS100 is a typical form of amorphous materials, whereas the pure drug showed the diffractographic profile of a crystalline material. When the nanoparticles were prepared with different polymer/drug ratios (F1, F2 and F3) it is clear that the nanoparticles with lower polymer concentration showed similar peaks as the blank nanoparticles. At high concentration of polymer and low concentration of drug some of the distinguishing peaks for VCM are detectable but with very low intensity due to the presence of lower concentration of drug in the sample in comparison with pure VCM sample. This confirms the results obtained from DSC.

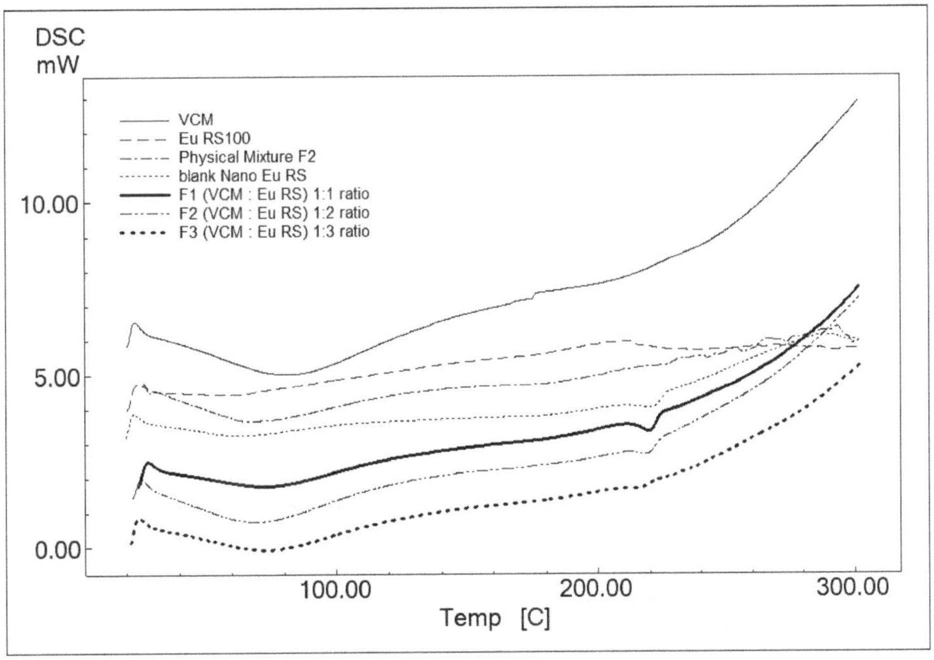

Figure 1. DSC thermogram of the VCM; RS100; PVA; physical mixture F_2; blank nanoparticles, VCM nanoparticles formulations as F_1, F_2 and F_3.

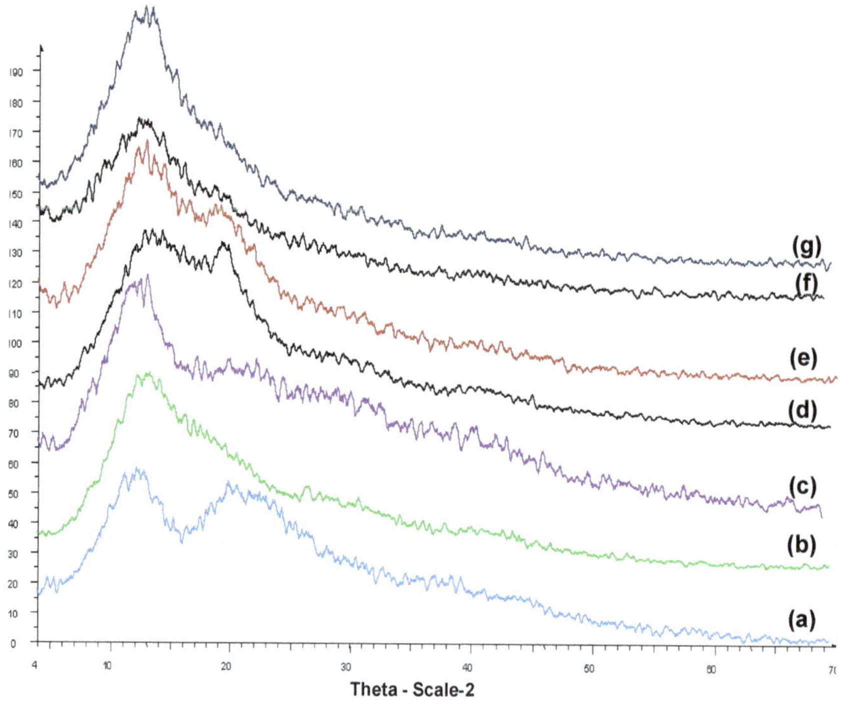

Figure 2. X-ray diffraction a) VCM; b) RS100; c) Physical Mixture F2; d) blank nanoparticles; e) VCM : RS100 (1:1); f) VCM : RS100 (1:2); g) VCM RS100 (1:3).

FTIR Studies

The FTIR spectra of VCM, VCM-loaded RS-100 nanoparticles, physical mixture F_2 (1:1), and the individual components are portrayed in Figure 3. The FTIR of VCM showed phenolic OH at 3257.39 cm^{-1}, aromatic C=C stretching at 1652.7 cm^{-1} and C=O stretching at 1503.48 cm^{-1}. The peaks in the range between 2800 and 3100cm^{-1} pertain to the C—H stretching bands, the peak in the range between 1650 and 1800cm^{-1} is due to the C=O stretching vibrational groups, and the peak in the range between 1350 and 900 cm^{-1} corresponds to the C—O stretching vibration mode. The peaks within 2950–3000 cm^{-1} assigned to the stretching vibrations of CH2 and CH3, the peak at 1763 cm^{-1} conforms the C=O ester vibration, and the peak at 1153 cm^{-1} is fitted with the C—O ester vibration, respectively. Eudragit RS-100 has C=O stretching band at 1734.2 cm^{-1}. Nanoparticles F1, F2 and F3 have C=O stretching band at 1731.2, 1733.7, 1733.96 cm^{-1}, respectively (Figure 3). After VCM was encapsulated into the nanoparticles, the characteristic peaks for VCM showed by the stronger intensity peaks for of matrix materials. On the other hand, the C=O stretching bands of VCM in polymeric systems were merged, thus leading to a peak shifting from 1731.2 cm^{-1} to 1733.96 cm^{-1}.[51] The bands observed for nanoparticles spectrum showed similar unique peaks but with smaller intensity due to low concentration of drug in nanoparticles. No differences in the positions of the absorption bands were observed in spectra of the VCM physical mixture with RS-100, indicating that there are no chemical interactions in the solid state between the drug and the polymer. This suggests that there was no new chemical bond constructed between these functional groups in the drug and the polymer after preparing the nanoparticles and the results confirmed that the drug is physically dispersed in the polymer. FTIR investigations confirmed the compatibility of VCM and RS100.

In vitro release study

The mean cumulative release (%) versus time curves is shown in Figure 4. The rate of dissolution of physical mixture is quite fast, and more than 96% drug is dissolved in about 30 min and 100% by 60 min. The drug release from the nanoparticles manifested to have two components with an immediate release of about 10.78-12.27% at the first sampling time of 30 min. This was followed by a slower exponential release of the remaining drug over the next 6-8 h. The in vitro VCM release profiles from drug-loaded nanoparticles are also illustrated in Figure 4. Furthermore, Figure 4 clearly presentes that the rate of drug release from the nanoparticles depended on the polymer concentration in the system. A similar relationship was observed between polymer content and drug release rate from prepared nanoparticles. By decreasing the concentration of the polymer in the system, an increase was shown in the release rate of VCM. The difference was also not significant ($p > 0.05$) for 0.5 or 24 h. It is offered that a reduced diffusion path and increased tortuosity may have retarded the drug release rate from the matrix at the presence of polymer matrix.

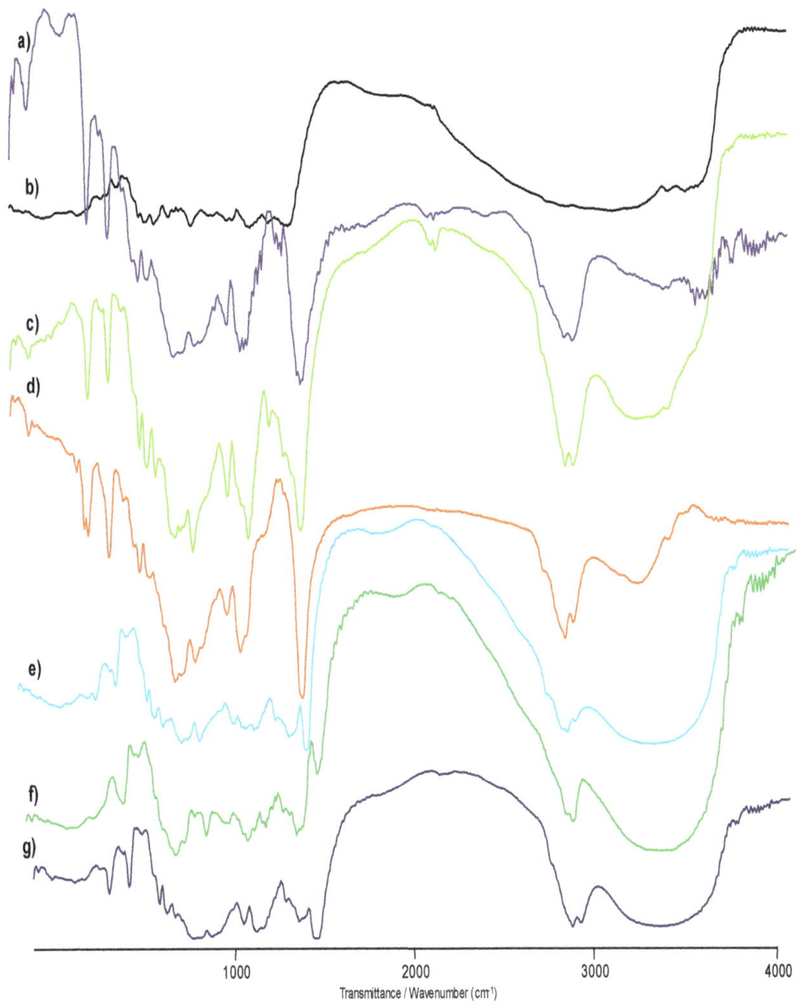

Figure 3. FTIR spectrum; a) RS100; b) VCM; c) Physical Mixture F_2; d) blank nanoparticles; e) VCM : RS100 (1:1), f) VCM : RS100 (1:2), g) VCM : RS100 (1:3).

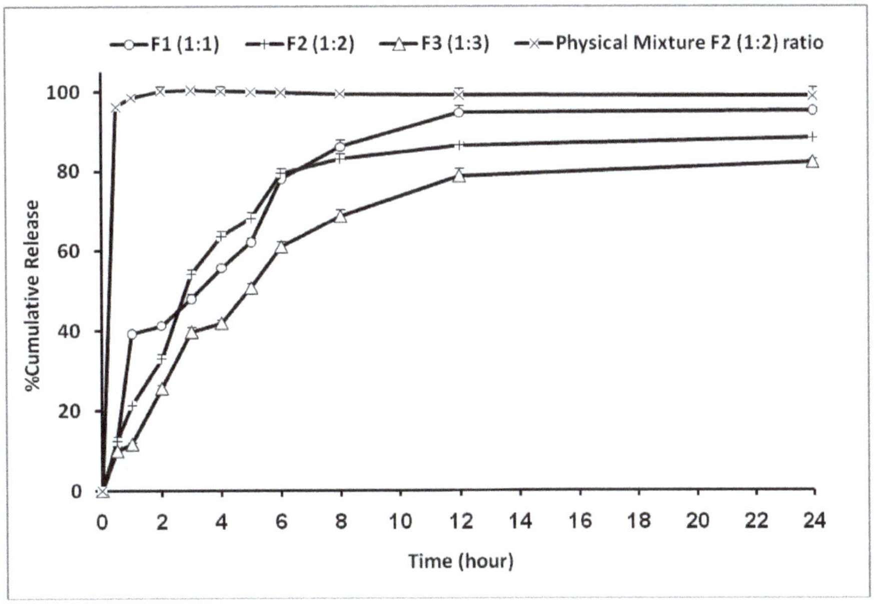

Figure4. Cumulative percent release of VCM nanoparticles prepared with different drug-to-polymer ratio and physical mixture F_2.

Nanoparticles containing 1:1 (F_1) released the drug more rapidly, wherease F_3 exhibited a relatively slower drug release profile. F_1, F_2 and F_3 nanoparticles showed higher dissolution efficiency of 81.44, 76. 25 and 66. 37%, respectively. Physical mixture of drug and polymer exhibited higher release in comparison with microspheres ($p < 0.05$) (Table 2 & Figure 4). The presence of Eudragit RS100 in the matrix of nanoparticles caused a slower and more advancing release of VCM during the time of the experiment.[52] The lowest dissolution efficiency was showed for F3 (66. 37%) and dissolution efficiency of the physical mixture was 98.03% ($p < 0.05$). The value of $t_{50\%}$ varies between 2.24 (F_2 formulation) to 4.85 h (F_3 formulation). The results of difference factor (f_2) observed that there is no similarity between the release profiles of nanoparticle formulations and physical mixture (Table 2). The in vitro release profiles were fitted to various kinetic models (Higuchi, first-order, zero-order, Peppas, Hixson crowell, square root of mass, three second root of mass, weibull, linear probability and log- probability) in order to determine the mechanism of drug release.[23] The dissolution rate constants were calculated from the slope of the respective plots and high correlation was observed for the Peppas models (Table 3). The data obtained were also put in Korsemeyer-Peppas model in order to find out n value, which particularizes the drug release mechanism. The n value of nanospheres of different drug to polymer ratio was between 0.392-0.569, indicating that the mechanism of the drug release were diffusion controlled.

Table 2. Comparison of various release characteristics of vancomycin from different nanoparticle formulations and physical mixture

Formulation	$^a t_{50\%}$ (h)	^{b}DE	$^c Q_{0.5}$	$^d Q_{24}$	Difference Factor (f_1)
F_1	3.25	81.44	11.44±0.99	95.03±2.17	38.11
F_2	2.24	76.25	12.27±1.25	88.27±0.77	40.52
F_3	4.85	66.37	9.95±0.49	82.23±0.78	52.55
Physical mixture	0.26	98.03	96.10±0.43	98.70±0.52	0.04

[a]dissolution time for 50% fractions. [b]Dissolution Efficiency. [c]amount of drug release after 0.5h.[d] amount of drug release after 24h

Intestinal permeability and oral fractional absorption data

In any in situ intestinal perfusion technique it is necessary to determine the magnitude of volume changes of the solution in the gut lumen during an experiment. For this purpose phenol red dye (200 μ g/ml) was added to drug solution in each experiment. Phenol red was used as a non-absorbable marker to detect gain or loss of water by the lumen. The determined mean P_{eff} values for different concentrations of vancomycin and its nanoparticles in PBS, oral fractional absorption and also the mean net water fluxes in the SPIP technique are listed in Table 4.

Discussion

The organic phase (O) behaves as a barrier between the two aqueous compartments. To control the methylene chloride elimination time and rate, we used a rotary evaporator method. Thus, the transfer of the drug into the external phase (W_2) was hampered. The particle formation itself is based on coacervation. The solvent is extracted from the polymer containing organic phase because of its initial diffusion into the continuous W_2 phase, motivating phase separation of the polymer. The organic solvent is eliminated by two steps; firstly by extraction and secondly by evaporation. In general, the solvent removal rate directly affects the encapsulation efficiency of a drug[53, 54] because the slow membrane formation rate may reduce the encapsulation efficiency as a result of improving the chances of drug molecules to be diffused out from the inner W_1 phase to outer W_2 water phase.[54,55] It is deduced that rapid membrane formation is an important criterion preventing the leakage of VCM to the W_2 phase. Generally, PVA is used as a surfactant in the $W_1/O/W_2$ emulsion method to comprise it onto the surface of RS-100 particles, thereby lowering the surface tension between the RS-100 surface and the W_2 phase.[54,56] However, because PVA cannot be washed away absolutely, it remains on the surface of RS-100.[54,57] PVA concentration in the external water phase is known to be a important factor to influence the size of nanoparticles.[43] The low drug incorporation efficiency may be ascribed to the water soluble nature of VCM hydrochloride. This led to its rapid partitioning into the aqueous phase and accordingly decreased entrapment into the nanoparticles during polymer deposition. The decreased drug entrapment with increasing theoretical drug loadings is due to an enhanced drug exudation into the aqueous phase at high loadings.

Table 3. Fitting parameters of the *in vitro* release data to various release kinetic models for nanoparticles

	ORDER	RSQ	Slope	intercept	MPE%	K
F_1	Zero order	0.627	0.036	0.341	3.1E+14	0.036
	First order	0.891	-0.152	-0.314	2.5E+14	-0.152
	Second order	0.950	1.320	-2.217	1.7E+15	1.320
	Higuchi	0.876	0.220	0.103	9.3E+13	0.220
	Peppas (Power Low)	0.999	0.569	-1.404	15.8656	1.767
	Hixson-Crowell	0.816	0.029	0.122	2.9E+14	0.029
	Square root of mass	0.770	0.034	0.184	3E+14	0.034
	Three-seconds root of mass	0.722	0.036	0.242	30.1957	0.036
	weibull	0.998	0.583	-0.857	15.6951	0.230
	Linear-probability	0.323	0.197	-1.446	5.5E+13	0.197
	Logarithmic-probability	0.911	0.160	0.198	59.8762	0.160
F_2	Zero order	0.543	0.034	0.335	3046748	0.034
	First order	0.714	-0.094	-0.459	3344353	-0.094
	Second order	0.855	0.353	0.497	3018450	0.353
	Higuchi	0.819	0.212	0.098	889793	0.212
	Peppas (Power Low)	0.995	0.393	-1.218	32.3218	1.481
	Hixson-Crowell	0.656	0.022	0.138	3271499	0.022
	Square root of mass	0.627	0.027	0.197	3222189	0.027
	Three-seconds root of mass	0.598	0.031	0.248	3167227	0.031
	weibull	0.986	0.410	-0.744	33.1694	0.163
	Linear-probability	0.339	0.142	-1.043	1349436	0.142
	Logarithmic-probability	0.868	0.155	0.066	61.8763	0.155
F_3	Zero order	0.686	0.034	0.226	2054809	0.034
	First order	0.834	-0.077	-0.238	1926127	-0.077
	Second order	0.925	0.213	0.102	841078	0.213
	Higuchi	0.905	0.199	0.016	149265	0.199
	Peppas (Power Low)	0.994	0.414	-1.515	30.4708	1.512
	Hixson-Crowell	0.788	0.019	0.080	2014231	0.019
	Square root of mass	0.763	0.025	0.119	2037665	0.025
	Three-seconds root of mass	0.738	0.029	0.157	2050986	0.029
	weibull	0.986	0.427	-1.179	34.4088	0.063
	Linear-probability	0.377	0.139	-1.359	791204	0.139
	Logarithmic-probability	0.871	0.155	-0.301	66.9204	0.155
Physical mixture	Zero order	0.081	0.012	0.828	7526441	0.012
	First order	0.016	0.072	-6.560	9078026	0.072
	Second order	0.042	-8796.400	153390.990	9090842	-8796.367
	Higuchi	0.261	0.112	0.669	6082596	0.112
	Peppas (Power Low)	0.982	0.508	-0.724	25.1718	1.662
	Hixson-Crowell	0.032	0.007	0.722	8895392	0.007
	Square root of mass	0.060	0.010	0.781	8656034	0.010
	Three-seconds root of mass	0.074	0.011	0.808	8326018	0.011
	weibull	0.973	0.574	0.991	4.88962	5.616
	Linear-probability	0.022	0.053	1.901	8830365	0.053
	Logarithmic-probability	0.837	0.281	2.517	10.1867	0.281

Table 4. Permeability coefficients and oral fractional absorption determined in rats for test and control groups

Group	C_{in}	Mean Puff ($\times 10^5$ cm/sec)	Oral fractional absorption	Mean NWF (ml/min/cm)
Control	200	6.11(± 2.66)	0.37(± 0.17)	-0.0003(± 0.0002)
	300	3.87(± 2.45)	0.53(± 0.09)	0.0006(± 0.0003)
	400	2.54 (± 1.64)	0.28(± .012)	0.0004(± 0.0001)
Test	200	17.88 (± 2.61)	0.45(± 0.15)	-0.0005(± 0.0002)
	300	16.63(± 2.98)	0.77(± 0.13)	0.0004(± 0.0002)
	400	15.75(± 4.47)	0.42(± 0.20)	-0.0006(± 0.0003)

Zeta potential results (Table 1) showed that drug-loaded formulations carried a positive charge, which assists particle stability because the repulsive forces prevent aggregation with aging. It has been reported that the positive charge of RS-100 nanoparticles is due to positive charge of VCM,.[58] because VCM is cationic drug and changed the charge of nanoparticles. Drug-free RS-100 nanoparticles had a positive surface charge of 15. 7 mV, which can be attributed to the presence of carboxyl groups and quaternary ammonium of the polymer on the nanoparticles.[30] Zeta potential measurements showed a insignificant increase in positivity (from 18.1 mV to 25.7 mV) with an decrease in theoretical drug loadings. These findings are concuring to what was expected, for instance a decrease in the surface positivity due to interaction of carboxyl groups and the cationic drug on the particle surface. The increase in nanoparticle size with decreases in the theoretical drug loading of VCM (Table 1) may possibly have influenced the surface charge of the RS-100 nanoparticles.[59] From the data it is obvious that all the formulations are almost unstable in the colloidal state. This indicates that the particles should not be stored in a liquid suspension form and rather they should be stored in a lyophilized state.[59]The rapid initial release of VCM was probably due to the drug which was adsorbed or near to the surface of the nanoparticles and the large surface to volume ratio of nanoparticle geometry because of their size. [30] It may also be due to the water soluble nature of VCM. The exponential delayed release may be attributed to diffusion of the dissolved drug within the RS-100 core of the nanoparticle into the dissolution medium. Similar observations were reported by other researchers working. [60,61] Loading of VCM into the nanoparticles prompts to a modification of in vitro drug release, depending on their combination . The data obtained were also put in Korsemeyer-Peppas model in order to perceive the n value, which describes the drug release mechanism. The n value of nanospheres of different drug:polymer ratio was between 0.39-0.56, indicating that the drug release was diffusion controlled (Table 3). On the other hand, from the acquired results in rats it is demonstrated that the intestinal permeability oral fractional absorption of VCM is significantly increased using its nanoparticles in all three concentrations which were used ($P < 0.05$). The stable water fluxes and permeability coefficients in each perfusion, as a function of time, for tested compounds indicated that intestinal barrier function was maintained during the methodology. The intestinal permeability of VCM was determined to be in the range of 1.96 (±1.09)$\times 10^{-5}$cm/sec to 4.66 (±1.32)$\times 10^{-5}$ cm/sec in control groups. regardless, the drug permeability in test groups' intestinal segments which were perfused by VCM nanoparticles in PBS, ranged between 3.68 (±2.82)$\times 10^{-5}$ cm/sec and 10.06 (±2.61)$\times 10^{-5}$ cm/sec. There were statistical differences among the P_{eff} values in different concentrations. The maximum permeability, was seen at doses of 300 μg/ml. Therefore, it seems that the intestinal permeability of VCM is not concentration-dependent. The oral fractional absorption of VCM was determined to be in the range of 0.28 (±0.12) to 0.53 (±0.09) in control groups, while the test group was determined to be in the range of 0.42 (±0.20) to 0.77 (±0.13) (Table 4). In view of the hydrophilicity and high molecular weight of the peptidic drug, VCM, the higher intestinal permeability after nanonization is probable due to enhanced paracellular passage and endocytotic uptake, because the particles with small size are absorbed by intestinal enterocytes through endocytosis. Coating of VCM nanoparticles with PVA, a bioadhesive material, can also be a tactic to increase nanoparticle uptake by intestinal enterocytes. Nanoparticles coated with bioadhesive materials were contemplated to develop mucoadhesion. Adhesion of a carrier system to the mucus may improve residence time and drug contact with the underlying epithelium, thus increasing drug intestinal permeability which was demonstrated in the present study.

Conclusion

VCM-loaded RS-100 nanoparticles were successfully provided by using $W_1/O/W_2$ double-emulsion solvent evaporation method. Drug release from nanoparticles was more sustained than physical mixture. Moreover, the intestinal permeation and fractional absorption of VCM were improved using its nanoparticles and this may allow more efficient therapy compared to VCM formulations present in the market.

Acknowledgments
The financial support from biotechnology center, Tabriz University of Medical Sciences, is greatly acknowledged.

Conflict of interest
The authors report no conflicts of interest in this work.

References

1. Robles-Piedras AL, Gonz‹lez-Lpez EH. Therapeutic Drug Monitoring of Vancomycin. Proc West Pharmacol Soc 2009;52:21-3.
2. Moellering RC Jr. Monitoring Serum Vancomycin Levels: Climbing the Mountain Because It Is There? *Clinical infectious diseases* 1994;18:544-6.
3. Cook FV, Farrar WE. Vancomycin revisited. Annals of internal medicine 1978; 88(6): 813-8.
4. Bryan CS, White WL. Safety of oral vancomycin in functionally anephric patients. *Antimicrobial Agents and Chemotherapy* 1978; 14(4): 634-35.
5. Geraci JE, et al. Some laboratory and clinical experiences with a new antibiotic, vancomycin. Antibiot Annu 1956-1957:90-106.
6. Florence AT. Nanoparticle uptake by the oral route: Fulfilling its potential? *Drug discovery today: technologies* 2005; 2(1):75-81.
7. Yallapu MM, et al. Fabrication of curcumin encapsulated PLGA nanoparticles for improved therapeutic effects in metastatic cancer cells. *Journal of colloid and interface science* 2010; 351(1): 19-29.
8. Kumar GS, et al. Synthesis and characterization of bioactive hydroxyapatite-calcite nanocomposite for biomedical applications. *Journal of colloid and interface science* 2010; 349(1): 56-62.
9. Nouvel C, et al. Biodegradable nanoparticles made from polylactide-grafted dextran copolymers. *Journal of colloid and interface science* 2009; 330(2): 337-43.
10. Han DP, et al. Spectrum and susceptibilities of microbiologic isolates in the Endophthalmitis Vitrectomy Study. *American journal of ophthalmology* 1996; 122(1): 1-17.
11. Jelvehgari M, et al. Formulation, characterization and in vitro evaluation of theophylline-loaded Eudragit RS 100 microspheres prepared by an emulsion-solvent diffusion/evaporation technique. *Pharmaceutical Development and Technology* 2011;16:637-44.
12. Valizadeh H, et al. A simple and rapid high-performance liquid chromatography method for determining furosemide, hydrochlorothiazide, and phenol red: applicability to intestinal permeability studies. *J AOAC Int* 2006; 89(1): 88-93.
13. Zakeri-Milani,P, et al. Biopharmaceutical classification of drugs using intrinsic dissolution rate (IDR) and rat intestinal permeability. *Eur J Pharm Biopharm* 2009; 73(1): 102-6.
14. Zakeri-Milani P, et al. Investigation of the intestinal permeability of ciclosporin using the in situ technique in rats and the relevance of P-glycoprotein. *Arzneimittelforschung* 2008; 58(4): 188-92.
15. Zakeri-Milani P, et al. Predicting human intestinal permeability using single-pass intestinal perfusion in rat. *J Pharm Pharm Sci* 2007; 10(3): 368-79.
16. Zakeri-Milani P, et al. The utility of rat jejunal permeability for biopharmaceutics classification system. *Drug Dev Ind Pharm* 2009; 35(12): 1496-502.
17. Dashevsky A, Zessin G. The effect of ethylcellulose molecular weight on the properties of theophylline microspheres. *Journal of microencapsulation* 1997; 14(3): 273-80.
18. Saravanan M, et al. Ibuprofen-loaded ethylcellulose/polystyrene microspheres: an approach to get prolonged drug release with reduced burst effect and low ethylcellulose content. *Journal of microencapsulation* 2003; 20(3): 289-302.
19. Benichou A, Aserin A, Garti N. Polyols, high pressure, and refractive indices equalization for improved stability of W/O emulsions for food applications. *Journal of dispersion science and technology* 2001; 22(2-3): 269-80.
20. Fagerholm U, Johansson M, Lennernas H. Comparison between permeability coefficients in rat and human jejunum. *Pharmaceutical research* 1996; 13(9): 1336-42.
21. Shantha Kumar TR, et al. Validated HPLC analytical method with programmed wavelength UV detection for simultaneous determination of DRF-4367 and Phenol red in rat in situ intestinal perfusion study. *Journal of pharmaceutical and biomedical analysis* 2005; 38(1): 173-9.
22. Favetta P, et al. New sensitive assay of vancomycin in human plasma using high-performance liquid chromatography and electrochemical detection. *Journal of Chromatography B: Biomedical Sciences and Applications* 2001; 751(2): 377-382.
23. Hoffart V, et al. Low molecular weight heparin-loaded polymeric nanoparticles: formulation, characterization, and release characteristics. *Drug Dev Ind Pharm* 2002; 28(9): 1091-9.
24. Hasan AS, et al,.. Effect of the microencapsulation of nanoparticles on the reduction of burst release. *Int J Pharm* 2007; 344(1-2): 53-61.
25. Couvreur P, et al. Nanocapsule technology: a review. *Critical reviews in therapeutic drug carrier systems* 2002; 19(2): 99-134.
26. Agnihotri SM, Vavia PR. Diclofenac-loaded biopolymeric nanosuspensions for ophthalmic application. *Nanomedicine* 2009; 5(1): 90-5.

27. Foster KA, Yazdanian M, Audus KL. Microparticulate uptake mechanisms of invitro cell culture models of the respiratory epithelium. *Journal of pharmacy and pharmacology* 2001, 53(1): 57-66.
28. Mehnert W, Mäder K. Solid lipid nanoparticles: Production, characterization and applications. *Advanced Drug Delivery Reviews* 2001; 47(2-3): 165-96.
29. Mohanraj V, Chen Y. Nanoparticles-a review. *Tropical Journal of Pharmaceutical Research* 2007; 5(1): 561-73.
30. Govender T, et al. PLGA nanoparticles prepared by nanoprecipitation: drug loading and release studies of a water soluble drug. *Journal of Controlled Release* 1999; 57(2): 171-85.
31. Govender T, et al. Defining the drug incorporation properties of PLA-PEG nanoparticles. *International journal of pharmaceutics* 2000; 199(1): 95-110.
32. Panyam J, et al .Solidstate solubility influences encapsulation and release of hydrophobic drugs from PLGA/PLA nanoparticles. *Journal of pharmaceutical sciences* 2004; 93(7): 1804-14.
33. Gavini E, et al. PLGA microspheres for the ocular delivery of a peptide drug, vancomycin using emulsification/spray-drying as the preparation method: in vitro/in vivo studies. *European journal of pharmaceutics and biopharmaceutics* 2004; 57(2): 207-12.
34. Mukherjee B, et al. A comparison between povidone-ethylcellulose and povidone-eudragit transdermal dexamethasone matrix patches based on in vitro skin permeation. *European journal of pharmaceutics and biopharmaceutics* 2005; 59(3): 475-83.
35. Lin SY Yu HL. Microscopic fourier transform infrared/differential scanning calorimetry system used to study the different thermal behaviors of polymethacrylate copolymers of Eudragits RS, RL, E 30D, or E. *Journal of applied polymer science* 2000; 78(4): 829-35.
36. Gribb AA ,Banfield JF. Particle size effects on transformation kinetics and phase stability in nanocrystalline TiO2. *American Mineralogist* 1997; 82(7): 717-28.
37. Kumar GS, et al. Synthesis and characterization of bioactive hydroxyapatite-calcite nanocomposite for biomedical applications. *J Colloid Interface Sci* 2010; 349(1): 56-62.
38. Fagerholm U, Johansson M, Lennernas H. Comparison between permeability coefficients in rat and human jejunum. *Pharm Res* 1996; 13: 1336-1342.
39. Amidon GL, et al. A theoretical basis for a biopharmaceutic drug classification: the correlation of in vitro drug product dissolution and in vivo bioavailability. *Pharmaceutical research* 1995; 12(3): 413-20.
40. Olfert ED, et al. Guide to the care and use of experimental animals. Vol. 1. 1993: Canadian Council on Animal Care Ottawa, Ontario, Canada.
41. Danzer L. Liquid-chromatographic determination of cephalosporins and chloramphenicol in serum. *Clinical chemistry* 1983; 29(5): 856-8.
42. Swenson ES, Milisen WB, Curatolo W. Intestinal permeability enhancement: efficacy, acute local toxicity, and reversibility. *Pharmaceutical research* 1994; 11(8): 1132-42.
43. Youan BBC, et al. Protein release profiles and morphology of biodegradable microcapsules containing an oily core. *Journal of controlled release* 2001; 76(3): 313-26.
44. Pignatello R, et al. Properties of tolmetin-loaded Eudragit RL100 and Eudragit RS 100 microparticles prepared by different techniques. *STP pharma sciences* 1997;7(2): 148-57.
45. Malamataris S, Avgerinos A. Controlled release indomethacin microspheres prepared by using an emulsion solvent-diffusion technique. *International Journal of Pharmaceutics* 1990; 62(2-3): 105-11.
46. Alex R, Bodmeier R. Encapsulation of water-soluble drugs by a modified solvent evaporation method. I. Effect of process and formulation variables on drug entrapment. *Journal of Microencapsulation* 1990; 7(3): 347-55.
47. Xie J, Wang CH. Self-assembled biodegradable nanoparticles developed by direct dialysis for the delivery of paclitaxel. *Pharmaceutical research* 2005; 22(12): 2079-90.
48. Ceschel G, et al. Degradation of components in drug formulations: a comparison between HPLC and DSC methods. *Journal of pharmaceutical and biomedical analysis* 2003; 32(4-5): 1067-72.
49. Jelvehgari M, et al. Control of encapsulation efficiency in polymeric microparticle system of tolmetin. *Pharmaceutical development and technology* 2010; 15(1): 71-9.
50. Aaltonen,J, et al. Polymorph screening using near-infrared spectroscopy. *Analytical Chemistry* 2003; 75(19): 5267-73.
51. Gupta M, Saini T. preformulation parameters characterization to design, development and formulation of vancomycin hydrochloride tablets for psudomembranous colitis. *international Journal of pharmaceutical reaserch and development* 2009; 1(9):1-7.
52. Jelvehgari M, et al. Preparation and Evaluation of Poly (-caprolactone) Nanoparticles-in-Microparticles by W/O/W Emulsion Method. *Iranian Journal of Basic Medical Sciences* 2010; 13(3): 1-8.
53. Capan Y, et al. Preparation and characterization of poly(D,L-lactide-co-glycolide) microspheres for controlled release of human growth hormone. *AAPS Pharm Sci Tech* 2003; 4(2): E28.
54. Yang YY, Chung TS, Ping Ng N. Morphology, drug distribution, and in vitro release profiles of

biodegradable polymeric microspheres containing protein fabricated by double-emulsion solvent extraction/evaporation method. *Biomaterials* 2001; 22(3): 231-41.
55. Wu JC, et al. Effect of the solvent-non-solvent pairs on the surface morphology and release behaviour of ethylcellulose microcapsules prepared by non-solvent-addition phase separation method. *J Microencapsul* 1994; 11(3): 297-308.
56. Wickramasinghe R, Liow JL, Leong YK. Nanobiotech congress. 2007; Available from: http://www.aiche.org/uploadedfiles/SBE/events/Tuesday07.pdf.
57. Martin A, Bustamante P, Chun AH. Physical Pharmacy and Pharmaceutical Sciences. Fifth edition ed. Philadelphia: Lippincott Williams & Wilkins, 2006.
58. Mondal S, et al. Flocculation of yeast suspension by a cationic polymer: Characterization of flocculent-cell interaction. 2011. American Institute of Chemical Engineers.
59. Mukherjee B, et al. Preparation, characterization and in-vitro evaluation of sustained release protein-loaded nanoparticles based on biodegradable polymers. *Int J Nanomedicine* 2008; 3(4): 487-96.
60. Fonseca C, Simoes S, Gaspar R. Paclitaxel-loaded PLGA nanoparticles: preparation, physicochemical characterization and in vitro anti-tumoral activity. *J Control Release* 2002; 83(2): 273-86.
61. Ahlin P, et al. Investigation of polymeric nanoparticles as carriers of enalaprilat for oral administration. *Int J Pharm* 2002; 239(1-2): 113-20.

6

Effect of Taurine on the antimicrobial efficiency of Gentamicin

Mina Islambulchilar [1,2,4], Mohammad Reza Sattari[2,3], Mohammad Sardashti[2,4], Farzaneh Lotfipour[2,5*]

[1]*School of Pharmacy, Zanjan University of Medical Sciences, Zanjan, Iran*

[2]*Faculty of Pharmacy, Tabriz University of Medical Sciences, Tabriz, Iran*

[3]*Infectious & Tropical diseases research center, Tabriz University of Medical Sciences, Tabriz, Iran*

[4]*Student Research Committee, Tabriz University of Medical Sciences, Tabriz, Iran*

[5]*Hematology and Oncology Research Center, Tabriz University of Medical Sciences, Tabriz, Iran*

ARTICLE INFO

Keywords:
Taurine
antimicrobial activity
Gentamicin

ABSTRACT

Context: Gentamicin is mainly used in severe infections caused by gram-negatives. However toxicity including nephrotoxicity and ototoxicity is one of the most important complications of its treatment. The production of free radicals seems to be involved in gentamicin toxicity mechanism. Taurine, a major intracellular free β-amino acid, is known to be an endogenous antioxidant. So potentially the co-therapy of taurine and gentamicin would reduce the adverse effects of the antibiotic. ***Objectives:*** In this study, we wished to know the effect of taurine on the antibiotic capacity of gentamicin. ***Methods:*** strainsof *P. aeruginosa*, *E. coli, S. aureus* and *S. epidermidis* were used as test organisms. Minimum inhibitory concentrations of gentamicin in the presence and absence of taurine at quantities from 40 to 2 mg/L were determined using macro-dilution method. ***Results:*** MICs were determined in the various concentrations of taurine for bacterial indicators. The MIC values of gentamicin for *P. aeruginosa, S. aureus* and *E. coli* remained unchanged in the values of 2.5, 5 and 20 µg/ml respectively in the absence and presences of different concentrations of taurine. The bactericidal activity of gentamicin against *S. epidermidis* was increased by addition of taurine in the concentrations higher than 6 mg/L. ***Conclusion:*** According to our study the antibacterial activity of gentamicin against the indicator microorganisms were not interfere with taurine at selected concentrations. Further in vivo studies are needed to establish if a combination of gentamicin and taurine would have the same effect.

Introduction

Aminoglycosid antibiotics including gentamicin are used mainly in severe infections caused by gramnegatives especially pseudomonas, enterobacter, serratia, proteus, acinetobacter, and klebsiella and they produce synergistic bactericidal effects against enterococci, streptococci, and staphylococci.[1,2] The major complications of gentamicin treatment are nephrotoxicity and irreversible ototoxicity.[3] However, the exact mechanisms leading to gentamicin induced cell injury and cell death are unknown at present. Present evidences support the concept that reactive oxygen metabolites including free radical species are important mediators of gentamicin nephrotoxicity and outotoxicity.[4-8]

Several free radicals are produced in the body as byproducts of normal metabolism and also upon exposure to radiation and various environmental pollutants. They are highly reactive, causing damage to cellular components and leading to a variety of diseases. These free radicals are also known as reactive oxygen species (ROS) and include super oxide (O_2^-), hydroxyl radical (OH^-) and hydrogen peroxide (H_2O_2). They contribute towards cytotoxicity, morphological and metabolic changes, changes in the CNS, and increased muscle proteolysis.[9] To prevent injury from oxidative stress, aerobic organisms have evolved a system of chemical and enzymatic antioxidants.

Among the antioxidant enzymes are superoxide dismutase (SOD), glutathione peroxidase (GPx) and catalase (CAT). SOD catalyzes the dismutation of the superoxide radical anion to hydrogen peroxide and oxygen. CAT and GPx convert H_2O_2 to H_2O.[10]

***Corresponding author:** Farzaneh Lotfipour (PhD), E-mail: lotfipoor@tbzmed.ac.ir

Antioxidants play an important role in health maintenance. Significant increase in lipid peroxidation and reduction of antioxidant enzymes after the treatment of gentamicin indicated the generation of free radicals and the involvement of oxidative stress to nephrotoxicity[11-13] and ototoxicity[14-16] caused by gentamicin treatment. Later in vivo experiments confirmed that several radical scavengers may attenuate aminoglycoside-induced ototoxicity and nephrotoxicity.[17-25]
Taurine (2-aminoethanesulfonic acid), a sulphur-containing amino acid, is found naturally in food, especially in seafood and meat (figure 1). It is a conditionally essential amino acid that is present at millimolar concentrations in many animal tissues, especially nervous tissue, retina and neutrophils.[9,26-30]

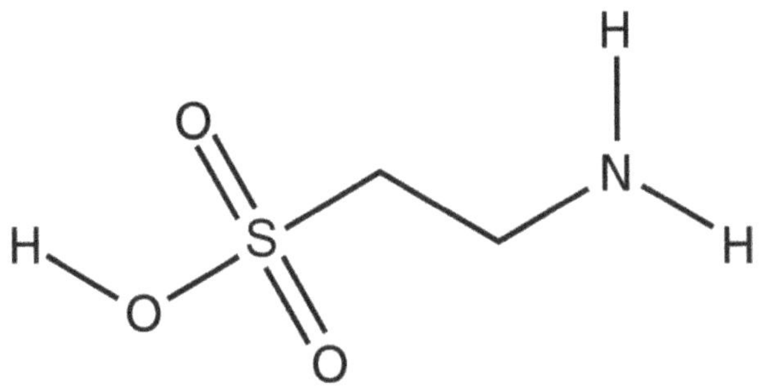

Figure 1. Taurine structure.

Mammals are able to endogenously synthesize taurine, but some species such as humans are more dependent on dietary sources of taurine.[31] It is not incorporated into proteins, but is found free in many tissues. Taurine is involved in a number of physiological processes including bile acid conjugation,[32-33] (osmoregulation, detoxification of xenobiotics, cell membrane stabilization (2001), modulation of cellular calcium flux, and modulation of neuronal excitability.[34-35] Low levels of taurine have been associated with retinal degeneration,[36] growth retardation, and cardiomyopathy (2001). Taurine has been used clinically in the treatment of cardiovascular diseases,[37-38] hypercholesterolemia, seizure disorders,[39] ocular disorders, diabetes,[40-42] Alzheimer's disease,[43-44] hepatic disorders,[26] cystic fibrosis,[45] acetaminophen toxicity,[46] and alcoholism.[47] Taurine is reported to exhibit direct anti-oxidant properties by lowering ROS and/or as an indirect antioxidant by preventing changes in membrane permeability due to oxidant injury.[48]
Taurine has been recognized as an antioxidant long time ago, scavenging both ROS and nitrogeneous radicals.[26]
In view of the importance of gentamicin in treatment of a wide variety of systemic infections, several researches focused on the possibility of lowering its toxicities. In this regard, various studies have been investigated the mitigating effect of antioxidants, such as D-methionine,[21] aspirin,[32] vitamins E & C,[49] N-acetylcysteine,[50] deferoxamine and 2,3-dihydroxybenzoate[51] on gentamicin-induced ototoxicity or nephrotoxity.
As we mentioned above, taurine can act as an antioxidant so potentially it could prevent the development of gentamicin-induced toxicities. But first of all it should be determined if or whether cotreatment of taurine and gentamicine is compatible with gentamicin's antibacterial activity or not. The purpose of this study was to ascertain the interaction of taurine on the antibiotic capacity of the aminoglycosides.

Materials and methods

Bacteria

The microorganisms used in this study included *Staphylococcus aureus* ATCC 29737, *Pseudomonas aeruginosa* ATCC 9027, *Staphylococcus epidermidis* ATCC 12228, and *Escherichia coli* ATCC 8739all were stocks of the Department of Pharmaceutical and Food Control, School of Pharmacy, Tabriz University of Medical Sciences.

Antibiotic and Taurine

Gentamicin sulfate (Merck, Germany) and taurine (Aviforme, UK) were provided as pure powders of stated potency and stored at 4°C.

Media and Buffers

The bacterial culture media included Soybean-Casein Digest Broth medium (SCDB) purchased from Merck Co. (Germany). For preparing buffer (buffer NO. 3) 16.73 g of dibasic potassium phosphate and 0.523 g of monobasic potassium phosphate dissolved in 1000 ml of distilled water and its pH was adjusted with 18N phosphoric acid or 10 N potassium hydroxide to 8.0 ± 0.1.

Gentamicin and Taurine stock solution

To prepare a stock solution, 1000 mg of gentamicin sulfate powder were accurately weighed and dissolved in the 1000 ml of buffer NO.3, stored in refrigerator. To prepare a stock solution, 800 mg of taurine powder were accurately weighed and dissolved in the 1000 ml of sterile distilled water, stored in refrigerator.

Inoculum preparation

Inocula were obtained from an overnight agar culture of the test organisms. Inoculum for the MIC test was prepared by transferring at least one to two well-isolated colonies of the same morphology from an agar plate culture into a tube containing 4 ml of Soybean-Casein Digest Broth. The broth culture was incubated for 24 h at 35° C. The turbidity of the actively growing broth culture was adjusted with sterile broth on a spectrophotometer set at a wavelength of 580 nm to achieve a turbidity equivalent to a 0.5 McFarland standard. This results in a suspension containing approximately 1 to 2 x 10^8 CFU/ml.

Minimum inhibitory concentrations (MICs)

Standard antibiotic solutions were prepared in sterile buffer No.3 for using at the same day. MICs were determined using broth macro-dilution MIC method; twofold serial dilutions of gentamicin yielding the concentrations of 40-0.156 mg/L were prepared in 4-ml volumes in the absence or presence of taurine (extending from 40-2 mg/L, a few concentrations more and less than it's serum concentrations: 22-8 mg/L). Bacterial inocula (100 µl) were transferred to the tubes; accordingly all tubes were incubated for 24 h ± 1 h at 35 ° C, finally turbidity of the cultures was assessed visually by comparison to uninoculated controls. The MIC was recorded as the lowest concentration of antibiotic at which visible growth was inhibited as detected by the unaided eye. All experiments were performed in independent triplicate occasions.

Results

To demonstrate if the in vitro activity of gentamicin could be affected by the concentration of dissolved taurine in the broth media, MICs were determined in the absence and presence of various concentrations of taurine in growth media for bacterial indicators.

First of all, potential antibacterial activity of taurine powder against the selected strains was evaluated. To this end susceptibility testing of our indicator bacteria for taurine were performed with diminution of taurine in broth. Based on the results taurine didn't show any antibacterial activity against all four strains.

In the second step, the MIC values of gentamicin alone against *P. aeruginosa, S. aureus* and *E. coli* were determined that were 2.5, 5 and 20 µg/ml respectively. Furthermore the MIC values of gentamicin against *P. aeruginosa, S. aureus* and *E. coli* measured in the presence of different concentrations of taurine (40, 32, 20, 16, 8, 6 µg/ml), had no significant changes in comparison with those obtained in the absence of taurine.

Surprisingly, as it can be seen in table 1, the inhibitory activity of gentamicin against *S. epidermidis* was increased by the addition of taurine. Taurine at quantities higher than 6 mg/L amelioratedgentamicin's antibacterial activity against *S.epidermidis*. The lower concentrations of tuarine (≤ 6µg/ml) did not alter the MIC values of gentamicin against the bacterium. The results of this experiment are summarized in Table 1.

Table 1. MIC values of gentamicin ± Taurine

Concentration of taurine	MIC values of gentamicin against *S.pidermidis*(µg/ml)	MIC values of gentamicin against *S.aureus* (µg/ml)	MIC values of gentamicin against *P.aeruginosa*(µg/ml)	MIC values of gentamicin agains *E. coli* (µg/ml)
40 µg/ml	0.312	5	2.5	20
32 µg/ml	0.312	5	2.5	20
20 µg/ml	0.312	5	2.5	20
16 µg/ml	0.312	5	2.5	20
8 µg/ml	1.25	5	2.5	20
6 µg/ml	5	5	2.5	20
0 µg/ml	5	5	2.5	20

Discussion

Gentamicin has been extensively used for the prophylaxis and the treatment of severe infectious diseases. The clinical application of this antibiotic has been limited by nephrotoxicity & outotoxicity that is related in part by its enhancing effect on the production of free radicals. In order to test the hypothesis that taurine may become useful in quenching the gentamicin's side effects, at first it should be investigated whether taurine hampers gentamicin's bactericidal activity. For this reason, we have tried to evaluate the possible interactions between taurine at serum level concentrations and the antibacterial action of gentamicin.

According to our study the MIC values of gentamicin against S. *aureus, P. aeruginosa, S. epidermidis,* and *E. coli* resembled those of gentamicin plus taurine against bacterial indicators. In the present study taurine can even augment gentamicin's antibacterial activity against *S. epidermidis*. Previous studies also showed that N-chlorotaurine exhibit antibacterial, antiviral, antifungal, antiamoebic and vermicidal activity.[52-57] According to Grisham et al. NH_2Cl is responsible for N-chlorotaurine's antioxidant and bactericidal effects.[58] Taurine, or 2-aminoethanesulfonic acid, is a derivative of the Cysteine, a sulfur-containing amino acid. It appears to be one of the naturally occurring sulfonic acids. Taurine contains sulfonate group instead of carboxylic acid group but it is often called an amino acid, even it is called an amino sulfonic acid. It is of interest that sufonic acid and sulfonates has already been proven to be moderately bactericidal, viricidal and fungicidal. Sucrose octa-sulphate suspension has shown inhibitory and antibacterial activity against 85% of 128 strains of Gram-negative bacilli.[59] Poly sulfonated compounds have shown microbicidal activity against human papillomavirus (HPV).[60] It has reported that substituted 8-quinolinol sulfonic acids have antifungal activity.[61] According to Zaneveld et al. T-PSS (poly (sodium 4-styrenesulfonate)) gel was an effective inhibitor of the infectivity of STD-causing microbes (HIV, HSV-1, HSV-2, *C. trachsomatis* and the multiplication of *N. gonorrhea*).[62]Another study indicated that several sulfunated compounds showed antiviral activity against bovine papillomavirus type 1 (BPV-1).[60] Sulfunated Schiff bases had antibacterial activities against *E. coli, Klebsilla and S. aureus.*[63] In this study, we used pure taurine, so it may concluded that taurine's sulfonic acid moiety cause its microbicidal activity against *S. epidermidis.*

Conclusion

According to our study it was verified that Taurine alone did not produce inhibition of the microorganisms. In the same way, when gentamicin was used in combination with taurine the inhibition produced by this antibiotic was not decreased. As a result, it can be concluded that taurine does not interfere with the antibiotic capacity of Gentamicin against *S. aureus, P. aeruginosa, S. epidermidis,* and *E. coli.* Taurine can also ameliorate Gentamicin's microbicidal activity against *S. epidermidis*.

Further studies are needed to determine if a combination of gentamicin and taurine would have the same effect in vivo.

Acknowledgment

We are grateful to Dr. Maryam Hassan (Tabriz University of Medical Sciences) for her kind technical assistance through the experiment.

Conflict of interest

The authors report no conflicts of interest in this work.

References

1. Goodman LS, Gilman A, Brunton LL. Goodman & Gilman's Manual of Pharmacology and therapeutics. New York: McGraw-Hill; 2008.
2. Rudin A, Healey A, Phillips CA, Gump DW, Forsyth BR. Antibacterial activity of gentamicin sulfate in tissue culture. *Appl Microbiol* 1970;20:989-990.
3. Katzung BG. Basic & Clinical Pharmacology. 9th ed. New York: Lange Medical Books/ McGraw Hill; 2004.
4. Basnakian AG, Kaushal GP, Shah SV. Apoptotic pathways of oxidative damage to renal tubular epithelial cells. *Antioxid Redox Signal* 2002;4:915-924.
5. Priuska EM, Schacht J. Formation of free radicals by gentamicin and iron and evidence for an iron/gentamicin complex. *Biochem Pharmacol* 1995;50:1749-1752.
6. Sha SH, Schacht J. Formation of reactive oxygen species following bioactivation of gentamicin. *Free Radic Biol Med* 1999;26:341-347.
7. Sha SH, Schacht J. Stimulation of free radical formation by aminoglycoside antibiotics. *Hear Res* 1999;128:112-118.
8. Van der Harst MR, Bull S, Laffont CM, Klein WR. Gentamicin nephrotoxicity--a comparison of in vitro findings with in vivo experiments in equines. *Vet Res Commun* 2005;29:247-261.
9. Yu J, Kim AK. Effect of taurine on antioxidant enzyme system in B16F10 melanoma cells. *Adv Exp Med Biol* 2009;643:491-499.
10. Beatty S, Koh H, Phil M, Henson D, Boulton M. The role of oxidative stress in the pathogenesis of age-related macular degeneration. *Surv Ophthalmol* 2000;45:115-134.
11. Du XH, Yang CL. Mechanism of gentamicin nephrotoxicity in rats and the protective effect of zinc-induced metallothionein synthesis. *Nephrol Dial Transplant* 1994;9:135-140.
12. Martinez-Salgado C, Eleno N, Tavares P, Rodriquez-Barbero A, Garcia-criado J, Bolanos JP, Lopez-Novoa JM. Involvement of reactive oxygen species on gentamicin-induced mesangial cell activation. *Kidney Int* 2002;62:1682-1692.
13. Upaganlawar A, Farswan M, Rathod S, Balaraman R. Modification of biochemical parameters of gentamicin nephrotoxicity by coenzyme Q10 and green tea in rats. *Indian J Exp Biol* 2006;44:416-418.
14. Hirose K, Hockenbery DM, Rubel EW. Reactive oxygen species in chick hair cells after gentamicin exposure in vitro. *Hear Res* 1997;104:1-14.
15. Jeong SW, Kim LS, Hur D, Bae WY, Kim JR, Lee JH. Gentamicin-induced spiral ganglion cell death: apoptosis mediated by ROS and the JNK signaling pathway. *Acta Otolaryngol* 2010;130:670-678.
16. Takumida M, Anniko M, Shimizu A, Watanabe H. Neuroprotection of vestibular sensory cells from gentamicin ototoxicity obtained using nitric oxide synthase inhibitors, reactive oxygen species scavengers, brain-derived neurotrophic factors and calpain inhibitors. *Acta Otolaryngol* 2003; 123:8-13.
17. Devbhuti P, Saha A, Sengupta C. Gentamicin induced lipid peroxidation and its control with ascorbic acid. *Acta Pol Pharm* 2009;66:363-369.
18. Kadkhodaee M, Khastar H, Arab HA, Ghaznavi R, Zahmatkesh M, Mahdavi-Mazdeh M. Antioxidant vitamins preserve superoxide dismutase activities in gentamicin-induced nephrotoxicity. *Transplant Proc* 2007;39:864-865.
19. Maldonado PD, Barrera D, Medina-Campos ON, Hernandez-Pando R, Ibarra-Rubio ME, Pedraza-

Chaverri J. Aged garlic extract attenuates gentamicin induced renal damage and oxidative stress in rats. *Life Sci* 2003; 73:2543-2556.
20. Polat A, Parlakpinar H, Tasdemir S, Colak C, Vardi N, Ucar M, Emre MH, Acet A. Protective role of aminoguanidine on gentamicin-induced acute renal failure in rats. *Acta Histochem* 2006;108:365-371.
21. Sha SH, Schacht J. Antioxidants attenuate gentamicin-induced free radical formation in vitro and ototoxicity in vivo: D-methionine is a potential protectant. *Hear Res* 2000;142:34-40.
22. Shifow AA, Kumar KV, Naidu MU, Ratnakar KS. Melatonin, a pineal hormone with antioxidant property, protects against gentamicin-induced nephrotoxicity in rats. *Nephron* 2000; 85:167-174.
23. Sinswat P, Wu WJ, Sha SH, Schacht J. Protection from ototoxicity of intraperitoneal gentamicin in guinea pig. *Kidney Int* 2000;58:2525-2532.
24. Varalakshmi P, Sandhya S, Malarkodi KP. Evaluation of the effect of lipoic acid administered along with gentamicin in rats rendered bacteremic. *Mol Cell Biochem* 2003; 248:35-40.
25. Ye LF, Tao ZZ, Hua QQ, Xia BK, Zhou XH, Li J, Yuan YL. Protective effect of melatonin against gentamicin ototoxicity. *J Laryngol Otol* 2009; 123:598-602.
26. Gupta RC. Taurine analogues and taurine transport: therapeutic advantages. *Adv Exp Med Biol* 2006; 583:449-467.
27. Park E, Quinn MR, Wright CE, Schuller-Levis G. Taurine chloramine inhibits the synthesis of nitric oxide and the release of tumor necrosis factor in activated RAW 264.7 cells. *J Leukoc Biol* 1993; 54:119-124.
28. Saransaari P, Oja SS. Characteristics of taurine release in slices from adult and developing mouse brain stem. *Amino Acids* 2006; 31:35-43.
29. Saransaari P, Oja SS. Taurine release in mouse brain stem slices under cell-damaging conditions. *Amino Acids* 2007; 32:439-446.
30. Wright CE, Tallan HH, Lin YY, Gaull GE. Taurine: biological update. *Annu Rev Biochem* 1986;55:427-453.
31. Bouckenooghe T, Remacle C, Reusens B. Is taurine a functional nutrient. *Curr Opin Clin Nutr Metab Care* 2006; 9:728-733.
32. Chen Y, Huang WG, Zha DJ, Qiu JH, Wang JL, Sha SH, Schacht J. Aspirin attenuates gentamicin ototoxicity: from the laboratory to the clinic. *Hear Res* 2007; 226:178-182.
33. Nishimura N, Yamamoto T, Ota T. Taurine feeding inhibits bile acid absorption from the ileum in rats fed a high cholesterol and high fat diet. *Adv Exp Med Biol* 2009; 643:285-291.
34. Taurine - monograph. *Altern Med Rev* 2001;6:78-82.
35. Foos TM, Wu JY. The role of taurine in the central nervous system and the modulation of intracellular calcium homeostasis. *Neurochem Res* 2002; 27:21-26.
36. Heller-Stilb B, van Roeyen C, Rascher K, Hartwiq HG, Huth A, Seeliqer MW, Warskulat U, Haussinger D. Disruption of the taurine transporter gene (taut) leads to retinal degeneration in mice. *FASEB J* 2002;16:231-233.
37. Oudit GY, Trivieri MG, Khaper N, Husain T, Wilson GJ, Liu P, Sole MJ, Backx PH. Taurine supplementation reduces oxidative stress and improves cardiovascular function in an iron-overload murine model. *Circulation* 2004;109:1877-1885.
38. Xu YJ, Arneja AS, Tappia PS, Dhalla NS. The potential health benefits of taurine in cardiovascular disease. *Exp Clin Cardiol* 2008;13: 57-65.
39. El Idrissi A, Messing J, Scalia J, Trenkner E. Prevention of epileptic seizures by taurine. *Adv Exp Med Biol* 2003;526:515-525.
40. Chauncey KB, Tenner TE Jr, Lombardini JB, Jones BG, Brooks ML, Warner RD, Davis RL, Raqain RM. The effect of taurine supplementation on patients with type 2 diabetes mellitus. *Adv Exp Med Biol* 2003; 526:91-96.
41. Franconi F, Loizzo A, Ghirlanda G, Seghieri G. Taurine supplementation and diabetes mellitus. *Curr Opin Clin Nutr Metab Care* 2006; 9:32-36.
42. Hansen SH. The role of taurine in diabetes and the development of diabetic complications. *Diabetes Metab Res Rev* 2001; 17:330-346.
43. Louzada PR, Paula Lima AC, Mendonca-Silva DL, Noel F, De Mello FG, Ferreira ST. Taurine prevents the neurotoxicity of beta-amyloid and glutamate receptor agonists: activation of GABA receptors and possible implications for Alzheimer's disease and other neurological disorders. *FASEB J* 2004; 18:511-518.
44. Santa-Maria I, Hernandez F, Moreno FJ, Avila J. Taurine, an inducer for tau polymerization and a weak inhibitor for amyloid-beta-peptide aggregation. *Neurosci Lett* 2007; 429:91-94.
45. De Curtis M, Santamaria F, Ercolini P, Vittoria L, De Ritis G, Garofalo V, Ciccimarra F. Effect of taurine supplementation on fat and energy absorption in cystic fibrosis. *Arch Dis Child* 1992; 67:1082-1085.
46. Waters E, Wang JH, Redmond HP, Wu QD, Kay E, Bouchier-Hayes D. Role of taurine in preventing acetaminophen-induced hepatic injury in the rat. *Am J Physiol Gastrointest Liver Physiol* 2001; 280:G1274-1279.
47. Kerai MD, Waterfield CJ, Kenyon SH, Asker DS, Timbrell JA. Taurine: protective properties against ethanol-induced hepatic steatosis and lipid peroxidation during chronic ethanol consumption in rats. *Amino Acids* 1998;15:53-76.
48. Schuller-Levis GB, Park E. Taurine and its chloramine: modulators of immunity. *Neurochem Res* 2004; 29:117-126.

49. Kavutcu M, Canbolat O, Ozturk S, Olcat E, Ulutepe S, Ekinci C, Gokhun IH, Durak I. Reduced enzymatic antioxidant defense mechanism in kidney tissues from gentamicin-treated guinea pigs: effects of vitamins E and C. *Nephron* 1996; 72:269-274.
50. Ali BH, Al-Salam S, Al-Husseini I, Nemmar A. Comparative protective effect of N-acetyl cysteine and tetramethylpyrazine in rats with gentamicin nephrotoxicity. *J Appl Toxicol* 2009; 29:302-307.
51. Song BB, Anderson DJ, Schacht J. Protection from gentamicin ototoxicity by iron chelators in guinea pig in vivo. *J Pharmacol Exp Ther* 1997; 282:369-377.
52. Furnkranz U, Nagl M, Gottardi W, Kohsler M, Aspock H, Walochnik J. Cytotoxic activity of N-chlorotaurine on Acanthamoeba spp. *Antimicrob Agents Chemother* 2008; 52:470-476.
53. Nagl M, Hengster P, Semenitz E, Gottardi W. The postantibiotic effect of N-chlorotaurine on Staphylococcus aureus. Application in the mouse peritonitis model. *J Antimicrob Chemother* 1999;43:805-809.
54. Nagl M, Hess MW, Pfaller K, Hengster P, Gottardi W. Bactericidal activity of micromolar N-chlorotaurine: evidence for its antimicrobial function in the human defense system. *Antimicrob Agents Chemother* 2000; 44:2507-2513.
55. Nagl M, Larcher C, Gottardi W. Activity of N-chlorotaurine against herpes simplex- and adenoviruses. *Antiviral Res* 1998; 38:25-30.
56. Nagl M, Lass-Florl C, Neher A, Gunkel A, Gottardi W. Enhanced fungicidal activity of N-chlorotaurine in nasal secretion. *J Antimicrob Chemother* 2001; 47:871-874.
57. Yazdanbakhsh M, Eckmann CM, Roos D. Killing of schistosomula by taurine chloramine and taurine bromamine. *Am J Trop Med Hyg* 1987; 37:106-110.
58. Grisham MB, Jefferson MM, Melton DF, Thomas EL. Chlorination of endogenous amines by isolated neutrophils. Ammonia-dependent bactericidal, cytotoxic, and cytolytic activities of the chloramines. *J Biol Chem* 1984; 259:10404-10413.
59. Bragman SG, Pankhurst CL, Casewell MW. Activity of sucralfate (sucrose octa-sulphate), an anti-ulcer agent, against opportunistic gram-negative bacilli. *J Antimicrob Chemother* 1995; 36:703-706.
60. Christensen ND, Reed CA, Culp TD, Hermonat PL, Howett MK, Anderson RA, Zaneveld LJ. Papillomavirus microbicidal activities of high-molecular-weight cellulose sulfate, dextran sulfate, and polystyrene sulfonate. *Antimicrob Agents Chemother* 2001; 45:3427-3432.
61. Gershon H, Gershon M, Clarke DD. Antifungal activity of substituted 8-quinolinol-5- and 7-sulfonic acids: a mechanism of action is suggested based on intramolecular synergism. *Mycopathologia* 2002; 155:213-217.
62. Zaneveld LJ, Waller DP, Anderson RA, Chany C2nd, Rencher WF, Feathergill K, Diao XH, Doncel GF, Herold B, Cooper M. Efficacy and safety of a new vaginal contraceptive antimicrobial formulation containing high molecular weight poly(sodium 4-styrenesulfonate). *Biol Reprod* 2002; 66:886-894.
63. Ibrahim MN, Sharif SAI, El-Tajory AN, Elamari AA. Synthesis and Antibacterial Activities of Some Schiff Bases. *E-Journal of Chemistry* 2011; 8:212-216.

7

Antioxidant and Antimicrobial activity of *Pedicularis sibthorpii Boiss.* and *Pedicularis* wilhelmsiana *Fisch ex.*

Laleh khodaie[1, 2, 3*], Abbas Delazar[1, 3], Farzaneh Lotfipour[3], Hossein Nazemiyeh[3]

[1] *Drugs Applied Research Center, Tabriz University of Medical Sciences, Tabriz, Iran.*

[2] *Student Research Committee, Tabriz University of Medical Sciences, Tabriz, Iran.*

[3] *Faculty of Pharmacy, Tabriz University of Medical Sciences, Tabriz, Iran.*

ARTICLE INFO

Keywords:
Pedicularis sibthorpii
Pedicularis wilhelmsiana
Antimicrobial
Antioxidant
Methanolic extract

ABSTRACT

Purpose: This research paper presents antioxidant and antimicrobial activities of *Pedicularis sibthorpii* and *Pedicularis wilhelmsiana* which grow in Azerbaijan/Iran with claimed a lot of therapeutic effects. ***Methods:*** DPPH assay and agar well diffusion method were carried out to determine antioxidant and antimicrobial activities respectively. ***Results:*** Methanolic extract showed better antioxidant activity compared to other crude extracts (n-hexane and dichloromethane). Methanolic extracts of both *Pedicularis sibthorpii* and *Pedicularis wilhelmsiana* were found to have antibacterial activity especially against gram positive strains of *S. ureus, S.epidermidis*. No antifungal activity was observed in the tested extracts. ***Conclusion:*** Existence of some phenolic compounds in methanolic extracts, such as phenylethanoids and flavonoids (found in other species of *Pedicularis*), which cause both antioxidant and antibacterial activities, is probable. Antimicrobial and antioxidant activity of the methanolic extracts supports further studies related to phytochemical investigation and bioassay of different fractions to isolate pure compounds of plants.

Introduction

As a folk medicinal herb *Pedicularis* is one of the most widely used groups of medicinal plants which have different therapeutic effects on cardiac problems, exhaustion, spontaneous sweating and digestion problems.[1] There has been no biological research on *Pedicularis sibthorpii* and *Pedicularis wilhelmsiana* which grow in Azerbaijan/Iran. Pedicularis species are also traditionally used in India for some clinical disorders such as cold, cough and fever.[2] Since these traditional applications can be attributed in part to the antimicrobial and antioxidant activity of the plant, in this study we intended to evaluate experimentally the invitro antibacterial effects of *P.sibthorpii* and *P.wilhelmsiana* against some clinically important species and antioxidant activity of these two plants were evaluated by DPPH test.

Materials and Methods

Plant material and extraction

The arial parts of *Pedicularis sibthorpii Boiss* and *Pedicularis wilhelmsiana Fisch ex.* were collected from Lighvan and Arasbaran region respectively in East Azerbaijan province, Iran in 2009. Voucher specimens for this collection (TBZ FPI 701, TBZ FPI 700) have been deposited in the Herbarium of the Faculty of Pharmacy, Tabriz, Iran.

Arial parts of plant were air dried and powdered. A 200g amount of powder of sample was extracted by n-hexane (8hours), dichloromethane (10hours) and methanol (8hours) in soxhlet extractor. Solvents removed by rotary evaporator and resulting extracts were used for further examinations.

DPPH assay

For determining antioxidant activity of the extracts, bleaching of purple colored methanol solution of 1, 1-diphenylpycryl hydrazyl (DPPH) was measured by spectrophotometric assay. In order to obtain different sample concentrations dilutions series were prepared. 50 µl of each concentration of methanolic extract were added to 5ml of 0.004% methanolic solution of DPPH. After incubation of solutions at room temperature for 30 min, bleaching of DPPH was monitored at 517 nm against a blank. Inhibition of DPPH was calculated as RC_{50}, extrapolated from dose-response curve. Tests were carried out in duplicate .[3,4]

Antimicrobial assay

Bacterial cultures of gram negative species *Pseudomonas aeroghinosa* (ATCC 9027), *Escherichia coli* (ATCC 8739), *Salmonella paratyphi* (ATCC 4420), as well as gram positive species namely

***Corresponding author:** Laleh Khodaei, Faculty of Pharmacy, Tabriz University of Medical Sciences, Tabriz, Iran.
E-mail: khodaiel@gmail.com

Staphylococcus epidermidis (ATCC 12228), *Bacillus cereus* (ATCC 9372), *Staphylococcus aureus* (ATCC 6538), *Micrococcus luteus* (ATCC 10240) and a fungi (*Candida albicans*) were used to evaluate antimicrobial properties of the methanolic extract. The bacterial strains in lyophilized form purchased from institute of pasture, Iran. Centrifuged pallets of bacteria from 24 hours cultures were mixed with distilled water, and the turbidity was corrected by adding sterile distilled water until 0.5 McFarland's turbidity standard [10^8 colony forming units (CFUs) per ml] was obtained. Then these inoculums were used for seeding the Muller Hinton agar (MERCK). Autoclaved Muller Hinton agar medium was allowed to cool up. Then it was seeded with 10 ml of prepared inoculums (10^6CFUs per ml). The antimicrobial activity of tested extract was monitored using agar diffusion method, which is highly recommended method for routine assessment of preliminary antimicrobial screening. Using Muller Hinton plates, inoculated with a 0.5McFarland's standard of selected bacteria, 5 wells for test samples, two for solutions of extract and different fractions, and one for vehicle control (DMSO), were applied to each Petri plate. For incubation and analysis, by micropipette 100µl of test solution was poured in respective well. Petri plate was incubated at 37°C. After 24 hours of incubation, diameter of the clear zones, showing no bacterial growth, around each well (excluding well diameter) was measured with the help of venire calipers. Triplet plates were prepared for each sample.[5-7] Compounds that have shown significant antibacterial activity, at this concentration were further assayed for their minimum inhibitory concentration. Serial two-fold dilutions of fractions were prepared in broth. Cultures containing only sterile nutrient broth, which did not influence bacterial growth, were used as controls. To each test tube an equal volume of the adjusted inoculums was added. After incubation at 37 °C for 24 h the MIC was read. The minimal inhibitory concentration (MIC) was defined as the lowest concentration of a fraction which was able to completely inhibit the growth of each bacterial strain.[8]

Results

Results of antioxidant test

Table 1 demonstrated antioxidant activities of n-hexane, dichloromethane and methanolic extracts of *P.sibthorpii* and *P.wilhelmsiana* by DPPH test.

Results of antimicrobial test

The results for antibacterial activity of the methanolic extract as Mean Inhibition Zone diameters (MIZD) as well as the MIC values against susceptible strains have been shown in table 2. N-hexan and dichloromethane esxtracts of two plants did not show any antimicrobial activity.

Table 1: antioxidant activities of the extracts of *Pedicularis sibthorpii* and *Pedicularis wilhelmsiana*

Extracts of P.s.*	RC_{50} (mg/ml)	Extracts of P.w.*	RC_{50} (mg/ml)
hexan	2.098	hexan	1.26
dichloromethane	No activity	dichloromethane	No activity
methanol	0.033	methanol	0.159

*P.s.: *Pedicularis sibthorpii*, *P.w.: *Pedicularis wilhelmsiana*

Table 2: Antibacterial activity of the methanolic extracts as Mean Inhibition Zone Diameter±SD (MIZD) and Minimum Inhibitory Concentration (MIC) of the extract against different strains (n=3).

MO*		*E.coli*	*P. aeroginosa*	*S. paratyphi*	*S. epidermidis*	*B. cereus*	*S.aureus*	*M. luteus*	*Candida albicans*
M.E. of P.S*	MIZD±SD (mm)	-	11.6± 0.28	-	15.6± 0.57	-	8.5±0.5	-	-
	MIC (mg/ml)	-	200	-	200	-	200	-	-
M.E. of P.W*	MIZD±SD (mm)	-	14.3± 0.47	-	15.6± 0.6	-	8.5±0.4	15.6±0.53	-
	MIC (mg/ml)	-	200	-	200	-	200	200	-

MO*: microorganisms, M.E. of P.S*: Methanolic Extract of *Pedicularis sibthorpii*, M.E. of P.W*: Methanolic Extract of *Pedicularis wilhelmsiana*

As it can be seen from table 2, the total methanolic extract of *P.sibthorpii* demonstrated inhibitory activity against some strains (*P. aeroginosa, S. epidermidis, S. aureus,*), and methanolic extract of P.wilhelmsiana showed inhibitory activity against *P. aeroginosa, S. epidermidis, S. Aureus* and *M.luteus.* Methanolic extracts did not show any inhibitory activity against gram-negative strains (*E.coli, S. Paratyphi and B.cereus*) except *P.aeroginosa.* Moreover methanolic extracts of *P.sibthorpii* and *P.wilhelmsina* were not active against *C.albicans* as well.

Discussion

The results of DPPH test as it can be seen in table 1 indicate that RC_{50} of methanolic extracts of two plants are lower than n-hexane and dichloromethane extracts, which shows methanolic extracts are potent antioxidants. These results reveals existence of phenolic compounds such as phenylethanoids and flavonoids (found in other species of *Pedicularis*) in both methanolic extracts, which are powerful antioxidants and have good radical scavenging activities.[9,10] Moreover, the current study found that methanolic extract of *P.sibthorpii* is more potent antioxidant than methanolic extract of *P.wilhelmsina.* This finding suggests that compounds with antioxidant activity (phenolic compounds) are found more in methanolic extract of *P.sibthorpii* than methanolic extract of *P.wilhelmsina.*

The results of in vitro antimicrobial assay of methanolic extract of *P.sibthorpii*, shown in table 2, demonstrates that methanolic extract of this plant is active against *P.aeroginosa, S.epidermidis* and *S.aureus.* Methanolic extract of *P.sibthorpii* is more active against *S.epidermidis* than other susceptible species. The results of well diffusion assay of methanolic extract of *P.wilhelmsina* shown in table 2, indicates that the extract is active against *P.aeroginosa, S.epidermidis, S.aureus* and *M. luteus.* This extract was more active against *S.epidermidis* and *M. luteus* than other strains. None of these two extracts were active against *C. albicans* by well diffusion method. According to results shown in table 2, methanolic extract of *Pedicularis wilhelmsiana* is more potent than methanolic extract of *Pedicularis sibthorpii* against susceptible strains. Furthermore the results of this study is in agreement with previous results which show that, the most susceptible strains, were gram-positive microorganisms (*S.aureus ,S.epidermidis* and *M.luteus*).[5,11,12] It could be due to several possible reasons; one is the presence of multilayer structure of membrane surrounding each gram-negative bacteria cell, whereas, gram –positive bacteria consist of a single layer, accounting for why gram-negative bacteria are more resistant to antibiotics than other gram-positive bacteria.[13-15] Among them *S. epidermidis* which cause serious infections in human and other animals, was more susceptible to both methanolic extracts than other susceptible strains. Contrary to expectations, methanolic extracts of *P.sibthorpii* and *P.wilhelmsiana* were active against *P.aeroginosa* a gram-negative strain and methanolic extract of *P.wilhelmsiana* was more active than methanolic extract of *P.sibthorpii.* Due to multi resistance feature of *P.aeroginosa* finding an effective antimicrobial agent against this microorganism is a difficult task.[16] Insusceptibility of *Candida albicans* to the tested extracts may be Due to lipophylic characteristic of fungi structure such as *C. Albicans*. Methanolic extracts of these two plants containing hydrophilic compounds were not active against this strain. [17-19]

According to the findings, it can be concluded that existence of some phenolic compounds in methanolic extracts, such as phenylethanoids and flavonoids (found in other species of *Pedicularis*), which cause both antioxidant and antibacterial activity, is probable. Antibacterial and antioxidant activity of methanolic extracts supports further studies like isolation and purification of phenolic compounds, which will be carried out in further investigations and the relationship between biological activities of the extracts with isolated compounds will be revealed.

Acknowledgments

This article was written based on a dataset of PhD thesis, registered with the number of 43 at pharmacy faculty in Tabriz University of Medical Sciences.

Conflict of interest

The authors report no conflicts of interest.

References

1. Jiang TF, Ou QY, Shi YP. Separation and determination of phenylpropanoid glycosides from Pedicularis species by capillary electrophoresis. *J Chromatogr A* 2003;986(1):163-167.
2. Ballabh B, Chaurasia OP. Traditional medicinal plants of cold desert Ladakh--used in treatment of cold, cough and fever. *J Ethnopharmacol* 2007;112(2):341-349.
3. Goupy P, Bautista-Ortin AB, Fulcrand H, Dangles O. Antioxidant activity of wine pigments derived from anthocyanins: hydrogen transfer reactions to the dpph radical and inhibition of the heme-induced peroxidation of linoleic acid. *J Agric Food Chem* 2009;57(13):5762-5770.
4. Fagali N, Catala A. Antioxidant activity of conjugated linoleic acid isomers, linoleic acid and its methyl ester determined by photoemission and DPPH techniques. *Biophys Chem* 2008;137(1):56-62.
5. Aqil F, Ahmad I. Antibacterial properties of traditionally used Indian medicinal plants. *Methods Find Exp Clin Pharmacol* 2007;29(2):79-92.
6. Perumal Samy R, Ignacimuthu S, Sen A. Screening of 34 Indian medicinal plants for antibacterial properties. *J Ethnopharmacol* 1998;62(2):173-182.
7. Essawi T, Srour M. Screening of some Palestinian medicinal plants for antibacterial activity. *J Ethnopharmacol* 2000;70(3):343-349.
8. Bussmann RW, Malca-Garcia G, Glenn A, Sharon D, Chait G, Diaz D, et al. Minimum inhibitory concentrations of medicinal plants used in Northern Peru as antibacterial remedies. *J Ethnopharmacol* 2010;132(1):101-108.
9. Ono M, Oda E, Tanaka T, Iida Y, Yamasaki T, Masuoka C, et al. DPPH radical-scavenging effect on some constituents from the aerial parts of Lippia triphylla. *J Nat Med* 2008;62(1):101-106.

10. Lee OH, Lee BY. Antioxidant and antimicrobial activities of individual and combined phenolics in Olea europaea leaf extract. *Bioresour Technol* 2010;101(10):3751-3754.
11. Dulgar B, Hagioglu N. Evaluation of Antimicrobial Activity of Two Endemic Scrophulariaceae Members. *Asian Journal of Chemistry* 2008;20(8):6385-6390.
12. Dulger B. Antimicrobial Activity of Some Endemic Scrophulariaceae from Turkey. *Pharmaceutical Biology* 2006;44(6):672-676
13. Tortora GJ, Funke BR, Case CL. *Microbiology: an introduction*: Benjamin Cummings. San Francisco; 2001.
14. J. Y, R. M. *Antibacterial agents. In: Murray P, Baron E, Pfaller M, Tenover F, Yolken R, Manual of clinical microbiology*: Washington DC: ASM press; 1995.
15. Ali-Shtayeh MS, Yaghmour RM, Faidi YR, Salem K, Al-Nuri MA. Antimicrobial activity of 20 plants used in folkloric medicine in the Palestinian area. *J Ethnopharmacol* 1998;60(3):265-271.
16. Giamarellos-Bourboulis EJ, Grecka P, Dionyssiou-Asteriou A, Giamarellou H. In vitro interactions of gamma-linolenic acid and arachidonic acid with ceftazidime on multiresistant Pseudomonas aeruginosa. *Lipids* 1999;34: 151-152.
17. Edris AE, Farrag ES. Antifungal activity of peppermint and sweet basil essential oils and their major aroma constituents on some plant pathogenic fungi from the vapor phase. *Molecular Nutrition food research* 2003;47(2):117-21.
18. Oriente FT, Sanmartin EI, Fransisco A. Antifungal phloroglucinol Derivatives and lipophylic flavonoids from Helichr Ysum Decumbens. *Phytochemistry* 1988;28(6):1613-1615.
19. Guleria S, Kumar A. Antifungal activity of some Himalayan medicinal plants using direct bioautography. *Journal of Cell and Molecular Biology* 2006;5:95-98.

Application of lactobionic acid and nonionic surfactants as solubilizing agents for parenteral formulation of clarithromycin

Parvin Zakeri-Milani[1,2], Niaz Mousavian-Fathi[1,3], Saeed Ghanbarzadeh[1,4], Mohammad-Hosein Zarrintan[1], Hadi Valizadeh[1,5]*

[1] *Faculty of Pharmacy, Tabriz University of Medical Sciences, Tabriz, Iran.*

[2] *Liver and Gastrointestinal Diseases Research Center, Tabriz University of Medical Sciences, Tabriz, Iran.*

[3] *Student Research Committee, Tabriz University of Medical Sciences, Tabriz, Iran.*

[4] *Drug Applied Research Center, Tabriz University of Medical Sciences, Tabriz, Iran.*

[5] *Research Center for Pharmaceutical Nanotechnology, Tabriz University of Medical Sciences, Tabriz, Iran.*

ARTICLE INFO

Keywords:
Clarithromycin
Lactobionic acid
Nonionic surfactants
Solubility
Parenteral

ABSTRACT

Purpose: The purpose of this paper is to enhance the solubility of clarithromycin (CLR) using nonionic surfactants and some type of acids for preparation of the new formulations. ***Methods***: Myrj 52 and chremophor (2.5 and 5% w/v) were used in two concentrations. To investigate solubility, the formulations were shaken for 48 hours at room temperature. For stability test, lyophilized samples were maintained in refrigerator at 4° C, and in oven at 40° C. Drug analysis was performed by reverse phase high performance liquid chromatography (HPLC) with ultraviolet detection. ***Results***: Solubility tests indicated that lactobionic acid was the most effective to increase clarithromycin solubility and chremophor showed higher enhancing effect than myrj 52 on CLR solubility. The stability tests results also confirmed that shelf-lives of all formulations have been the equivalent to 24 months. ***Conclusion***: On the whole, formulations described in this article may be very suitable for industrial-scale manufacturing and clinical application.

Introduction

Clarithromycin is a relatively new, second-generation, semi synthetic macrolide antibiotic with a methoxy group (OCH3) attached to the C6 position of erythromycin. This derivatization makes clarithromycin more acid stable than erythromycin. [1,2] Clarithromycin has broad-spectrum activity against gram-positive and gram-negative aerobes, atypical bacterial pathogens of the respiratory tract, mycobacterium species, Legionella and helicobacter pylori. [3] Many dosage forms of clarithromycin, such as immediate and extended release tablets, capsules, dry suspensions, liposome-encapsulated, microspheres, cyclodextrin-compressed and IV formulation have been developed due to its wide antibacterial spectrum. [2,4-9] Nevertheless considering adverse effects of oral dosage forms such as gastrointestinal disorders and low bioavailability which doesn't exceed 55%, and the existence of some situations such as unconscious patients for whom the only usable dosage form is parenteral form and also the absence of generic intravenous dosage form in Iran, there is considerable interest in the development of a parenteral formulation of clarithromycin. However, the main problem related with clarithromycin intravenous form is its practical insolubility in water. Clarithromycin has the dimethylamino moiety as the only ionizable group (pK8.8) and hence its aqueous solubility at pH 7.0 is only about 500 μg/ml. [2,10] Using binary systems with a hydrophilic carrier by mixing, melting or solvent methods emulsion formulations for its IV use have been studied. However, leaving residual solvent, thermal degradation of clarithromycin during thermal sterilization and complication of these processes has limited the application of these methods. [2,10] Therefore it is necessary to develop a new formulation to improve its solubility for intravenous administration of clarithromycin. [11] We hypothesized that surfactants and gluconic acids can enhance clarithromycin solubility. [10] Based on this hypothesis myrj52 and chremophor (in different proportions) and lactobionic acid were investigated and results were compared and the best formulations were reported.

***Corresponding author:** Hadi Valizadeh (PhD), Department of Pharmaceutics, Faculty of Pharmacy, Tabriz University of Medical Sciences, Tabriz, Iran. 51664. E-mail: valizadeh@tbzmed.ac.ir

Materials and Methods

Materials

Clarithromycin (Elder Nerul, Pawane and Patalg, India), Lactobionic acid (Sigma – Aldrich, Co. St. Louis , MO , USA), Chremophor (BASF Florham Park, New Jersey), Myrj 52 (Atlas San Diego, USA), Anhydride citric acid(Merck Dermstadt, Germany), Sulfuric acid (Merck Dermstadt, Germany), Stearic acid (Merck Dermstadt, Germany), Boric acid (Merck Dermstadt, Germany), Hydrochloric acid (Merck Dermstadt, Germany), Phosphoric acid (Merck Dermstadt, Germany), Salicylic acid (Merck Dermstadt, Germany), NaOH (Merck Dermstadt, Germany), Sodium dihydrogen phosphate (Merck Dermstadt, Germany), Acetonitril (Merck Dermstadt, Germany), Tartaric acid (Seelze- Hannover Riedel _ Dehaen AG , Germany).

Formulation

To increase clarithromycin solubility in water to prepare an injectable solution, above mentioned acids were used. Results indicated that lactobionic acid is the only acid which can improve drug solubility. Nonionic surfactants, myrj 52 and chremophor also were used for solubilization. To produce 5 formulations, different concentrations of two surfactants were selected, added to appropriate amount of double distilled water and were sonicated (Julabo USR 3 Labortechnik, Germany) until complete dissolution. Then 500 mg of clarithromycin was added up and agitation was continued for 15 min. Acid solution was then added and after 5 minutes of stirring, pH was measured (Metrohm, Switzerland). Acid addition was continued until a clear solution was achieved. However to increase stability the pH was kept above 4.8. pH of solutions were adjusted using phosphoric acid 85% and NaOH 1N in the range of 5 to 6.5. Then the solutions were filtered through the 0.22μ membrane filter. To prepare samples for stability tests, 20 vials of each formulation were prepared. The samples were dried and lyophilized for 48 hours in the freezer (- 20°C), and then were maintained in refrigerator at 4°C.

Solubility study

CLA solubility samples were prepared in glass tubes at serial concentrations for all five solvent systems developed. For each system ten glass tubes with different concentration of drug were prepared. Then the samples were shaken for 48 hours at room temperature. The first tube in each series in which the fine un-dissolved drug particles were seen, was detected by visual inspection and finally the range of drug solubility were determined.

Drug analysis

A reverse phase high performance liquid chromatography (HPLC) (Knauer, Germany) analytical method with ultraviolet detection was employed for drug analysis. The mobile phase consisted of acetonitrile- sodium dihydrogen phosphate (2:3 v/v) containing phosphoric acid (3M) and NaOH (1N) to adjust the pH on 4.5. The flow-rate was 2 ml/min and the detection wavelength was set at 205nm. Column (Shimadzu C18:250mm×4.6mm, 4μm) temperature was maintained at 59°C using oven (Memmert, Germany) and the injection volume was 20μL.

Method validation

In this study a reverse phase HPLC method with ultraviolet detection was used. Standard solutions of 3.125 to 50 mg/ml were prepared in water, and linearity range and correlation coefficient were obtained. To evaluate the inter-assay precision and accuracy, samples were analyzed for 3 consecutive days, while intra-assay precision and accuracy were evaluated through analysis of samples at three different concentrations in the same run. Relative standard deviation (RSD) and the accuracy were calculated using the experimental concentration and the nominal concentration for each sample.

Stability tests

To investigate the short-term storage stability of clarithromycin in formulations and determine the shelf life, at least 6 vials of each formulation were kept for 6 month in undesirable conditions including constant relative humidity of 75% and temperature of 40° C which equals maintaining for 2 years in ambient conditions. Other lyophilized formulations were kept in -20° C. For stability study of newly prepared and ready to use injection solution of formulations, a sample of each formulation was tested over 120 h at 4° C.

For determination remained drug in formulations, monthly a vial from samples in oven and freezer was taken and was brought to volume 10ml with double distilled water. Samples were shaken and sonicated for 5 minutes and injected to HPLC column in triplicate. This test was also performed for ready to use solution within 5 days. Monthly a calibration curve was taken.

Differential Scanning Calorimetry (DSC)

Differential Scanning Calorimetry is a rapid and exact way to examine drug and excipient compatibility and provides the most information about possible interactions. Samples (5 mg) were sealed in aluminum pans and heated at a rate of 20° C per minute from 30° C to 300° C (DSC-60, Shimadzu, Japan). Thermal behaviors of clarithromycin and exipients, the complex and the physical mixture of them were determined and compared.

Results

To examine the effect of different acids on CLR solubility, various acids such as lactobionic acid, anhydride citric acid, sulfuric acid, stearic acid, boric acid, hydrochloric acid, phosphoric acid, salicylic acid and tartaric acid were used. Lactobionic acid showed the best result in improving drug solubility in water and forming a soluble dosage form suitable for injection. The results obtained for used surfactants, myrj 52 and chremophor were illustrated in Table 1.

Table 1. CLR solubility in the presence of surfactants, chremophor and myrj 52 in two concentration levels.

Surfactant	Formulation code	Surfactant concentration (w/v)	Solubility (mg/ml)
-	1	-	65-70
Myrj 52	2	2.5	70-75
	3	5	75-80
Chremophor	4	2.5	75-80
	5	5	80-85

To determine shelf lives of various formulations that were kept under undesired conditions for 6 months, and also frozen samples, residual drug was determined monthly using HPLC method. Representative chromatograms of serial concentration of clarithromycin were shown in Figure 1. The method was linear under the reported conditions between 3.125 and 50 mg/ml with a correlation coefficient of 0.9995. Calibration curve was taken monthly. Relative standard deviation (RSD) and recoveries were calculated from the theoretical and experimental concentrations in order to determine the precision and accuracy of the method. The with-in-day and day-to-day RSD values were determined to be 0 .096 and 0.103 respectively. The accuracy for with-in-day and day-to-day were determined as 107% and 108% respectively. The half-lives of various pharmaceutical formulations from accelerated tests were obtained from division of the respective area under curve in the chromatogram, on the area under the curve of that concentration in standard calibration curve taken on that month. The consequence results indicated that all formulations had shelf lives more than 24 months. Hence, it can be concluded that the formulated IV products had sufficient physicochemical stability for storage at room temperature for 24 months. Drug remained in various formulations kept in oven or freezer, was determined monthly and illustrated in Table 2. In order to check the stability of drug in ready to use form, the reconstituted product was kept for five days in refrigerator (4°C). For content analysis, HPLC method was also applied. The results indicated that for all formulations remained drug after five days were more than 90%. To screen drug and excipient compatibility, DSC was used and polymorph types and melting points of individual substances were determined. The melting points of lactobionic acid and myrj 52 were 61.75° C and51.78° C respectively. The clarithromycin endothermic peak temperature was 228.51° C, which had not been changed significantly in physical mixture of drug and excipients and also in formulations. An example of the thermograms of CLR, lactobionic acid and Formulation (F_2) is given in Figure 2.

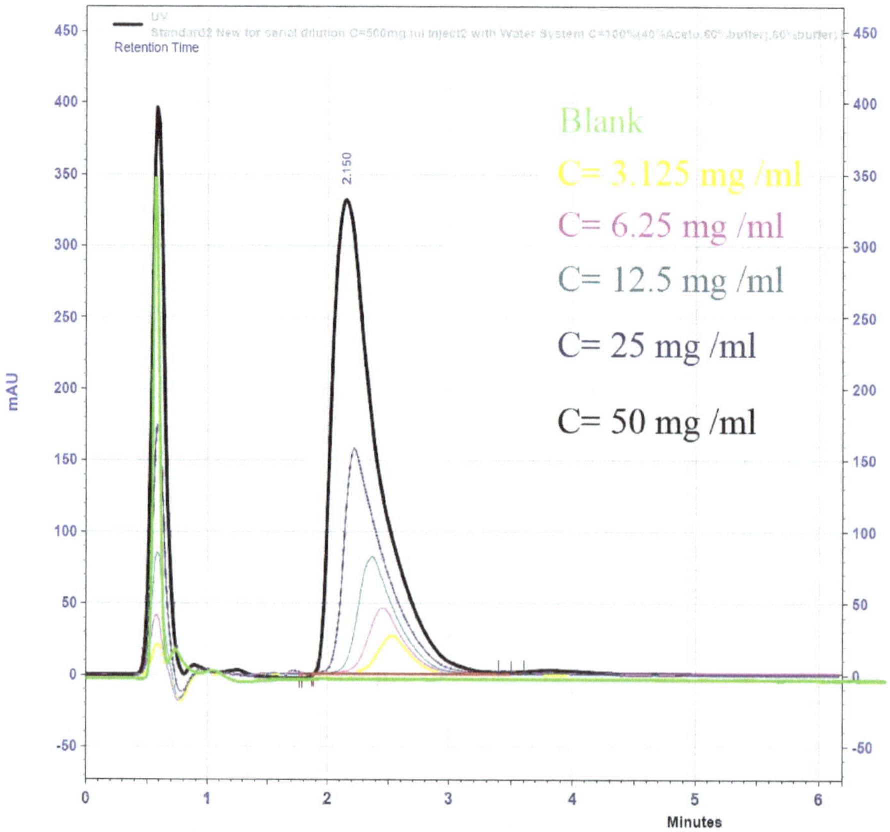

Figure1. HPLC chromatograms of different concentration of clarithromycin

Table 2. The percent drug remained in formulations kept in oven or freezer.

Formulation code	Month 4		Month 5		Month 6	
	Oven	Freezer	Oven	Freezer	Oven	Freezer
1	91.81	96.43	102.9	90.97	98.31	92.69
2	99.17	95.37	97.99	90.69	102.40	100.84
3	104.74	98.13	102.63	97.17	101.76	90.96
4	97.23	105.18	94.92	104.57	90.60	98.11
5	103.13	96.15	97.13	95.37	105.95	102.77

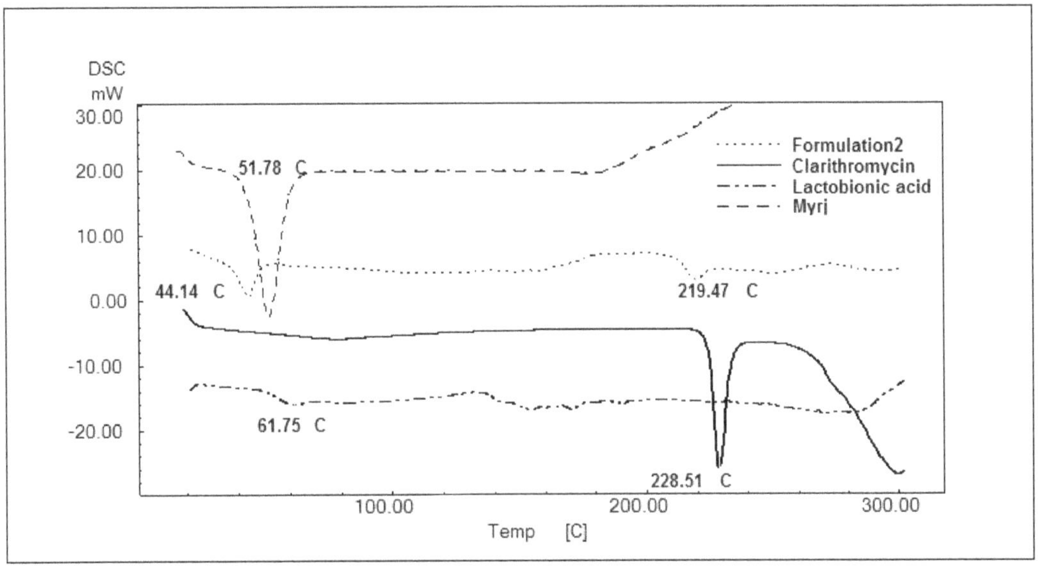

Figure 2. Thermograms of CLR, lactobionic acid and formulation (F_2) kept in the freezer - 20° C for 6 months.

Discussion

As stated before, clarithromycin is a drug that its solubility is very low (0.33 mg/ml) and it is practically insoluble in water. [12] Suitable form for intravenous injection of clarithromycin is a soluble form. Solubility tests for nine different acids with the aim of increasing the water solubility of clarithromycin were performed, and lactobionic acid found the most effective to increase clarithromycin solubility. In a similar study on erythromycin and clarithromycin, lactobionic acid was the best acid to increase their solubility [10], and in another study ascorbic acid 2-glucoside improved clarithromycin solubility. [13] Concerning the structural similarity of erythromycin with clarithromycin, and also the similarity of ascorbic acid 2-glucoside and lactobionic acid this result seems to be reasonable. On the other hand obtained results showed that drug solubility in formulations containing surfactants was higher than those without surfactants (65-70 mg/ml and 70-85 mg/ml respectively). Myrj 52 with concentrations of 2.5% and 5% w/v could increase CLR solubility 5 and 10 mg/ml respectively. Moreover chremophor showed higher enhancing effect than myrj 52 on CLR solubility (5mg/ml more increase in obtained solubility using the same concentrations). It has been suggested that formation of the stronger hydrogen bonds in chremophor than myrj is may be the reason of it's tough emulsification power. [10] Furthermore DSC technique was used to check the compatibility of drug and excipients. As illustrated in Figure 2, there is no significant difference in melting point peak of clarithromycin in formulations, and pure clarithromycin. This indicated that its polymorphism has not been changed by manufacturing process. From the sample analysis point of view, although previous studies have presented several HPLC methods with electrochemical, fluorescent, ultraviolet, and mass spectrometric detectors for CLA analysis [8,9,14-17], in the present study we have developed a simple reverse-phase HPLC method with acceptable precision and accuracy. The results of this study also illustrated that (Table 2) shelf-lives of all formulations have been the equivalent to 24 months. In previous studies CLR shelf life of 48 months was reported. [18] Hence, it can be concluded that the prepared formulations in this study have sufficient physicochemical stability for storage at -20° C for 24 months. There are situations such as kidney or liver failure or drug therapy in children, where administration of less than a vial dose is needed, Therefore the storage of prepared solution and its stability over the storage time is of importance, which was determined to be at least 120 hours in this investigation. The acceptance criterion was remaining at least 90% of initial dose in the formulations. In similar studies, the stability of the drug solution, kept at 2 to 8°C (refrigerator temperature) was reported to be 24 hours. [19] Although ready for injection drug solutions were stable until 5 days, however for reason of sterility consideration, it is recommended to limit the time elapsed between reconstituting and administration to 24 hours.

Conclusion

Based on obtained results using nonionic surfactants such as myrj52 and chremophor and gluconic acid derivatives like lactobionic acid can enhance clarithromycin solubility without any complication in manufacturing in industrial scale. The results obtained proved that clarithromycin had sufficient physicochemical stability in the prepared formulations. Therefore IV dosage form of clarithromycin can be a good candidate to be made in an industrial scale.

Acknowledgements

We are grateful to authorities in Faculty of Pharmacy, Tabriz University of Medical Sciences for providing analytical facilities. This paper is based on Pharm D thesis (number 3517) was performed in Faculty of Pharmacy, Tabriz University of Medical Sciences.

Conflict of interest

There is no conflict of interest in this study.

References

1. Adam D, Glaser-Caldow E, Wachter J, et al. Comparative efficacy of clarithromycin modified-release and clarithromycin immediate-release formulations in the treatment of lower respiratory tract infection. *Clin Ther* 2001;23(4):585-595.
2. Lovell MW, Johnson HW, Hui HW, Cannon JB, Gupta PK, Hsu CC. Less-painful emulsion formulations for intravenous administration of clarithromycin. *Int J Pharm* 1994;109(1):45-57.
3. Zakeri-Milani P, Valizadeh H, Ghanbarzadeh S, Nemati M. Pharmacokinetics and comparative bioavailability study of two clarithromycin suspensions following administration of a single oral dose to healthy volunteers. *Arzneim-Forsch/Drug Res* 2009;59(8):429-432.
4. Li J, Nie S, Yang X, Wang C, Cui S, Pan W. Optimization of tocol emulsions for the intravenous delivery of clarithromycin. *Int J Pharm* 2008;356(1-2):282-290.
5. Allin D, James I, Zachariah J, et al. Comparison of once- and twice-daily clarithromycin in the treatment of adults with severe acute lower respiratory tract infections. *Clin Ther* 2001;23(12):1958-1968.
6. Weiss K, Vanjaka A. An open-label, randomized, multicenter, comparative study of the efficacy and safety of 7 days of treatment with clarithromycin extended-release tablets versus clarithromycin immediate-release tablets for the treatment of patients with acute bacterial exacerbation of chronic bronchitis. *Clin Ther* 2002;24(12):2105-2122.
7. Salem II, Duzgunes N. Efficacies of cyclodextrin-complexed and liposome-encapsulated clarithromycin against Mycobacterium avium complex infection in human macrophages. *Int J Pharm* 2003;250(2):403-414.
8. Davey PG. The pharmacokinetics of clarithromycin and its 14-OH metabolite. *J Hosp infect* 1991;19 Suppl A:29-37.
9. Lu Y, Zhang Y, Yang Z, Tang X. Formulation of an intravenous emulsion loaded with a clarithromycin-phospholipid complex and its pharmacokinetics in rats. *Int J Pharm* 2009;366(1-2):160-169.
10. Inoue Y, Yoshimura S, Tozuka Y, et al. Application of ascorbic acid 2-glucoside as a solubilizing agent for clarithromycin: Solubilization and nanoparticle formation. *Int J Pharm* 2007;331(1):38-45.
11. Lu Y, Wang Y, Tang X. Formulation and thermal sterile stability of a less painful intravenous clarithromycin emulsion containing vitamin E. *Int J Pharm* 2008;346(1-2):47-56.
12. *The United State Pharmacopeia. United State Pharmacopeia Convention Inc, Rockville.* Vol 2. 31 ed, 2008.
13. Serdoz F, Voinovich D, Perissutti B, et al. Development and pharmacokinetic evaluation of erythromycin lipidic formulations for oral administration in rainbow trout (Oncorhynchus mykiss). *Eur J Pharm Biopharm* 78(3):401-407.
14. Amini H, Ahmadiani A. Sensitive determination of clarithromycin in human plasma by high-performance liquid chromatography with spectrophotometric detection. J Chromatogr B Analyt Technol Biomed Life Sci 2005;817(2):193-197.
15. Chu S-Y, Sennello LT, Sonders RC. Simultaneous determination of clarithromycin and 14(R)-hydroxyclarithromycin in plasma and urine using high-performance liquid chromatography with electrochemical detection. *J Chromatog B: Biomed Sci Appl* 1991;571(1-2):199-208.

16. Guay DR, Gustavson LE, Devcich KJ, Zhang J, Cao G, Olson CA. Pharmacokinetics and tolerability of extended-release clarithromycin. *Clin Ther* 2001;23(4):566-577.
17. Shin J, Pauly DF, Johnson JA, Frye RF. Simplified method for determination of clarithromycin in human plasma using protein precipitation in a 96-well format and liquid chromatography-tandem mass spectrometry. J Chromatogr B Analyt Technol Biomed Life Sci 2008;871(1):130-134.
18. Lovell MW, Johnson HW, Gupta PK. Stability of a less-painful intravenous emulsion of clarithromycin. *Int J Pharm* 1995;118(1):47-54.
19. Erah PO, Barrett DA, Shaw PN. Ion-pair high-performance liquid chromatographic assay method for the assessment of clarithromycin stability in aqueous solution and in gastric juice. *J Chromatogr B Biomed Sci Appl* 1996;682(1):73-78.

Utilization of thin film method for preparation of celecoxib loaded liposomes

Eskandar Moghimipour, Somayeh Handali *

Nanotechnology Research Center, Ahvaz Jundishapur University of Medical Sciences, Ahvaz, Iran.

ARTICLE INFO

Keywords:
Celecoxib
Liposome
Thin film method
Differential scanning calorimeter
Transmission electron microscopy
Particle size

ABSTRACT

Purpose: Celecoxib is nonsteroiddal anti-inflammatory drug that has been used extensively to treat patients with arthritis. The aim of the present study was to formulate and characterize liposomal vesicles loaded with celecoxib. ***Methods:*** Liposomes were prepared by thin film method using soya lecithin and cholesterol. The release of drug was determined using a dialysis membrane method. Liposomes were characterized by Differential Scanning Calorimetery (DSC), Transmission Electron Microscopy (TEM) and their particle size was also determined. ***Results:*** The results showed that the drug encapsulation efficiency was 67.34% and there was 67.16% release after 0.5, 1, 2, 3, 4, 5, 6, 7, 8 and 24 h. Results of particle size determination showed a mean size of 677nm and nanoparticles were spherical as shown by TEM. The DSC curve of lecithin, cholesterol and celecoxib were different from celecoxib containing liposome. ***Conclusion:*** The results of characterization of the vesicles indicated the potential application of celecoxib loaded liposome as carrier system.

Introduction

Celecoxib is a non-steroiddal anti-inflammatory drug (NSAID) that acts on cyclooxygenase-2 (COX-2). It has been used extensively to safely treatment patients with arthritis and also treatment patients with familial adenomatous polyposis and to induce apoptosis in colon, stomach, prostate cancer cells and have antitumor activity in lung, colon and pancreatic cancer.[1,2]

Liposomes are used as drug carrier for a wide range of drugs including analgesics and anti-inflammatory drug.[3] Liposome is a spherical vesicle composed of a bilayer membrane [4] and commercially important drug delivery system for their biodegradability and biocompatibility.[5]liposomes have been used to administer drugs by several routs such as oral, parenteral and topical.[4] Several studies have showed that encapsulation of drug in liposome may enhance the drug permeation into the skin.[5]

The aim of this study was to prepare and evaluate celecoxib loaded liposomes and to study their in vitro release behavior.

Materials and Methods

Soya lecithin and cholesterol were purchased from Acros, USA and Merck, Germany respectively. Celecoxib was kindly donated by Exir pharmaceutical Co., Iran. All of the solvents were of the analytical grade.

Preparation of liposome

Liposomes were prepared by thin film method. Briefly soya lecithin and cholesterol were dissolved in chloform-methanol (1:1) and 5 mg celecoxib was added in the solution, then the mixture was evaporated in a rotary evaporator. The thin film formed in the round-bottomed flask was hydrated with phosphate buffer. The suspension was agitated by vortex for 30 min and then sonicated for an hour.[4,5]

Evaluation of the loading efficacy

The liposomal suspension was centrifuged at 20000 rpm for 30 min. The supernatant was analyzed at 260 nm using spectrophotometer (Biochrom WAP Biowave II).

In vitro drug release studies

In vitro celecoxib release from the liposome was determined using dialysis membrane method. 5 g of each formulation was put in a dialysis bag (BETAGEN, width 40 mm). The receptor phase was 25 ml ethanol 80% and was continually using a magnet stirred at 37°C. An aliquot of 2 ml of sample was withdrawn from each batch at definite time intervals (0.5, 1, 2, 3, 4, 5, 6, 7, 8 and 24 h) and replaced with the same amount of ethanol to maintain sink condition. Then, the concentration of drug released was monitored using a UV spectrophotometer at 260 nm.

***Corresponding author:** Somayeh Handali, Nanotechnology Research Center, Ahvaz Jundishapur University of Medical Sciences, Ahvaz, Iran. Email: handali_s81@yahoo.com

Differential Scanning Calorimetry (DSC)

The calorimetric analysis was performed in order to determine the differences in properties of lecithin and cholesterol previously structured in the liposome and the effect of the celecoxib on these properties. The DSC curves were recorded using a DSC-1 Mettler Toledo oven with a temperature range of 30 to 200°C for 6 min.

Particle size determination

The average diameter and polydispersity index (PDI) of liposomes were determined using a particle sizer Qudix, ScatterO Scope I system (Korea) at 25 °C.

Transmission Electron Microscopy (TEM)

The morphology of the liposomes were observed under Transmission Electron Microscope (Philips- CM-10) operated at HT-100 KV. The samples were stained with 25% (w/v) Formuar and placed on copper grids with films for viewing.

Results

The encapsulation of celecoxib in liposome was 67.34%. Celecoxib release from the liposome formulation was 67.16%. Sonication time was affected the liposomal particle size. By increasing the sonication time from 30 min to 1 h, the particle size decreases from 969 nm to 677 nm that had shown in Figure 1a and b (P>0.05), but the particles had polydispersity as shown in Figure 1b. So it suggested the sonication time is an important parameter in the liposome preparation because the increasing the time of sonication is necessary to decrease the polydispersity. The PDI the liposomes were 2.5 ± 0.0.

The results of DSC of cholesterol, lecithin, celecoxib and celecoxib containing liposome are shown in Figure 2a, b, c and d respectively. The DSC curve of cholesterol, lecithin and celecoxib containing liposome showed two endothermic peaks in the regions 70-80 and 110-120°C for cholesterol, 190-200°C for lecithin and 130-140, 140-150°C for celecoxib containing liposome (Figure 2a, b, d), while the DSC curve of celecoxib showed single endothermic peak at 160-170°C (Figure 2c).

Figure 3, shows the TEM photograph of liposome, denoting shape of the nanoparticles. It is evident that the particles are spherical in shape and also shows that the liposomes have polydispersity and monodispersity.

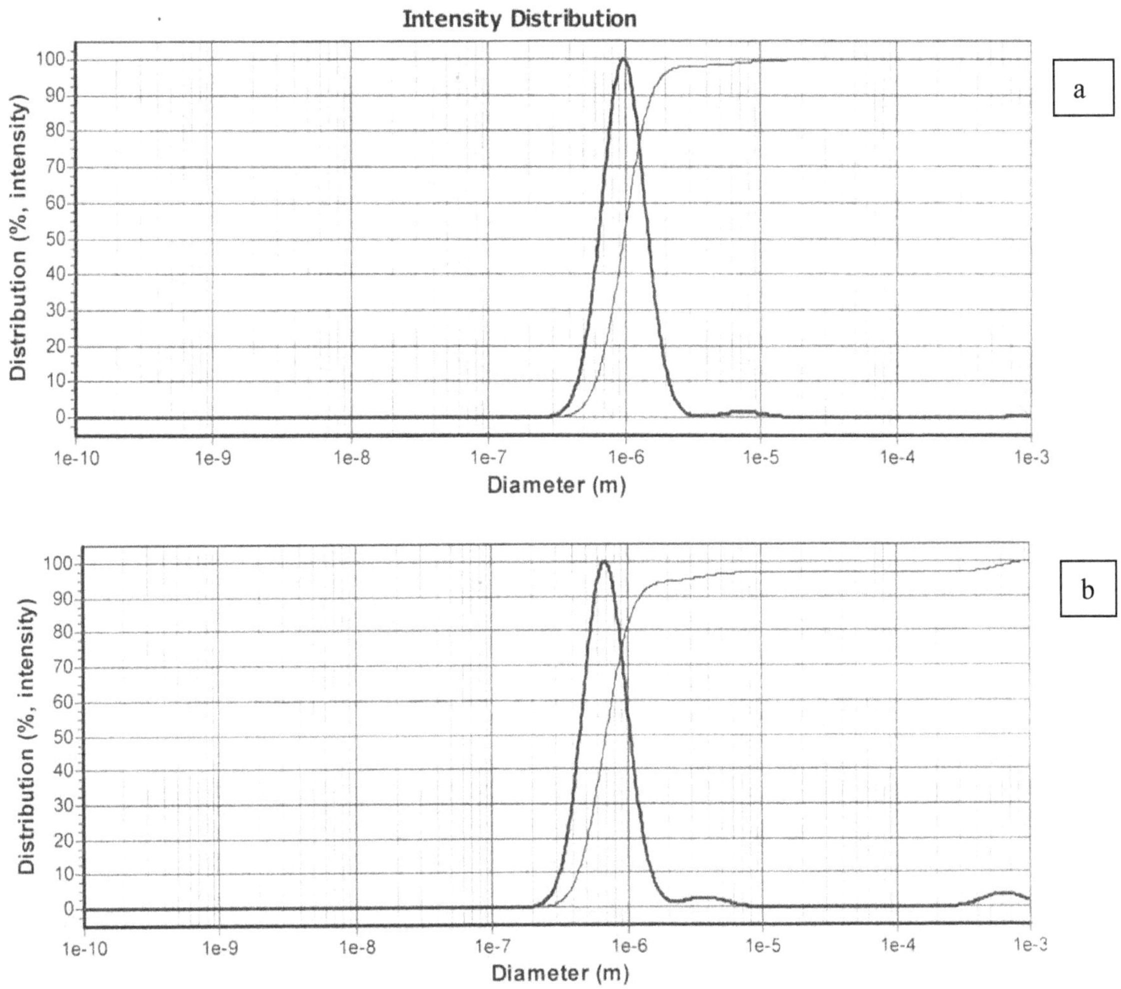

Figure 1. a) Particle size of liposomes containing celecoxib after 30 min sonication.
b) Particle size of liposomes containing celecoxib after 1 h sonication.

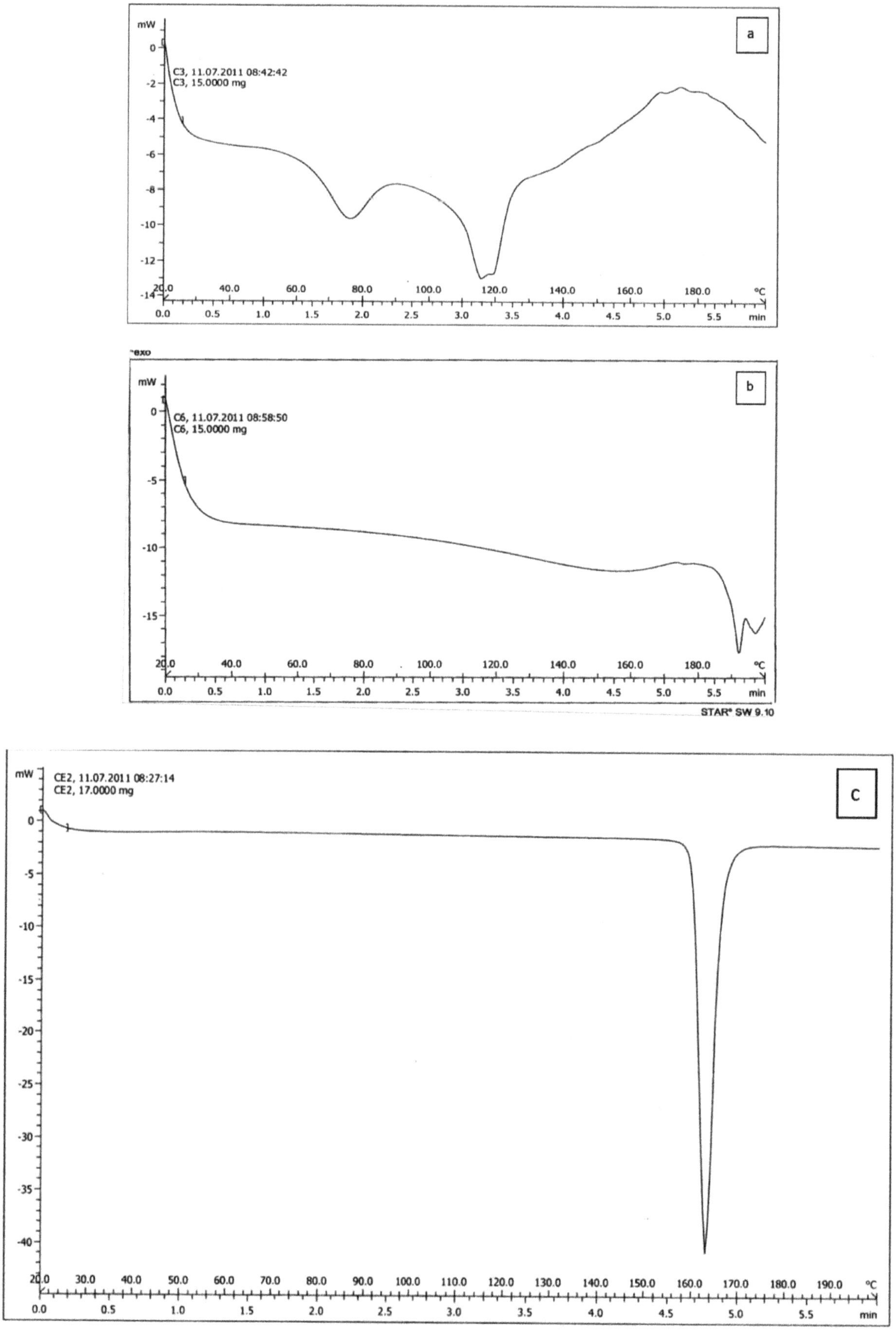

Figure 2. a) Differential Scanning Calorimetry of cholesterol. b) Differential Scanning Calorimetry of lecithin. c) Differential Scanning Calorimetry of celecoxib.

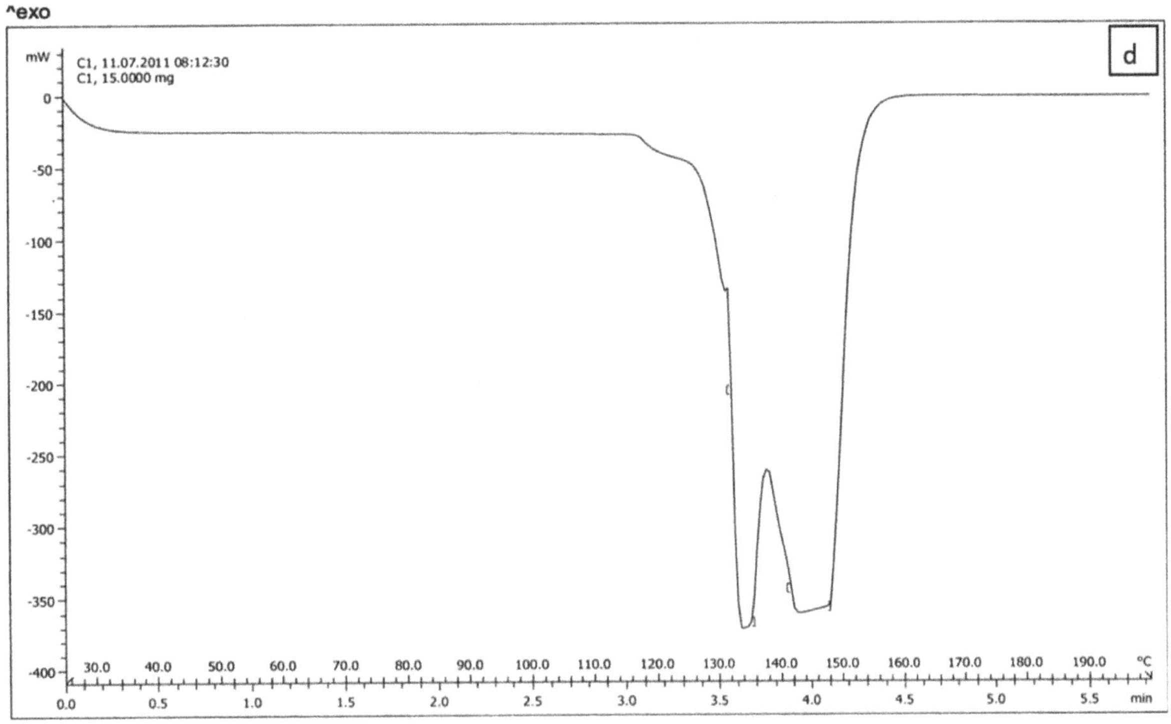

Figure 2. d) Differential Scanning Calorimetry of celecoxib containing liposome.

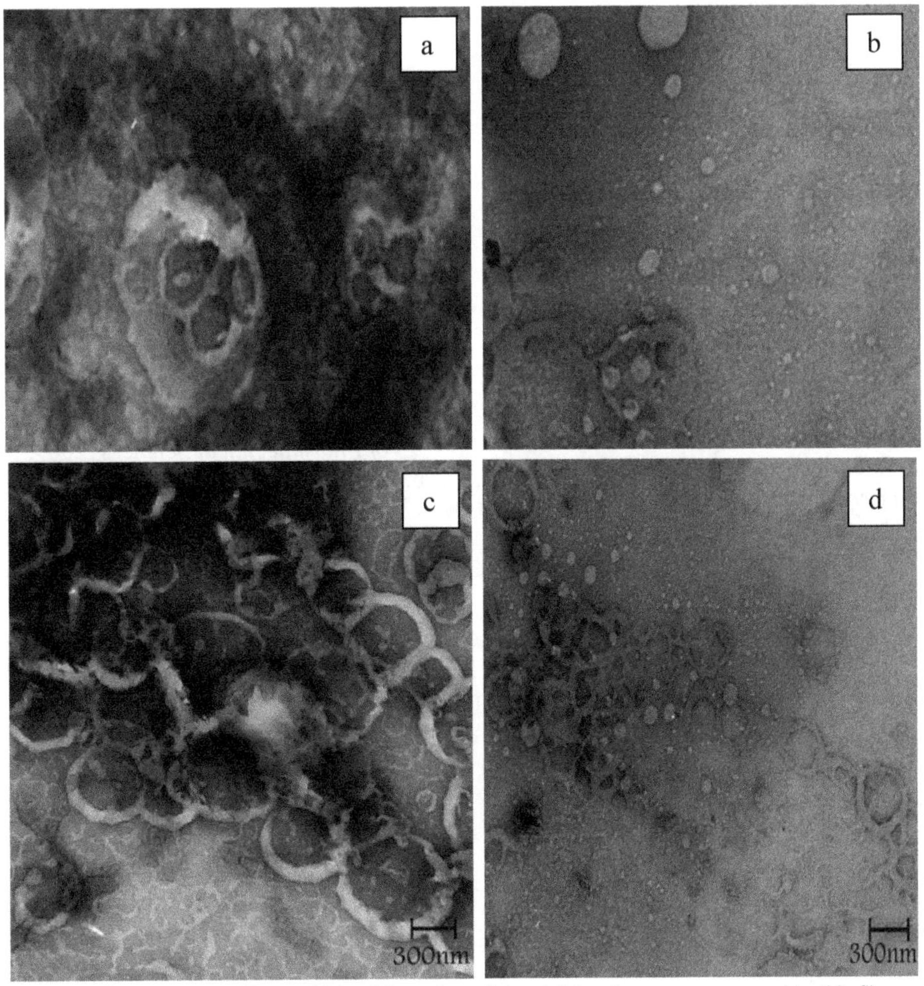

Figure 3. TEM image in different fields of the celecoxib containing liposomes prepared by thin film method (a-d).

Discussion

Celecoxib is a new anti-inflammatory drug that acts on cyclooxygenase-2 and also has been shown to have antitumor properties.[1,2] Liposomes are used as drug carriers for a wide range of drugs and are importante in pharmaceutical field due to decrease of side effects.[3] Liposome incorporates hydrophilic drugs through an aqueous core or entraps hydrophobic drugs using phospholipid bilayers which surround the aqueous core.[6]

According to our results, the loading drug and release drug was 67.34% and 67.16% respectively. Many other studies indicated that the liposomes were suitable systems for loading drugs, for example, Glavas *et al* showed that the percentage of Lidocaine HCL encapsulation into liposome gels was over 72%.[7] Another study showed that cyproterone acetate containing liposomes had 74±6.11% loading efficiency and the liposomal formulation has better penetration potential than conventional cyproterone acetate formulation.[5] In another study, the results of the skin retention studies showed fairly high miconazol retention with liposomes when compared with commercial creams of the drug.[8] Also, quantitative analysis of encapsulated carvacrol in liposome vesicles showed that only a small amount 4.16% of the starting quantity of carvacrol was incorporated.[9]

The results of DSC curve of lecithin, cholesterol and celecoxib were very different from celecoxib containing liposomes. On the other hand, the DSC curve of lecithin, cholesterol can be dependent on the previous organization of these molecules to form liposome bilayer and also the results of Figure 2 indicated that celecoxib can interact with lecithin and cholesterol during the preparation of the liposomes. When celecoxibe was added to lipid phase during the liposome preparation, The DSC curve was shifted. The absence of flattened peaks indicated the homogeneity in the lipids forming the liposome.

The sonication time is an important parameter in the liposome preparation because the size of liposome decreased (Figure 1). Reduction in the particle size is a key factor for improving the performance of poorly soluble drugs .[10] The results of a study demonstrated that the size of the drug loaded liposome decreased significantly from 188 ±1.2 nm to 73 ±7.8 nm when the drug-lipid ratio was decreased from 1:10 to 1:1.[6] TEM image analysis of celecoxib containing liposome showed the spherical structure. TEM imaging showed the small vesicles began to emerge until finally aggregated and vesicle formed the multilamellar vesicle (Figure 3a). Also Figure 3b and 3d showed liposomes of various shapes and TEM image confirmed that liposomes are vesicle having phospholipids bilayer. Many other TEM studied also indicated that TEM is a suitable instrument for investigating the morphology of liposomes prepared by thin film method.[4]

Conclusion

Loaded of celecoxib in liposomes were found to have the appropriate size and exhibited improved release properties. Also, celecoxib containing liposome would be a suitable means for protecting and permeation of the drug.

Acknowledgments

The work was financially supported by Nanotechnology Research Center, Ahvaz Jundishapur University of Medical Sciences, Ahvaz, Iran.

Conflict of interest

The authors report no conflicts of interest.

References

1. Yang HM, Kim HS, Park KW, You HJ, Jeon SI, Youn SW, et al. Celecoxib, a cyclooxygenase-2 inhibitor, reduces neointimal hyperplasia through inhibition of Akt signaling. Circulation 2004;110(3):301-8.
2. Guirguis M.S, Sattari S, Jamali F. Pharmacokinetics of celecoxib in the presence and absence of interferon induced acute inflammation in the rat: application of a novel HPLC assay. *J. Pharm Pharmaceut Sci* 2001; 4(1):1-6.
3. Lopes L.B, Scarpa V.M, Pereira L.N, De Oliveira L.C, Gomes Oliveira A. Interaction of sodium diclofenac with freeze-dried soya phosphatidylcholine and unilamellar liposomes. *Brazilian J of Pharmaceutical Sciences* 2006; 42(4):497-504.
4. Chetanachan P, Akarachalanon P, Worawirunwong D, Dararutana P, Bangtrakulonoth A, Bunjop M, Kongmuang S. Ultrastructural characterization of liposome using transmission electron microscope. *Advanced Materials Research* 2008;55-57:709-711.
5. Mohammadi Samani S, Montaseri H, Jamshidnejad M. Preparation and evaluation of cyproterone acetate liposome for topical drug delivery. *Iranian J of Pharmaceutical Sciences* 2009; 5(4):199-204.
6. Ramana LN, Sethuraman S, Rauga U, Krishnan UM. Development of a liposomal nanodelivery system for nevirapine. *J of Biomedical Science* 2010;17(57): 1-9.
7. Dodov M.G, Simonska M, Goracinova K. Formulation and characterization of topical liposome gel bearing Lidocaine HCL. *Bullention of the Chemists and Technologists of Macedonia* 2005;24(1): 59-65.
8. Agarwal R, Katare OP, Vyas SP. Preparation and in vitro evaluation of liposomal/niosomal delivery systems for antipsoriatic drug dithranol. International journal of pharmaceutics. 2001;228(1-2):43-52.

10

Anti-bacterial performance of azithromycin nanoparticles as colloidal drug delivery system against different gram-negative and gram-positive bacteria

Morteza Azhdarzadeh[1,2], Farzaneh Lotfipour[3,4], Parvin Zakeri-Milani[3,5], Ghobad Mohammadi[6], Hadi Valizadeh[1, 3*]

[1] *Research Center for Pharmaceutical Nanotechnology, Tabriz University of Medical Sciences, Tabriz, Iran.*

[2] *Students Research Committee, Tabriz University of Medical Sciences, Tabriz, Iran.*

[3] *Faculty of Pharmacy, Tabriz University of Medical Sciences, Tabriz, Iran.*

[4] *Biotechnology Research Center, Tabriz University of Medical Sciences, Tabriz, Iran.*

[5] *Liver and Gastrointestinal Diseases Research Center, Tabriz University of Medical Sciences, Tabriz, Iran.*

[6] *Faculty of Pharmacy, Kermanshah University of Medical Sciences, Kermanshah, Iran.*

ARTICLE INFO

Keywords:
Azithromycin
PLGA
Nanoparticle
Modified quasi emulsion solvent-diffusion
Minimum inhibitory concentration

ABSTRACT

Purpose: Azithromycin (AZI) is a new macrolide antibiotic with a better activity against intracellular gram negative bacteria in comparison with Erythromycin. The purpose of this research was to prepare AZI nanoparticles (NPs) using PLGA polymer and to compare the effectiveness of prepared nanoparticles with untreated AZI solution. ***Methods***: AZI NPs were prepared by Modified Quasi-Emulsion Solvent Diffusion method. The antibacterial activities of prepared NPs in comparison with AZI solution were assayed against indicator bacteria of *Escherichia coli (PTCC 1330), Haemophilus influenzae (PTCC 1623) and Streptococcus pneumoniae (PTCC 1240)* using agar well diffusion. Inhibition zone diameters (IZD) of nano-formulation were compared to the corresponding untreated AZI. Mean Inhibitory Concentration (MIC) values of AZI were also determined using serial dilution method in nutrient broth medium. ***Results***: Mean IZD of nano-formulations for all indicator bacteria were significantly higher than that of untreated AZI ($P<0.01$). The enhanced antibacterial efficacy was more dominant in the gram positive species. The MIC values of NPs against the tested bacteria were reduced 8 times in comparison to those of untreated AZI. ***Conclusion***: These results indicated an improved potency of AZI NPs which could be attributed to the modified surface characteristics as well as increased drug adsorption and uptake.

Introduction

Nanoparticles as one of the most recent novel drug delivery carriers have been shown to improve drug efficiency via targeting the delivery of drugs, improving the bioavailability and either sustaining the release of the drugs or solubilizing them for systemic delivery. Additional advantage of this novel technology is the lower enzymatic as well as environmental degradation of pharmaceutical active ingredients. [1-5] The main features of nanoparticles, making them ideal candidates for drug delivery, are small size and use of biodegradable materials in their preparation. Indeed the nano-sized character of these particles causes their extravagation through the endothelium in inflammatory sites, epithelium, tumors, or penetrate microcapillaries and consequently allows for efficient uptake by a variety of cell types and selective drug accumulation at target sites. [2,5-8] The use of biodegradable materials for nanoparticles preparation allows for sustained drug release within the target site over a period of days or even weeks and thus increases the therapeutic benefit, while minimizing side effects. The best-known class of biodegradable materials for controlled release is the poly lactide-co-glycolides (PLGAs). PLGAs are biocompatible and biodegradable polymers that are hydrolytically degraded into nontoxic oligomers or monomers, lactic acid and glycolic acid. [9-12]

There have been numerous studies in recent years, especially based on nanoparticle systems, in order to the targeted the delivery of antibiotics toward the infected cells as well as enhancing their physicochemical properties. Fawaz and coworkers showed that Ciprofloxacin-loaded nanoparticles were

***Corresponding author:** Hadi Valizadeh (PhD), Faculty of Pharmacy, Tabriz University of Medical Sciences, Tabriz, Iran.
E-mail: valizadeh@tbzmed.ac.ir

more active in human macrophages infected with *Mycobacterium avium* than free drug. [13] In the other study it has been found by Fattal and coworkers that the efficacy of ampicillin is increased by 120-fold in murine salmonellosis by loading the drug into the nanoparticles. [14] Moreover Italia and coworkers proved that biodegradable nanoparticles improve oral bioavailability of amphotericin B and show reduced nephrotoxicity. [15]

Azithromycin (AZI) is a new macrolide antibiotic (Figure 1) that is similar in structure to erythromycin with a broader gram-negative antibacterial spectrum. This drug acts by binding to the 50s ribosomal subunit of susceptible microorganism and interfering with microbial protein synthesis. [16,17] Antimicrobial spectrum of AZI is wide including aerobic gram-positive microorganism such as *Staphylococcus aureus, Streptococcus pneumoniae*, aerobic gram-negative microorganism such as *Haemophilus influenzae* and anaerobic microorganism such as *Clostridium perfingens* as well as Mycobacteria. It worth to note that *Haemophilus influenzae* and *Streptococcus pneumoniae* are responsible for a broad variety of infections such as lower respiratory tract diseases.

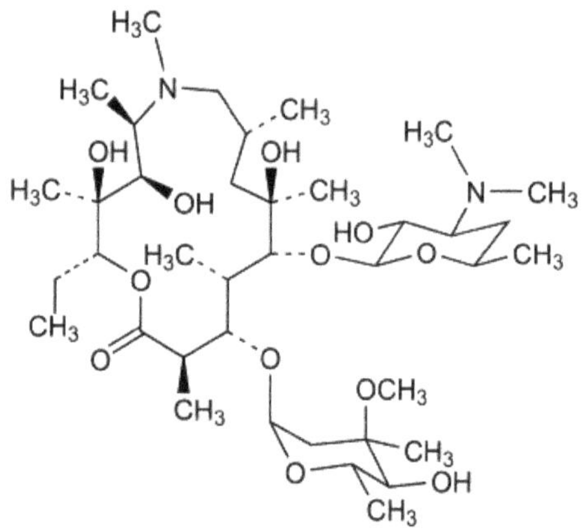

Figure 1. Chemical structure of azithromycin

In our previous study we developed AZI nanoparticles and evaluated their physicochemical properties. [18] In the present work we aimed to evaluate the antibacterial activity of selected formulations with appropriate physicochemical specifications against a group of most important AZI susceptible bacteria including *Escherichia coli, Haemophilus influenzae and Streptococcus pneumoniae* in comparison with untreated azithromycin.

Materials and Methods

Materials

AZI powder was obtained from Dr Reddy's pharmaceutical Company, India. Poly (D,L-lactide-co-glycolide) (PLGA) (50:50 D,L-lactide:glycolide) with average molecular weight of 12,000 g/mol (Resomer RG 502), was purchased from boehringer Ingelheim, Germany. Poly vinyl alcohol, PVA, with molecular weight of MW 95000 was obtained from Acros Organics (Geel, Belgium). *Escherichia coli (PTCC1330), Haemophilus influenzae* (PTCC 1623), *Staphylococcus aureus* (PTCC 1112) and *Streptococcus pneumoniae* (PTCC 1240) were purchased from Persian Type Culture Collection, Iran. Haemophilus Selective Agar, SoyBean Casein Digest Agar and Antibiotic assay Medium were purchased from Merck (Darmstadt, Germany). Blood Base Agar media was purchased from DIFCO, U.K. All other materials used were of analytical or HPLC grade.

Preparation of nanoparticles

Nanoparticles (Nanospheres) were prepared according to our previously published method. [18] Briefly NPs (nanospheres) with 1:3, 1:2 and 1:1 ratios of the drug to PLGA were prepared by nano-precipitation according to the modified quasi emulsion solvent diffusion technique. AZI and PLGA powders were co-dissolved in internal phase containing acetone, 2.5 ml, at room temperature (25°C). Typically, different ratios of drug and polymer, with the total amount of 100 mg, were co-dissolved in acetone. The resulting organic solution was injected at the constant rate of 0.5 ml/min in aqueous phase (40 ml) containing PVA 95000 (2% w/v), as a stabilizing agent. As water solubility of AZI decreases at higher pH, in order to gain higher drug loading, the pH of aqueous phase was adjusted to 8. The process was carried out under homogenization for 5 min using the Silent Crusher M (Heidolph, Germany). The agitation speed was 13000 rpm in an ice-water bath. Acetone was eliminated at the room temperature under stirring for 12 h. The final nano-suspension was centrifuged (Beckman Centrifuge, Avanti™J-25, USA) at 14000 rpm for 30 min and the precipitated NPs were washed twice with water, using the previously described centrifugation approach, and then lyophilized by using a lyophilizer (Christ Alpha 1-4; Germany). Final dry powder was taken out for anti bacterial investigations.

Physicochemical characterization of AZI loaded nanoparticles

The mean particle-size values of NPs were measured by using a laser diffraction particle-size analyzer (Sald 2101, Shimadzu, Japan) equipped with Wing software (version 1.20). The morphology of the NPs were investigated by scanning electron microscopy (SEM) (LEO 440i, Leo Electron Microscopy Ltd, Cambridge, UK) at an accelerating voltage of 20 kV. In order to determine the encapsulation efficiency of NPs, three samples were dissolved in acetone, after evaporation of the acetone the drug was dissolved in 100 ml sterile water. [3,5,19] The mixture was then centrifuged and the supernatant was drawn to measure their AZI contents microbiologically after appropriate dilution. A microbiological assay was adapted from the method described in the official US Pharmacopoeia (USP 2004) monograph. The X-ray powder diffraction (XRPD) of the drug, PLGA, NPs and physical mixture in the 1:2 drug to polymer ratio were recorded using an automated X-ray diffractometer (Siemens D5000, Munich, Germany). Drug release was performed in sink conditions according to our previously published method. [18]

Antibacterial activity of the nanoparticle suspensions

The NPs antimicrobial activity was compared with that of the free drug by means of well diffusion method as well as broth serial dilution method using *E. coli* (PTCC 1330), *H. influenzae* (PTCC 1623), *S. pneumoniae* (PTCC 1240) and *S. aureus* (PTCC 1112). All the bacteria were purchased from Persian type culture collection. The bacteria obtained in lyophilized form were activated according to their manufacturer's protocol. At first, their stock samples that contained 20% glycerol were prepared from activated bacteria and kept at freezer for further uses. The activated *E. coli*, *H. influenzae*, S. aureus and *S. pneumoniae* were cultured in Soy Bean Casein Digest Agar, Haemophilus Selective Agar, Nutrient Broth and Blood Base Agar medium respectively (24 hours before studies).

The antibacterial activity of the selected formulations as well as control samples was evaluated using agar well diffusion and broth dilution method. [20] In agar well diffusion method, firstly appropriate amount of prepared inoculum of each bacterium, were transferred into its selective medium. Soy Bean Casein Digest Agar medium was used for culturing *E. coli. Also H. influenzae* and *S. pneumoniae* were transferred on the surface of Haemophilus Selective Agar and Blood Base Agar respectively. Wells with 8-mm diameters were punched on the surface of agar media using a sterile cork borer. Aliquots of 100 µl of each sample (1:3, 1:2 and 1:1 AZI to PLGA nanoparticles) were transferred into the wells. After incubation at 37 °C for 24 hours, the inhibition zones around the wells were measured in using zone reader. In order to evaluate the MIC of NPs the mentioned nanoparticle suspensions were serially diluted. The tubes were inoculated with a 1ml of inoculums of tested bacterium (final concentration of 10^5-10^6 CFU/ml). After 24 h of incubation at 37°C, the tubes were screened for any evidence of bacterial growth. MIC was defined as the lowest concentration of AZI that completely suppressed the bacterial growth. [21] PLGA nanoparticles without AZI and untreated AZI were applied as positive and negative controls respectively.

Statistical analysis

One-way analysis of variance (ANOVA) was performed for comparison of the results. P values of 0 < 0.01 were considered significant.

Results and discussion

Physicochemical properties of AZI loaded nanoparticles

Based on our previously published paper, the submicron particles ranging from 212 to 252 nm with Narrow range of size (Figure 2), a relatively monodisperse distribution with spherical morphology (Figure 3) were achieved using modified quasi emulsion solvent diffusion technique. Results also indicated a maximum AZI loading of about 78.5% with an increasing manner with increase in the proportion of PLGA. This observation may be attributed to the higher viscosity of the internal organic phase for higher PLGA ratios, which in turn would decrease the diffusion coefficient of the drug. Furthermore at higher polymer ratio the extent of drug loss during washing procedure will be less.

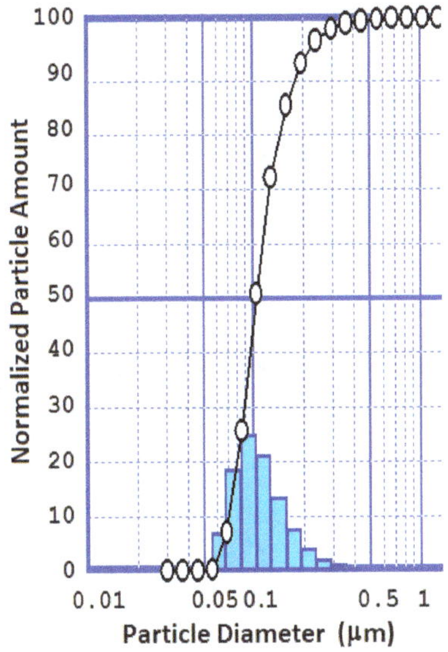

Figure 2. Particle size distribution of nanoparticles preparation with 1:3 ratios of the drug to PLGA ratio.

XRPD patterns of NPs were characterized by the complete absence of any diffraction peaks, suggesting a complete amorphization of AZI in the NPs. [18] Based on the results from release study the release rate of AZI from NPs was slower and more sustained than that of intact AZI that may be due to the presence of insoluble polymer (PLGA) in the NPs matrix body which in turn reduces the water penetration, hence dissolution and diffusion [22-24] (data not shown). [18]

Antimicrobial activity of AZI loaded nanoparticles

To evaluate the antibacterial activity of the selected nano formulations and untreated AZI samples, agar diffusion method and broth dilution method, that is highly recommended methods for testing of antimicrobial agents against fastidious organisms like Haemophilus spp. and streptococci, were performed based on NCCLS guideline with some modifications as described in material and method section. Mean inhibitory diameters related to each of the nano formulation of AZI were compared to their untreated counterparts in the same concentrations using ANOVA. Figure 4 to Figure 6 illustrate and compare mean inhibitory diameters related to AZI nonoparticles with untreated samples against *E. coli*, *H. influenzae* and *S. pneumoniae* respectively. As it can be seen there are

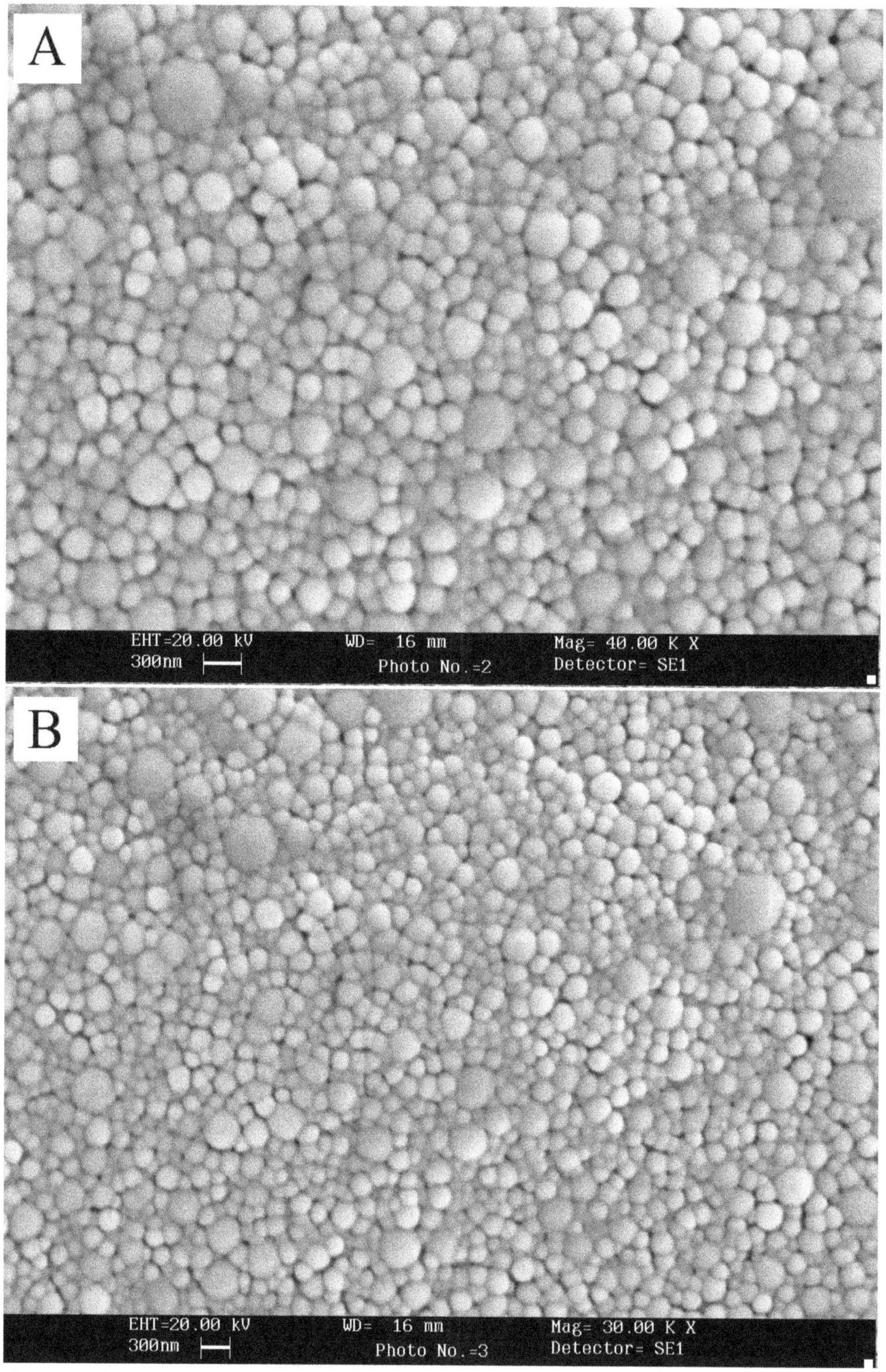

Figure 3. SEM images of azithromycin loaded nanoparticles of the (A) 1:2 (B) 1:3 drug to polymer ratios.

significant differences between inhibitory zone diameters of samples. For instance the concentration of 100 µg/ml of untreated AZI produced mean inhibitory diameter of about 20 mm, whereas AZI nanoparticles showed the same mean inhibitory diameter (20 mm) in the concentration of 12.5 µg/ml indicating 8 times reduction in the AZI concentration to achieve the same antibacterial activity against *E. coli* (Figure 4). In a same manner as shown in Figure 5 and 6 the activities of AZI nanoparticles were considerably enhanced against *H. influenzae* and *S. pneumoniae* compared to their untreated counterparts. As the first inhibitory diameters appear in the concentrations of 25 µg/ml and 3.12 µg/ml for untreated AZI against *H. influenzae* as well as *S. pneumoniae* respectively, they shift to 3.12 µg/ml and 0.19 µg/ml when AZI nanoparticles were applied, showing 8 and 16 times reductions in the required AZI concentrations for producing the same action against *H. influenzae* And *S. pneumoniae* respectively. Table 1 show the mean MIC of the nano formulation and untreated AZI against *E. coli* and *S. aureus*. The lowest inhibitory concentration were about 0.78 µg/ml and 0.39 µg/ml regardless of the ratio of drug:polymer in nanoparticle suspension, whereas the inhibitory concentration were about 6.25 µg/ml and 3.12 µg/ml for the corresponding Untreated AZI solution in *E. coli* and *S. aureus* respectively, indicating 8 times reduction in AZI MIC. Blank NPs indicated no antibacterial activity against indicated bacteria. Also the ratio of polymer used had no influence on the antibacterial activity of the nanoparticles, at least for the indicator bacteria examined here ($P>0.01$). It also worth to note that among three indicator bacteria tested in this study the activity of prepared nano formulations against gram positive *S. pneumoniae* were remarkably better than gram negative species of *E. coli* and *H. influenza.* This could be because of some possible mechanisms; one is the fact that presence of a double membrane could exclude certain structures from penetrating the cell, partially accounting for why gram negative bacteria are generally more resistant to antibiotics than other gram positive bacteria. [25]

Table 1. Minimum inhibitory concentration (MIC) of untreated AZI solution (AZI), physical mixtures (PM) and AZI-loaded nanoparticles with different drug:polymer ratios against E. coli and S. aureus

	MIC (µg/ml)	
Sample	***E. coli***	***S. aureus***
AZI	6.25	3.12
PM 1:1	6.25	3.12
PM 1:2	6.25	3.12
PM 1:3	6.25	3.12
NANO 1:1	0.78	0.39
NANO 1:2	0.78	0.39

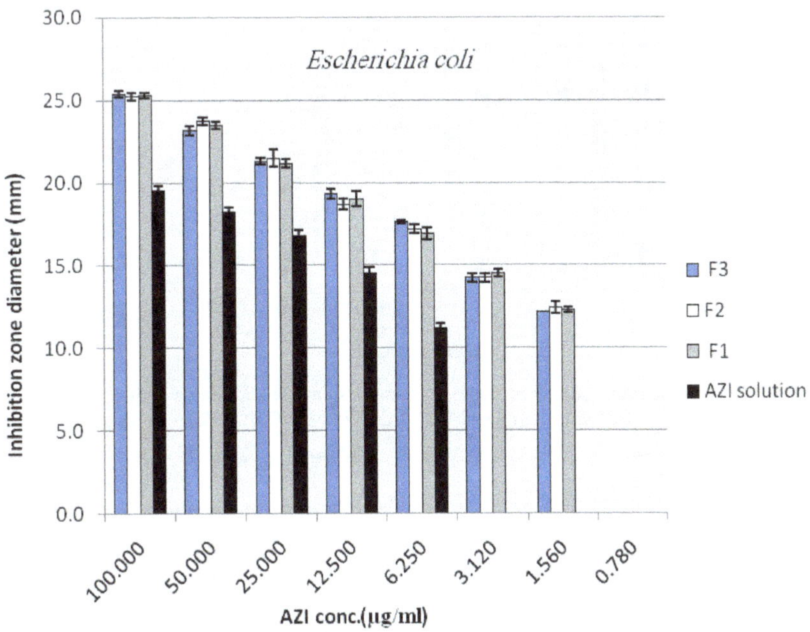

Figure 4. Inhibition zone diameter of azithromycin loaded nanoparticles in plates with *E.coli* inoculums (NANO 1:1 (F1), NANO 1:2 (F2), NANO 1:3 (F3))

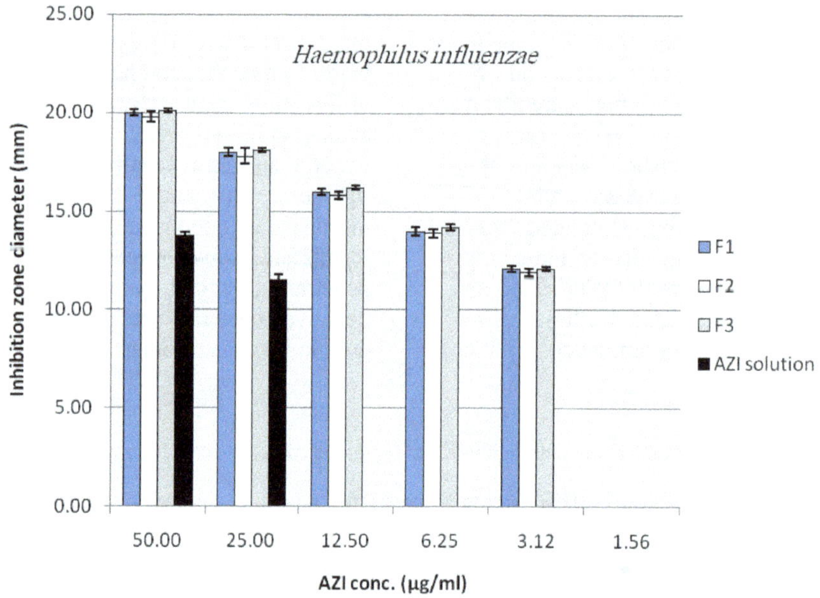

Figure 5. Inhibition zone diameter of azithromycin loaded nanoparticles in plates with *H. influenza* inoculums (NANO 1:1 (F1), NANO 1:2 (F2), NANO 1:3 (F3))

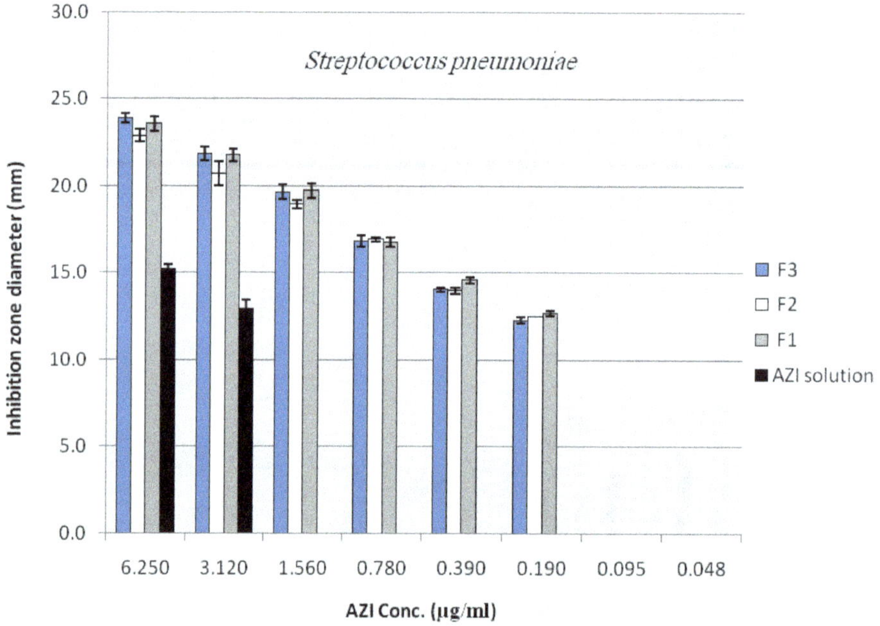

Figure 6. Inhibition zone diameter of azithromycin loaded nanoparticles in plates with S. pneumonia inoculum (NANO 1:1 (F1), NANO 1:2 (F2), NANO 1:3 (F3))

Conclusion

The present study was conducted to evaluate the antibacterial activity of AZI-PLGA nanoparticles against *E. coli*, *H. influenzae*, *S. aureus* and *S. pneumoniae* which are important species susceptible to AZI. The obtained results indicate that there is a significant enhancement in the efficacy of AZI loaded nano formulations in comparison with untreated AZI in the same concentration. The improved efficacy of pharmaceutical active products when prepared in nano formulations have been repeatedly reported so far. There are also numerous studies to enhance antibiotics efficacies against their indicator microorganisms exploiting the nano technology that showed better activities. [10,13,14] This may be due to the several reasons more dominantly facilitated penetration of drug in nano particle form into the bacterial cells; and better delivery of the drug to its site of action [10] as well as higher stability of the drug in nano encapsulated form against rapid enzymatic/hydrolytic degradation. [26]

Adhesion of the NPs to the bacterial cell wall can be another mechanism for greater antibacterial activity of the NPs in comparison with pure drug. This adhesion could provide a sustained antimicrobial activity of the drug incorporated against the target organisms.[27-29]

In conclusion, Azithromycin-loaded poly (lactide-co-glycolide) (PLGA) nanoparticles (NPs) were more effective than untreated AZI against *E. coli*, *H. influenzae*, *S. aureus* and *S. pneumonia*. Therefore, the clinical effectiveness of azithromycin might be enhanced if its nanoparticles are incorporated in the dosage forms e.g. aerosol, ocular, topical and oral preparations as colloidal drug delivery system compared to the conventional formulation of azithromycin present in the market.

Acknowledgments

The authors wish to thank *Research Center for Pharmaceutical Nanotechnology*, Tabriz, Iran for the financial support of this work.

Conflict of interest

All the authors report no conflicts of interest.

References

1. Ge H, Hu Y, Jiang X, Cheng D, Yuan Y, Bi H, et al. Preparation, characterization, and drug release behaviors of drug nimodipine-loaded poly(epsilon-caprolactone)-poly(ethylene oxide)-poly(epsilon-caprolactone) amphiphilic triblock copolymer micelles. *J Pharm Sci* 2002; 91: 1463-73.
2. Singh R, Lillard JW Jr. Nanoparticle-based targeted drug delivery. Exp Mol Pathol 2009; 86: 215-223.
3. Jelvehgari M, Barar J, Valizadeh H, Shadrou S, Nokhodchi A. Formulation, characterization and in vitro evaluation of theophylline-loaded Eudragit RS 100 microspheres prepared by an emulsion-solvent diffusion/evaporation technique. *Pharm Dev Technol* 2010;16(6):637-44.
4. Jelvehgari M, Nokhodchi A, Rezapour M, Valizadeh H. Effect of formulation and processing variables on the characteristics of tolmetin microspheres prepared by double emulsion solvent diffusion method. *Indian J Pharm Sci* 2010; 72: 72-78.
5. Jelvehgari M, Zakeri-Milani P, Siahi-Shadbad MR, Loveymi BD, Nokhodchi A, Azari Z, et al. Development of pH-sensitive insulin nanoparticles using Eudragit L100-55 and chitosan with different molecular weights. *AAPS PharmSciTech* 2010; 11: 1237-1242.
6. Desai MP, Labhasetwar V, Walter E, Levy RJ, Amidon GL. The mechanism of uptake of biodegradable microparticles in Caco-2 cells is size dependent. *Pharm Res* 1997; 14: 1568-1573.
7. Hajdo L, Szulc AB, Klajnert B, Bryszewska M. Metabolic limitations of the use of nucleoside analogs in cancer therapy may be overcome by application of nanoparticles as drug carriers: A review. *Drug Development Research* 2010; 71: 383-394.
8. Sunderland CJ, Steiert M, Talmadge JE, Derfus AM, Barry SE. Targeted nanoparticles for detecting and treating cancer. *Drug Development Research* 2006; 67: 70-93.
9. Barrera DA, Zylstra E, Lansbury PT, Langer R. Synthesis and RGD peptide modification of a new biodegradable copolymer: poly(lactic acid-co-lysine). *J Am Chem Soc* 1993; 115: 11010-11011.
10. Esmaeili F, Hosseini-Nasr M, Rad-Malekshahi M, Samadi N, Atyabi F, Dinarvand R. Preparation and antibacterial activity evaluation of rifampicin-loaded poly lactide-co-glycolide nanoparticles. *Nanomedicine* 2007; 3: 161-167.
11. Hou Z, Zhou C, Luo Y, Zhan C, Wang Y, Xie L, et al. PLA nanoparticles loaded with an active lactone form of hydroxycamptothecin: development, optimization, and in vitro–in vivo evaluation in mice bearing H22 solid tumor. *Drug Development Research* 2011;72(4):337-345. 12. Yadav KS, Chuttani K, Mishra AK, Sawant KK. Long circulating nanoparticles of etoposide using PLGA-MPEG and PLGA-pluronic block copolymers: characterization, drug-release, blood-clearance, and biodistribution studies. *Drug Development Research* 2010; 71: 228-239.
13. Fawaz F, Bonini F, Maugein J, Lagueny AM. Ciprofloxacin-loaded polyisobutylcyanoacrylate nanoparticles: pharmacokinetics and in vitro antimicrobial activity. *International Journal of Pharmaceutics* 1998; 168: 255-259.
14. Fattal E, Youssef M, Couvreur P, Andremont A. Treatment of experimental salmonellosis in mice with ampicillin-bound nanoparticles. *Antimicrob Agents Chemother* 1989; 33: 1540-1543.
15. Italia JL, Yahya MM, Singh D, Ravi Kumar MN. Biodegradable nanoparticles improve oral bioavailability of amphotericin B and show reduced nephrotoxicity compared to intravenous Fungizone. *Pharm Res* 2009; 26: 1324-1331.
16. Zakeri-Milani P, Ghanbarzadeh S, Lotfipoor F, Milani M, Valizadeh H. Pharmacokinetic study of two macrolide antibiotic oral suspensions using an optimized bioassay procedure. *Journal of Bioequivalence & Bioavailability* 2010; 2: 111-115.
17. Zakeri-Milani P, Valizadeh H, Islambulchilar Z, Damani S, Mehtari M. Investigation of the intestinal permeability of ciclosporin using the in situ technique in rats and the relevance of P-glycoprotein. *Arzneimittelforschung* 2008; 58: 188-192.
18. Mohammadi G, Valizadeh H, Barzegar-Jalali M, Lotfipour F, Adibkia K, Milani M, et al. Development of azithromycin-PLGA nanoparticles: physicochemical characterization and antibacterial effect against Salmonella typhi. Colloids Surf B *Biointerfaces* 2010; 80: 34-39.
19. Jelvehgari M, Valizadeh H, Rezapour M, Nokhodchi A. Control of encapsulation efficiency

in polymeric microparticle system of tolmetin. *Pharm Dev Technol* 2010; 15: 71-79.

20. National Committee for Clinical Laboratory Standards. Methods for dilution antimicrobial susceptibility tests for bacteria that grow aerobically, Approved Standard M7-A5. 5th ed. Wayne, PA: NCCLS; 2000.
21. No HK, Young Park N, Ho Lee S, Meyers SP. Antibacterial activity of chitosans and chitosan oligomers with different molecular weights. *International Journal of Food Microbiology* 2002; 74: 65-72.
22. Valizadeh H, Nokhodchi A, Qarakhani N, Zakeri-Milani P, Azarmi S, Hassanzadeh D, et al. Physicochemical characterization of solid dispersions of indomethacin with PEG 6000, Myrj 52, lactose, sorbitol, dextrin, and Eudragit E100. Drug *Dev Ind Pharm* 2004; 30: 303-317.
23. Azarmi S, Farid J, Nokhodchi A, Bahari-Saravi SM, Valizadeh H. Thermal treating as a tool for sustained release of indomethacin from Eudragit RS and RL matrices. *Int J Pharm* 2002; 246: 171-177.
24. Valizadeh H, Zakeri-Milani P, Barzegar-Jalali M, Mohammadi G, Danesh-Bahreini MA, Adibkia K, et al. Preparation and characterization of solid dispersions of piroxicam with hydrophilic carriers. *Drug Dev Ind Pharm* 2007; 33: 45-56.
25. Lotfipour F, Nazemiyeh H, Fathi-Azad F, Garaei N, Arami S, Talat S, et al. Evaluation of Antibacterial Activities of Some Medicinal Plants from North-West Iran. *Iranian journal of basic medicinal sciences* 2008; 11: 80-85.
26. Panyam J, Labhasetwar V. Biodegradable nanoparticles for drug and gene delivery to cells and tissue. *Adv Drug Deliv Rev* 2003; 55: 329-347.
27. Dillen K, Bridts C, Van der Veken P, Cos P, Vandervoort J, Augustyns K, et al. Adhesion of PLGA or Eudragit/PLGA nanoparticles to Staphylococcus and Pseudomonas. *Int J Pharm* 2008; 349: 234-240.
28. Lboutounne H, Chaulet JF, Ploton C, Falson F, Pirot F. Sustained ex vivo skin antiseptic activity of chlorhexidine in poly(epsilon-caprolactone) nanocapsule encapsulated form and as a digluconate. *J Control Release* 2002; 82: 319-334.
29. Sahoo SK, Panyam J, Prabha S, Labhasetwar V. Residual polyvinyl alcohol associated with poly (D,L-lactide-co-glycolide) nanoparticles affects their physical properties and cellular uptake. *J Control Release* 2002; 82: 105-114.

Phytochemical analysis and antioxidant activity of *Hyssopus officinalis L.* from Iran

Fatemeh Fathiazad[1*], **Masoumeh Mazandarani**[2], **Sanaz Hamedeyazdan**[1,3]

[1]*Department of Pharmacognosy, Faculty of Pharmacy, Tabriz University of Medical Sciences, Iran*

[2]*Islamic Azad University Gorgan Branch, Gorgan, Iran*

[3]*Student Research Committee, Tabriz University of Medical Sciences, Tabriz, Iran*

ARTICLE INFO

Keywords:
Hyssopus officinalis
Total phenols
Radical scavenging
Essential oil
Antioxidant
Culinary herb

ABSTRACT

Introduction: *Hyssopus officinalis* (L) (Hyssop, Family: Lamiaceae), one of the endemic Iranian perennial herb with a long history of medicinal use, was studied to detect some biologically active chemical constituents of the plant. ***Methods:*** The flavonoids of the hydromethanolic extract of the aerial parts of *Hyssopus officinalis (L.)* were studied by VLC and crystalisation of the major compound in subsequent fractions. Furthermore, the composition of its essential oil, total phenolic content and antioxidant activities were studied by GC-MS, Folin–Ciocalteau and DPPH reagents respectively. ***Results:*** Apigenin 7-*O*-β-D-glucuronide was isolated as the major flavonoid. All structural elucidation was performed by spectral means. A total of 20 compounds representing 99.97% of the oil have been identified. Myrtenylacetate, Camphor, Germacrene, Spathulenol were the main compounds The total phenol content of the n-butanol and ethylacetate extracts were determined spectrophotometrically according to the Folin–Ciocalteau procedure to be 246 mgGAE g^{-1} and 51 mgGAE g^{-1} in the aerial parts of *Hyssopus officinalis* . The antioxidant activities of apigenin 7-*O*-β-D-glucuronide, ethylacetate and *n*-butanol extracts were also determined by DPPH radical scavenging assay with IC_{50} values of 116×10^{-3}, 103×10^{-3}, 25×10^{-3} mg mL^{-1} respectively. The purified flavonoid showed weak radical scavenging activity (IC_{50} = 116×10^{-3}mg mL^{-1}). N-butanol extract, because of the highest content of total phenolic compounds (246 mgGAE100^{-1}g) had the best antioxidant activity (IC_{50} = 25mg mL^{-1}). ***Conclusion:*** On the whole, the findings of the study revealed that *Hyssop* possesses valuable antioxidant properties for culinary and possible medicinal use.

Introduction

In recent years, using traditional medicinal knowledge in drug discovery seems so promising that even large pharmaceutical companies have begun to show interest in this field.[1,2] The genus *Hyssopus* L. comprises about 10-12 species distributed mainly in the east Mediterranean to central Asia. *Hyssopus officinalis* (L) (Hyssop, Family: Lamiaceae), a perennial herb with a long history of medicinal use, is one of the endemic Iranian species of the genus *Hyssopus*.[3,4] Traditionally, *H. officinalis* named Zufa in Iran, have been used as a carminative, tonic, antiseptic, expectorant and cough reliever.[4] Despite having a slightly bitter taste, *H. officinalis* is often used as a minty flavor and condiment in food industries. The merit of the traditional use of *H. officinalis* has been supported by some prior studies from the genus *Hyssopus*, providing several biologically active constituents especially main compounds from essential oils.[5-7] Studies dealing with the antioxidant, anti-platelet, and anti-fungal activities of essential oil from *H. officinalis* have been previously reported.[5,7-9] Surveys such as that conducted by Miyazaki et al. have shown that *H. officinalis* extracts revealed alpha-glucosidase inhibitory effects on intestinal carbohydrate absorption, indicating significant activity against hyperglycemia.[10] Numerous studies refer to the composition of *H. officinalis* oil from different parts of the world.[4,11,12] However, a few studies have been conducted on flavonoid structures present in *H. officinalis.*[13-15] It is well known that phenolics and flavonoids from plants act as free radical scavenger. There is interest in knowing the phenolic content of fruits and vegetables in order to increase their potential use as nutraceuticals or functional foods. However, scientific information on antioxidant properties of various plants, particularly those that are used in culinary and medicine is still rather scarce.[16]

***Corresponding author:** Fatemeh Fathiazad (PhD), E-mail: fathiazad@tbzmed.ac.ir

Hence, the present study was carried out to detect some biologically active chemical constituents of the plant. This survey is an ongoing point in our study on the plants of Iranian flora.[12,17-19] Herein, we describe the analysis of essential oil, isolation and structural elucidation of a main flavonoid isolated from aerial parts of *H. officinalis*. The free radical scavenging activity of the flavonoid, essential oil and methanolic extract were also determined using (2,2-diphenyl-1-picrylhydrazyl) DPPH.

Materials and methods

General

All solvents and the Folin-Ciocalteu reagent used for the present work were purchased from Merck (Germany), DPPH (1,1-diphenyl-2- picryl-hydrazyl, 90%) was from Sigma (Germany).

UV spectra (λ max) were recorded on a Shimadzu 2100 spectrophotometer. 1H-NMR and 13C-NMR spectra were taken on a Bruker instrument 200 MHz (1H-NMR) and 50 MHz (13C-NMR) in MeOH-d_4.

Plant material

The aerial parts of Hyssopus officinalis were collected during flowering stage on June from north of Iran and authenticated by Dr. Mazandarani. Voucher specimens have been deposited at the herbarium of the Department of Pharmacognosy, Faculty of Pharmacy, Tabriz University of Medical Sciences, Tabriz, Iran.

Extraction and isolation of flavonoids

The dried aerial parts (200g) were ground and defatted with 1L n-hexane. The defatted powdered aerial parts were extracted with 2L 70% methanol in water by maceration at room temperature. The methanol of resultant hydroalcoholic extract was evaporated at 40°C under reduced pressure and affording the aqueous extract. Subsequently, the aqueous extract was partitioned with EtOAc (ETE) and n- butanol respectively. According to TLC analysis, the n-butanol flavonoid rich extract (NBE) was subjected to VLC on silica gel as the stationary phase and eluted with step-gradient EtOAc-MeOH mixtures (8:2, 7:3, 6:4, 5:5, 4:6, 3:7, 2:8, 1:9, each 200 ml) and MeOH (300 ml) providing nine fractions (A-I). All farctions were controlled by TLC on analytical Silica gel GF_{254} plate using a mixture of EtOAc-MeOH-H_2O (6:4:1) as eluent and 5% $AlCl_3$ reagent for detection. On separation, the fraction B and F, each containing one major flavonoid, were dried and dissolved in small volume of methanol and kept in refrigerator at +2°C.The crystals formed in fraction B and F, was separated by filteration and dried to provide Apigenin 7-*O*-glucuronide (compound **1**, 33.6 mg) and compound **2** (14.3 mg).

The structure of compound **1** was elucidated by interpretation and comparison of its spectral data (UV, 1H-NMR and 13C-NMR) with those published references. Due to the lack of sufficient and complete spectroscopic data, Compound **2** has not been identified.

Essential oil isolation and GC- MS analysis

Air-dried plant material was subjected to hydro distillation using a Clevenger-type apparatus for 3 h (1. 3% yield). The obtained essential oil was dried over anhydrous sodium sulphate and stored at +4 °C until tested and analyzed.

Analysis of the essential oil was performed using a Shimadzu, QP 5050A, (E.I Quadrapole) equipped with a FID detector and a DB-1 capillary column (60 m × 0.25 mm i.d.).

For GC–MS detection, an electron ionization system with ionization energy of 70 eV was used. Helium was the carrier gas, at a flow rate of 1 ml/min and split injection with split ratio 1:11. Injector, detector and MS transfer line temperatures were set at 250 °C, 280 °C and 290 °C, respectively. The program used was 60–200 °C at a rate of 1.5 °C/min, held isothermal for 10 min and finally raised to 250 °C at 5 °C/min. Diluted samples (1/100 v/v in methylene chloride) of 1.0 µl were injected manually. The components were identified based on the comparison of their relative retention times and mass spectra with those of standards, Nist 21, Nist 107 and Wiley 229 library data of the GC–MS system and literature data.[20]

Determination of Total Phenolic Content of Plant Extracts

Total phenolic content of ETE and NBE were measured according to the Folin-Ciocalteu assay.[21] Results were expressed as milligrams of gallic acid equivalents (GAE) per gram of dry weight. Briefly, 100 ml of crude extracts and the standard, previously dissolved in methanol, was diluted with water to 8 mL, 0.5 mL of Folin- Ciocalteu phenol reagent was added, and the flasks were shaken vigorously. After 8 min, 1.5 mL of 20% sodium carbonate solution was added, and the mixtures were mixed thoroughly again. The mixtures were allowed to stand for 1 h protected from light. The absorbance of the blue color produced was measured with a spectrophotometer (Shimadzu 2100) at 750 nm. The concentration of total phenolic compounds for each extract was calculated on the basis of a standard curve obtained using gallic acid.

DPPH radical-scavenging assay

DPPH was used to determine free radical-scavenging potential of copmpound**1**, ETE and NBE. DPPH solution in MeOH (80 g mL^{-1}) was used. IC_{50} (50% inhibitory concentrations) of compound **1** and extracts were calculated versus MeOH as a negative control and Quercetin was used as a positive control.[22]

Briefly, stock solutions of compound **1,** ETE and NBE were prepared in MeOH to achieve the concentration of 1mg mL^{-1}. Dilutions were made to obtain concentrations of 5×10^{-2}, 5×10^{-3},5×10^{-4},5×10^{-5},5×10^{-6}, 5×10^{-7} mg mL^{-1}. 2 ml of each solution was added to 2 ml of DPPH solution. The absorbance was measured at

517 nm after 30 min of reaction at 25°C. The experiments were performed in duplicate and the average absorption was noted for each concentration.

Results and discussion

The *n*-butanol extract (NBE) of *H. officinalis* was fractionated by using VLC on silica gel. Further purification was achieved by crystallization in methanol to give flavonoid compounds **1-2.** The structures of compound **1** was determined by ^{1}H NMR and ^{13}C NMR experiments and UV data. Compound 1 was obtained as yellow crystals. The UV spectra of compound I obtained in this study was as follows: UV, λmax (nm) (MeOH) 268.4, 332.4; (MeONa) 271.0, 300 sh, 386; (AlCl3) 273.6, 297.4, 345,381.8; ($AlCl_3$/HCl) 275.2, 297.4, 340, 379.2, 403; (NaOAc) 265.8, 389.4, 407; (NaOAc/H3BO3) 266.8, 341.8. These UV data were compared with published data (Mabry *et al.*, 1970 and Markham, 1982). The UV spectrum in methanol and its changes after the addition of the customary shift reagents suggested that compound 1 is a 7- substituted flavone with free hydroxyl groups at positions C-5and C-4′.

The ^{1}H NMR spectrum of 1 (Table 1) displayed signals corresponding to a momosubstituted B-ring of the flavonoid nucleus at δ 7.92 (d, J = 8.0) and 6.92 (d, J = 8.0 Hz) each integrating for two protons, which were assigned to H-2′ and H-6′, and H-3′ and H-5′, respectively. A typical flavone H-3 signal at δ 6.82 (1H, s) was observed. The A ring of flavonoid **1** showed two doublets (J =2.1 Hz, meta-coupling) at δ_H 6.43 and 6.77 attributed to hydrogen atoms H-6 and H-8, respectively.

The ^{1}H NMR spectrum suggested that compound **1** is a monosaccharide of apigenin on the basis of a signal in the sugar region at 5.15 (d, J = 7.1 Hz), corresponding to the anomeric protons of β- linked glycosidic bond. The remaining sugar protons appeared in the range δ 3.2- 4.3 ppm (Table 1).

The ^{13}C NMR spectrum of compound **1** (Table 1) revealed 21 carbon signals, 15 of which were assigned to an apigenin unit. The anomeric carbon absorbed at δ 100.35. Two signals at 182.78 ppm and 173.49 ppm attributed to C-4 of flavones skeleton and C-6″ of sugar moiety, respectively.[23-25]

The sugar moiety was determined to be β-D-glucuronide from analyses of 1H and ^{13}C-NMR spectroscopic data.[23,24] The structure of compound 1 is therefore established as apigenin 7-O-β-D-glucuronide (figure 1).

This flavonoid is determined to be the main flavonoid of the aerial parts of *H. officinalis.* Apigenin 7-O-β-D-glucuronide was previously isolated from the aerial parts from the study of Wang et al.[13]

The composition of the oil of *H. officinalis* is given in Table 2. Constituents were listed in order of their elution from the DB-1 capillary column. Nineteen components were identified, accounting for 99.97% of the sample collected in Iran. The main constituents of the oil were Myrtenyl acetate (74.08%), Camphor (6.76%), Germacrene (3.39%), Spathulenol (2.14%), Caryophyllen Oxide (2.13%) and β-Caryophyllene (2.10%) with lesser amts. of Cis- sabinol (1.75%), β-Bourbonene (1.47%), Bornyl acetate (1.42%).

Table 1. ^{1}H NMR and ^{13}C NMR data of compounds **1** in MeOH-d_4.

Position	δ_H (J in Hz)(ppm)	δ_C(ppm)
2	-	165.2
3	6.82	103.82
4	-	182.78
5	-	162.44
6	6.43(d, J=2.1)	100.35
7	-	163.80
8	6.77(d, J=2.1)	95.5
9	-	157.79
10	-	106
1′	-	121.60
2′	7.92(d, J=8.15)	129.35
3′	6.92(d, J=8.15)	116.86
4′	-	162.4
5′	6.92(d, J=8.15)	116.86
6′	7.92(d, J=8.15)	129.35
	β-D-glucuronide (at C-7)	
1″	5.15	100.35
2″	m*	73.77
3″	m	74.98
4″	m	72.78
5″	4.25(d, J=9)	77.2
6″	-	173.49

*multiple

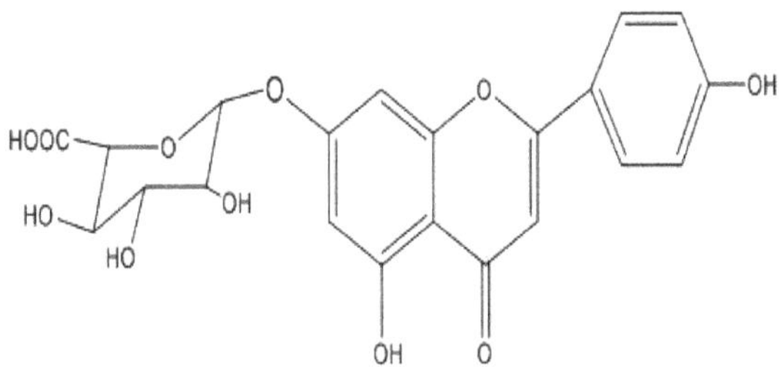

Figure1. Compounds 1 isolated from *H. officinalis* aerial parts n-butanol extract.

We could not find an explanation for the exceptionally large proportion of Myrtenylacetatein the *H. officinalis* from north of Iran. A review of the published literature indicates that the oil composition of *H. officinalis* may vary considerably within a single species from one growth season to another affected by climatic parameters and agrotechnical factors, such as fertilization, water supply, and harvesting, especially the phase of plant development at the time of harvest.[26]

Phenolic content of NBE extract was 246 mgGAE g^{-1}, while in ETE 51 mg GAEg^{-1}. This fact is in correlation with polarity of the solvents used for extraction and solubility of phenolic compounds in them.
The antioxidant activities of apigenin 7-glucuronide, ETE and NBE were examined by comparing them with the known antioxidant, quercetin, by employing the DPPH radical scavenging. The IC_{50} values for apigenin 7-glucuronide, ETE, NBE and quercetin were found to be 116×10^{-3}, 103×10^{-3}, 25×10^{-3} and 5.22×10^{-5} mg mL^{-1}. Our results showed a direct linear correlation between total phenolic content and antioxidant activities. This correlation suggests that the phenolic compounds contribute directly to the antioxidative action, but probably other compounds, to some extent, are also responsible for these activities.
Therefore, H. officinalis L. as a culinary herb and medicinal plant may be considered as natural food ingredients to replace synthetic antioxidants.

Table 2. Composition of *Hyssopus officinalis L.* essential oil.

Peak No.	Components	Composition (%)
1	1,8- Cineole	0.31
2	L- linalool	0.56
3	Cis- sabinol	1.75
4	Camphor	6.76
5	Terpineol-4	0.28
6	Myrtenal	0.43
7	Bornyl acetate	1.42
8	Myrtenyl acetate	74.08
9	α- Cubebene	0.53
10	β- Bourbonene	1.47
11	β-Caryophyllene	2.10
12	α- Caryophyllene	0.64
13	Germacrene	3.36
14	Cubenol	0.33
15	δ- Cadinene	0.47
16	Nerodiol Z and E	0.75
17	Spathulenol	2.14
18	Caryophyllene Oxide	2.13
19	Elemol	0.46
	Total	**99.97**

Acknowledgement
Authors are thankful to the staff of the Medicinal plants laboratory at the Drug Applied Research Center for their help in conducting GC-MS analysis.

Conflict of interest
The authors report no conflicts of interest in this work.

References

1. Do QT, Bernard P. Pharmacognosy and reverse pharmacognosy: a new concept for accelerating natural drug discovery. *IDrugs* 2004; 7: 1017-1027.
2. Vuorelaa P, Leinonenb M, Saikkuc P, Tammelaa P, Rauhad JP, Wennberge T, Vuorela H. Natural products in the process of finding new drug candidates. *Curr Med Chem* 2004; 11: 1375-1389.
3. Kazazi H, Rezaei K, Ghotb-sharif SJ, Emam-Djomeh Z, Yamini Y. Supercriticial fluid extraction of flavors and fragrances from Hyssopus officinalis L. cultivated in Iran. *Food Chemistry* 2007; 105: 805-811.
4. Khazaie HR, Nadjafi F, Bannayan M. Effect of irrigation frequency and planting density on herbage biomass and oil production of thyme (Thymus vulgaris) and hyssop (Hyssopus officinalis). *Industrial Crops and Products* 2008; 27:315-321.
5. Tognolini M, Barocelli E, Ballabeni V, Bruni R, Bianchi A, Chiavarini M, Impicciatore M. Comparative screening of plant essential oils: phenylpropanoid moiety as basic core for antiplatelet activity. *Life Sci* 2006; 78: 1419-1432.
6. De Almeida LF, Frei F, Mancini E, De Martino L, De Feo V. Phytotoxic activities of Mediterranean essential oils. *Molecules* 2010; 15: 4309-4323.
7. Ghfir B, Fonvieille JL, Koulali Y, Ecalle R, Dargent R. Effect of essential oil of Hyssopus officinalis on the lipid composition of Aspergillus fumigatus. *Mycopathologia* 1994; 126: 163-167.
8. Babovic N, Djilas S, Jadranin M, Vajs V, Ivanovic J, Petrovic S, Zizovic I. Supercritical carbon dioxide extraction of antioxidant fractions from selected Lamiaceae herbs and their antioxidant capacity. *Innovative Food Science & Emerging Technologies* 2010; 11: 98-107.
9. Ghfir B, Fonvieille JL, Dargent R. Influence of essential oil of Hyssopus officinalis on the chemical composition of the walls of Aspergillus fumigatus (Fresenius). *Mycopathologia* 1997; 138: 7-12.
10. Miyazaki H, Matsuura H, Yanagiya C, Mizutani J, Tsuji M, Ishihara C. Inhibitory effects of hyssop (Hyssopus officinalis) extracts on intestinal alpha-glucosidase activity and postprandial hyperglycemia. *J Nutr Sci Vitaminol (Tokyo)* 2003;49: 346-349.
11. Langa E, Cacho J, Palavra AMF, Burillo J, Mainar AM, Urieta JS. The evolution of hyssop oil composition in the supercritical extraction curve:Modelling of the oil extraction process. *The Journal of Supercritical Fluids* 2009; 49: 37-44.
12. Varga E, Hajdu Z, Veres K, Mathe I, Nemeth E, Pluhar Z, Bernath J. Investigation of variation of the production of biological and chemical compounds of Hyssopus officinalis L. *Acta Pharm Hung* 1998; 68: 183-188.
13. Wang N, Yang XW. Two new flavonoid glycosides from the whole herbs of Hyssopus officinalis. *J Asian Nat Prod Res* 2010; 12: 1044-1050.

14. Marin FR, Ortuno A, Benavente-Garcia O, Del Rio JA. Distribution of flavone glycoside diosmin in Hyssopus officinalis plants: changes during growth. *Planta Med* 1998; 64: 181-182.
15. Hilal S, El-Sherei M, El-Alfy T. Study of the flavonoid content of Hyssopus officinalis L. *Egyptian Journal of Pharmaceutical Sciences* 1979; 20: 271-278.
16. Miliauskas G, Venskutonis PR, Van Beek TA. Screening of radical scavenging activity of some medicinal and aromatic plant extracts. *Food Chemistry* 2004; 85: 231-237.
17. Modaressi M, Delazar A, Nazemiyeh H, Fathi-Azad F, Smith E, Rahman MM, Gibbons S, Nahar L, Sarker SD. Antibacterial iridoid glucosides from Eremostachys laciniata. *Phytother Res* 2009; 23: 99-103.
18. Fathiazad F, Khosropanah MK, Movafeghi A. Cycloartane-type glycosides from the roots of Astragalus caspicus Bieb. *Nat Prod Res* 2010; 24: 1069-1078.
19. Movafeghi A, Abedini M, Fathiazad F, Aliasgharpour M, Omidi Y. Floral nectar composition of Peganum harmala L. *Nat Prod Res* 2009; 23: 301-308.
20. Adams R. Identification of Essential Oils Components by GasChromatography Quadrupole Mass Spectroscopy. USA: Allured Publishing Corporation; 2001.
21. Sengul M, Yildiz H, Gungor N, Cetin B, Eser Z, Ercisli S. Total phenolic content, antioxidant and antimicrobial activities of some medicinal plants. *Pak J Pharm Sci* 2009; 22: 102-106.
22. Nahar L, Russell WR, Middleton M, Shoeb M, Sarker SD. Antioxidant phenylacetic acid derivatives from the seeds of Ilex aquifolium. *Acta Pharm* 2005; 55: 187-193.
23. Agrawal PK. Carbon-13 NMR of Flavonoids. The Netherlands: Elsevier Science Publishers; 1989.
24. Harborne JB. The Flavonoids: Advances in research since 1986. London: Chapman & Hall; 1994.
25. Mabry T J, Markham KR, Thomas MB. The Systematic Identification of Flavonoids. New York: Springer; 1970.
26. Kerrola K, Galambosi B, Kallio H. Volatile Components and Odor Intensity of Four Phenotypes of Hyssop (Hyssopus officinalis L.). *J Agric Food Chem* 1994; 42: 776-781.

12

Antiproliferative effect of *gynura procumbens (lour.) Merr.* Leaves etanolic extract on 7,12-dimethylbenz(*a*)antracene induced male rat liver

Fithriyatun Nisa, Adam Hermawan, Retno Murwanti, Edy Meiyanto*

Cancer chemoprevention research center, Faculty of pharmacy, universitas gadjah mada, Sekip Utara II, Yogyakarta 55281, Indonesia.

ARTICLE INFO

Keywords:
Liver cancer
Proliferation
Gynura procumbens
DMBA
AgNOR

ABSTRACT

Purpose: The leaves of *Gynura procumbens* (Lour.) Merr. has been traditionally used as anticancer. Ethanolic extract of *G. procumbens* leaves (EGP) showed cytotoxic activity and anticancer activity in animal cancer model. This study was conducted to observe antiproliferative effect using male rat's liver cells induced by 7,12-dimethylbenz(*a*)antracene (DMBA). ***Methods:*** Forty days old Sprague Dawley male rats were divided into 4 groups, (1) 0.5 % CMC Na, (2) 20 mg/kg BW DMBA p.o ten times in three weeks, (3) DMBA+300 mg/kg BW of EGP, and (4) DMBA+750 mg/kg BW of EGP. The extract was dissolved into 0.5 % CMC-and administered daily per oral one week before, during and terminated 1 week after the DMBA induction. After sixthteen week experiment, rat livers were sectioned and stained with Haematoxyllene and Eosin (H&E) and AgNOR. ***Results:*** Histopatology profile showed no primary liver tumor on DMBA group. mAgNOR value of DMBA+300 mg/kg BW EGP showed significant antiproliferative effect compared to DMBA group. ***Conclusion:*** Ethanolic extract of *G. procumbens* leaves showed antiproliferative activity on male rats liver induced by DMBA.

Introduction

Liver cancer is the world's fifth largest in man and the seventh largest in women of cancer deaths.[1] The number of deaths in the world caused by liver cancer showed more than one million deaths per year. Chemotherapy, surgery, hormonal therapy and radiotherapy has been developed, but remain several problems such as toxic effect on normal cells and drug resistance problem.[2] Discoveries and research have been developed to overcome those problem, including using natural products as an alternative for the prevention and treatment of cancers.[3]

One of the medicinal plants used traditionally as a cure for cancer is *Gynura procumbens* (Lour.) Merr. Previously, our research group named Cancer Chemoprevention Research Center (CCRC) Faculty of Pharmacy, Universitas Gadjah Mada, Yogyakarta, has explored several anticancer activity of *G. procumbens* leaves (EGP). Ethanolic extract of *G. procumbens* (EGP) showed inhibitory effect on carcinogenicity of mice lung tumor induced by benzo(a)pyrene (BAP) and also showed antimutagenic activity on *Salmonella typhimurium*.[4] The fraction XIX-XX of EGP has a cytotoxic activity on HeLa cervical cancer cells (IC_{50} 119 μg/ml), inhibited HeLa cell proliferation and induced apopotosis.[5] EGP is also reported to have antiangiogenic effects,[6] therefore the plant is potential as antimetastasis and anti-invasion. The Ethyl acetate fraction of *G. procumbens* leaves ethanolic extract increased the effectiveness of doxorubicin on MCF-7 and T47D breast cancer cells.[7] In vivo study of EGP on female rats induced by DMBA has been conducted. EGP performs chemopreventive effect to suppress breast cancer initiation,[8] and performs supression of breast cancer development on early state of female rats induced by DMBA.[9]

The aim of the present investigation was to examine the effect of EGP administration on carcinogenesis of DMBA on male rats liver. We would like to explore the effect of EGP on proliferation of male rats liver induced by DMBA. The results of this study is expected to be the scientific evidence of *G. procumbens* leaves as a chemopreventive agent and the development of subsequent research in cancer prevention.

***Corresponding author:** Prof. Dr. Edy Meiyanto, M.Si., Cancer chemoprevention research center, Faculty of pharmacy, universitas gadjah mada, Sekip Utara II, Yogyakarta 55281, Indonesia. Email : meiyan_e@ugm.ac.id

Materials and methods

Materials

G. procumbens leaves were harvested from Ngaglik, Sleman, Yogyakarta and determined in Department of Pharmaceutical Biology, Faculty of Pharmacy UGM. Extract was prepared by the soxhlet extraction procedure using 96% ethanol (Asia Lab, Yogyakarta), and concentrated using rotary evaporator. DMBA (7.12-dimetilbenz [a] anthracene) was obtained from Sigma (Saint Louis, MO). Sodium Carboxymethyl Cellulose (CMC-Na) (E. Merck) was used as suspending agent of the extract.

Animals

Sprague Dawley ale rats (*Rattus norvegicus*) (40 days old) weighed from 60 to 80 g were obtained from the Laboratory of Pharmacology and Toxicology, Department of Pharmacology and Clinical Pharmacy, Faculty of Pharmacy, Universitas Gadjah Mada, Yogyakarta, Indonesia. Animals were conditioned for one week before use, and were given standard pellet diet and water *ad libitum*, and kept on a 12:12 h light/dark cycle.

Forty rats were devided into four groups, 10 rats per group (Figure 1). In the beginning of 40 days age, solvent control (group 1) was administered with 0.5% CMC-Na, groups of animal (group 2, 3, and 4) intended for carcinogen were treated per oral with single dose of DMBA (Sigma) (20mg/kgBW), third a week for 3 weeks. DMBA was dissolved in CMC-Na and EGP was dissolved in 0.5% CMC-Na as vehicle. Group 3 and group 4 were administered per oral once a day by 300 mg/kgbw and 750 mg/kgbw, respectively for 5 weeks, started 1 week before DMBA initiation until 1 week after DMBA administration. Body weight were recorded weekly throughout the study. The animal handling protocols of this study were in accordance with the guidelines of the animal care of the Department of Pharmacology and Clinical Pharmacy, Faculty of Pharmacy, Gadjah Mada University, Indonesia, and approved by the committee for animal research.

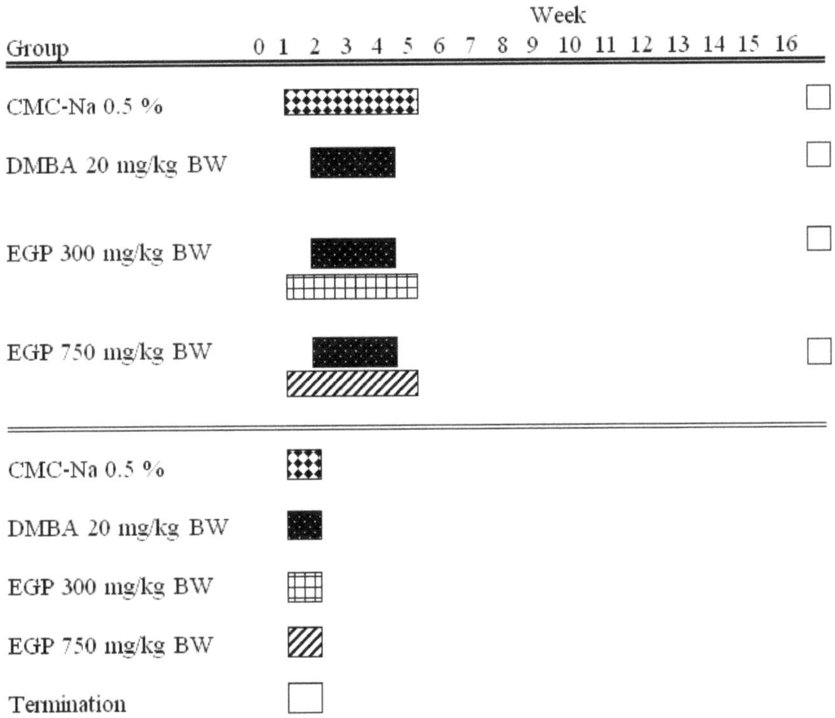

Figure 1. Experimental time line

H&E staining

At the end of the experiment (16 week) all rats were sacrificed by decapitation as scheduled. At autopsy, liver organ were removed and fixed in 10% buffered formalin. After 12-24 h of fixation, 3-5 μm tissue slices were embedded in paraffin, and stained with hematoxylin and eosin for microscopy.

AgNOR staining

AgNOR staining was performed according to the modified method.[10,11] The staining solution was prepared by mixing one part of 2% gelatin in 1% formic acid with two parts of 50% aqueous silver nitrate. All sections were cut to 3 μm in thickness from routinely processed paraffin blocks. Sections were immersed in sodium citrate buffered (pH 6.0) and incubated 20 min in autoclave (120°C,1.1-1.2 Bar). Sections then were covered with the AgNOR staining solution at room temperature in the dark for 15-20 min. The specimens were then washed with 5% sodium thiosulfate and distilled deionized water, dehydrated through graded ethanol to xylene, and mounted in synthetic medium.

AgNORs, which are appeared as dots both outside and within the nucleoli, were counted according to the description of previous report.[12] A minimum one hundred nuclei per specimen were observed randomly in three different views. Mean AgNOR (mAgNOR) was used as a parameter to evaluate antiproliferative activity. mAgNOR is a mean of black dots in a cell, computed from total amount of blackdots (min 100 cells) divided with amount of cells (min 100 cells). All specimens were observed on a binocular microscope (Olympus® DP12 *microscope digital camera system*, NY) with an immersion oil lens at magnification of x1000.

Statistical analyses

Statistically significant difference of body weight by ANOVA continued with LSD, while antiproliferative activity were evaluated by *Kruskal Wallis* continued with *Mann-Whitney*. Significance was set at $p < 0.05$ for all tests.

Results

Effect of EGP on body weight, survival rate and liver morphology of male rat

There was no direct evidence of toxicity due to EGP treatment. Body weight changes of the animal treated with CMC-Na, DMBA and DMBA+EGP were compared (Figure 2). In the beginning of the study and in the sixth week, the body weight changes of CMC-Na group was different from the other groups ($p<0.05$). Final body weight changes showed that DMBA was no significant different from other groups ($p<0.05$) (Table 1 and Figure 2). In general, treatment of EGP in low dose induced fluctuative body weight changes than EGP in high dose. The phenomenon is similar to DMBA control group. The survival curves for the DMBA and DMBA+EGP were practically identical before the 4th week of the experiment, then the survival curve of the DMBA group become higher compared to the EGP treatment group (Figure 3). The higher dose of EGP, the lower the lifespan of the rats. There were no macroscopic differences in morphology of liver organ (Figure 4).

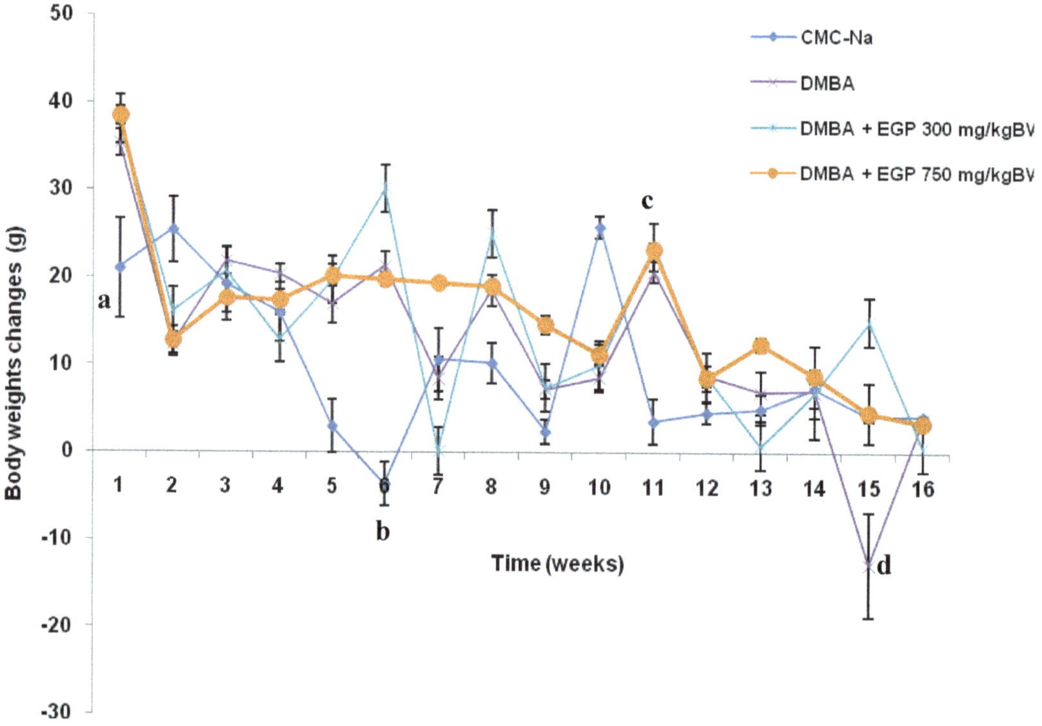

Figure 2. Body weight changes for animals. a=CMC-Na group significant different from DMBA, DMBA+EGP 300 mg/kgBW, and DMBA+EGP 750 mg/kgBW ($p<0.05$) in the first week, b= CMC-Na group significant different from DMBA+EGP 300 mg/kgBW ($p<0.05$) in the sixth week, c=CMC-Na group significant different from DMBA, DMBA+EGP 300 mg/kgBW, and DMBA+EGP 750 mg/kgBW ($p<0.05$) in the tenth week, d= CMC-Na group significant different from DMBA ($p<0.05$) in the fiftheen week.

Histopathological studies of liver

Histopathology profile of liver of DMBA and DMBA+EGP treated rats is depicted in figure 5. In general, hematoxylin and eosin staining showed no differences in morphology between DMBA and DMBA+EGP. There were no primary liver cancer i all of the rats. There was only one rat in DMBA group that showed lymphoblastic cells in the liver or lymphosarcoma (Figure 6).

Antiproliferative activity of EGP on male rat liver

AgNOR staining on rat liver (Figure 7) showed that DMBA group has higher blackdots than the other groups. mAgNOR score (Table 1) of CMC-Na and

DMBA are 1.49 ± 0.04 and 2.25 ± 0.170 respectively. Treatment of EGP 300 mg/kgbw exhibited significant antiproliferative activity of DMBA (Table 1) with mAgNOR score 1.72 ± 0.04 ($p<0.05$), while treatment EGP 750 mg/kgbw showed no significancy to DMBA group. In general, treatment of EGP inhibit proliferation on rat liver induced by DMBA. The higher dose of EGP, the lower proliferative activity of the extract.

Discussion

This study explored the effect of *G. procumbens* leaves ethanolic extract on DMBA induced male rats liver. In this study, EGP was given a week before, during and after induction of DMBA. EGP treatment was intended to prevent metabolic activation of DMBA and also prevent initiatition and progression of liver cancer.

Our present study showed that DMBA induced high proliferation compared to EGP treatment group. Treatment of EGP 300 mg/kgbw is significantly decreased proliferation of liver cells induced by DMBA. The results in similar to previous study [13] that reported treatment of EGP 300 mg/kgbw significantly ($p<0.05$) inhibited proliferation of mammary glands induced by DMBA. Antiproliferative activity of EGP is mediated by metabolic enzyme, CYP and GST.

Table 1. Effect of EGP on proliferation of DMBA-induced liver male rats

Treatment Group	Final Body Weight Changes (g)[1]	mAgNOR[2]
0.5 % CMC-Na	4.20 ± 2.77	1.49 ± 0.04
DMBA	10.00 ± 13.99	2.25 ± 0.17
DMBA + 300 mg/kg BW EGP	0.57 ± 5.79	1.72 ± 0.04*
DMBA + 750 mg/kg BW EGP	3.40 ± 2.96	1.95 ± 0.14

[1] Values represent means ± SD. [2] mAgNOR = mean AgNOR, * are statistically significant different from DMBA groups ($p< 0.05$) by *Kruskal Wallis* continued with *Mann-Whitney*

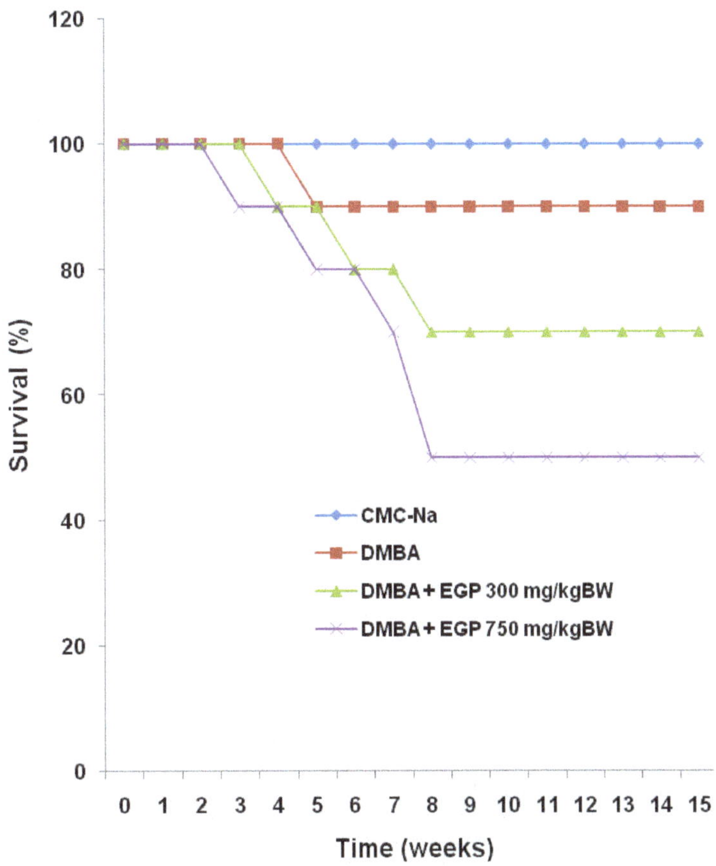

Figure 3. Survival curve of animals. The *y*-axis represents the number of rats (%) and the *x*-axis the time from the start of the experiment (week).

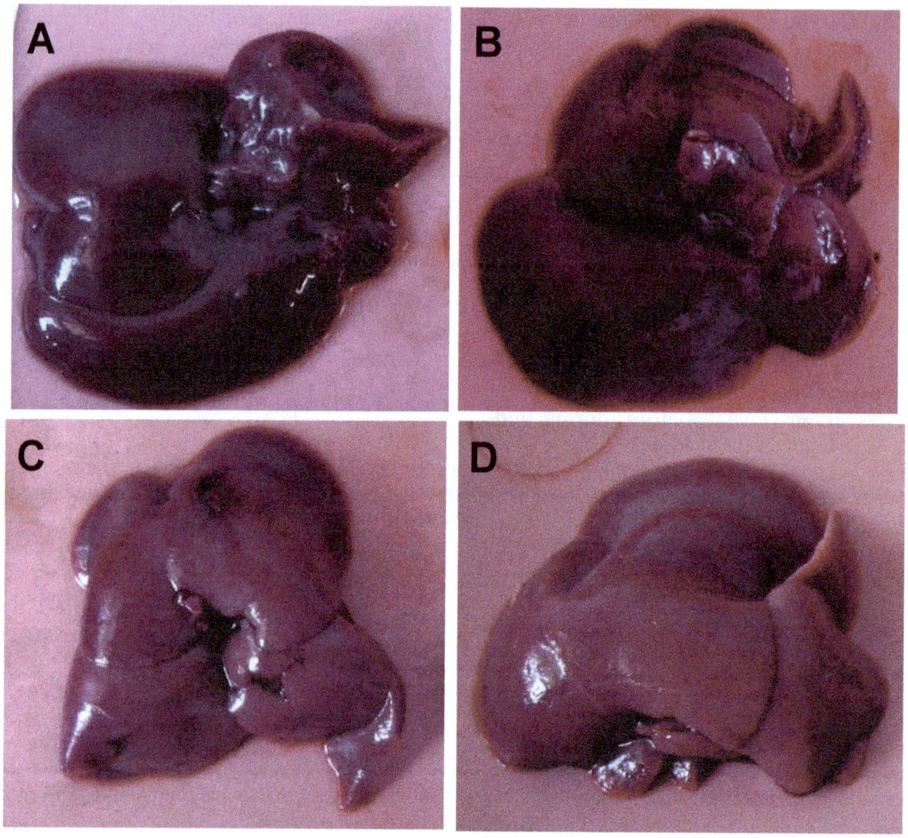

Figure 4. Morphology of liver treated with EGP in 7,12-dimethylbenz[*a*]nthracene-induced male rats liver. Rats were divided into 4 groups, (A) 0.5 % CMC-Na, (B) DMBA control group (20 mg/kgbW in CMC-Na), (C) DMBA+ 300 mg/kgBW EGP; (D) DMBA+750 mg/kgbw EGP. At autopsy, liver organ were removed and fixed in 10% buffered formalin.

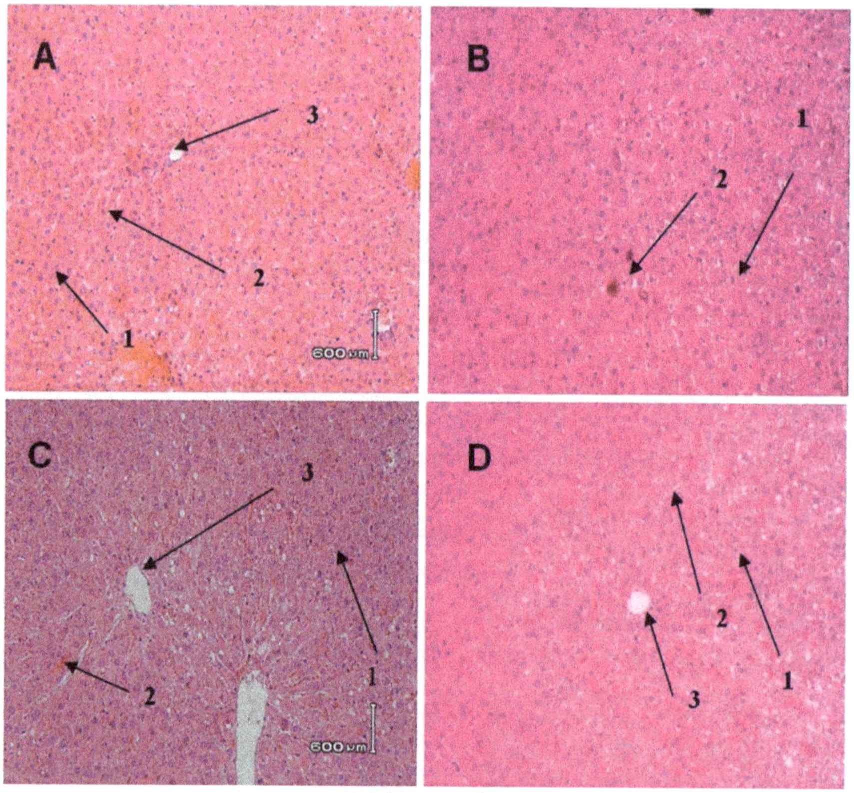

Figure 5. Histological evaluation in liver tissues of control and experimental group. Rats were divided into 4 groups, (A) 0.5 % CMC-Na, (B) DMBA control group (20 mg/kgbW in CMC-Na), (C) DMBA+ 300 mg/kgBW EGP; (D) DMBA+750 mg/kgbw EGP. At autopsy, liver organ were removed and fixed in 10% buffered formalin. 3-5 µm tissue slices were embedded in paraffin, and stained with hematoxylin and eosin (a1=hepatocyte, 2=sinusoid,3=central venous). Magnification x 400.

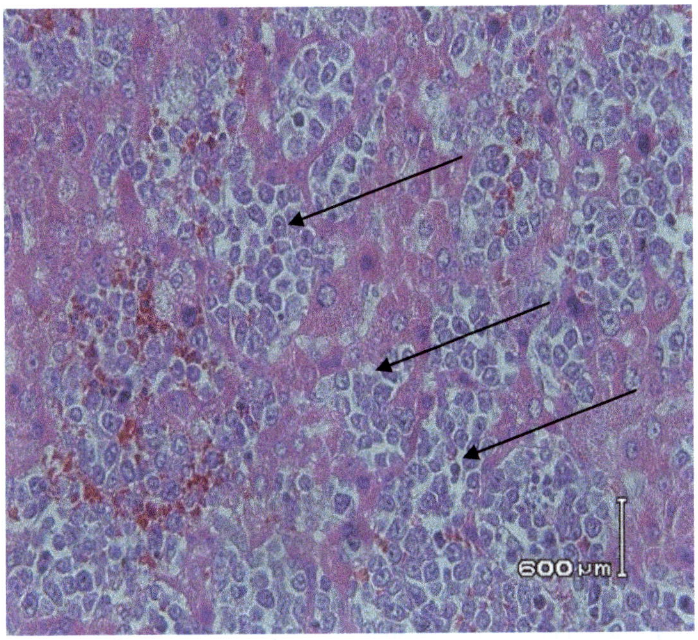

Figure 6. Hematoxylin and eosin stained of lymphoblastic cells in liver tissues of DMBA control group (20 mg/kgbW in CMC-Na). At autopsy, liver organ were removed and fixed in 10% buffered formalin. 3-5 µm tissue slices were embedded in paraffin, and stained with hematoxylin and eosin. Lymphoblastic cells are pointed by black arrow. Magnification x 400.

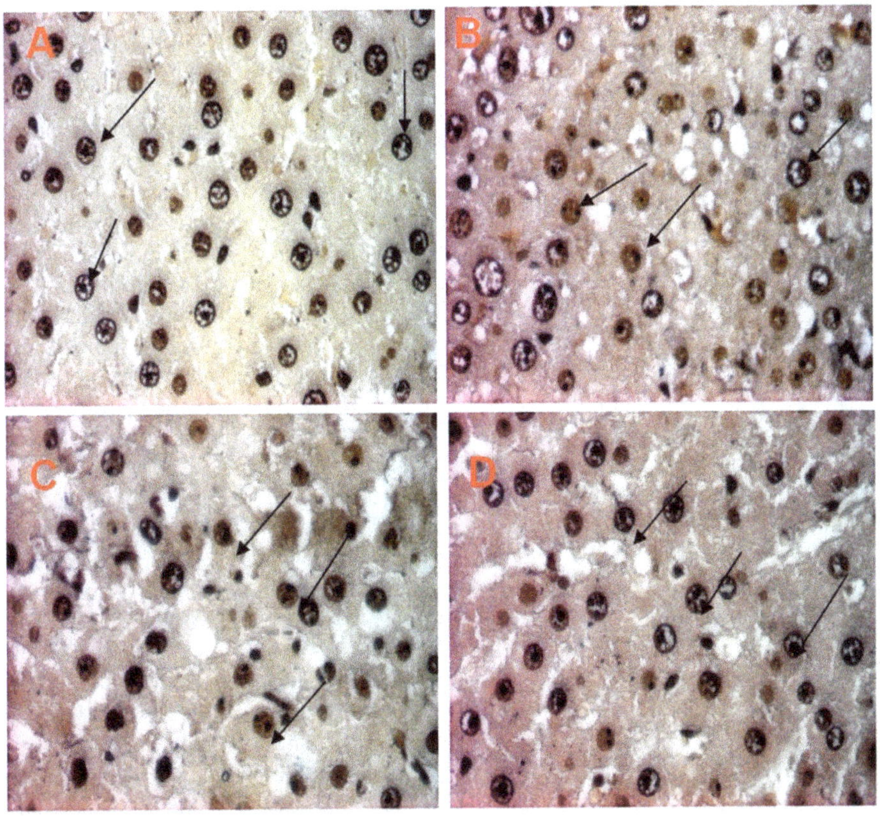

Figure 7. $AgNO_3$ stained liver tissues of control and experimental group. Rats were divided into 4 groups, (A) 0.5 % CMC-Na, (B) DMBA control group (20 mg/kgbW in CMC-Na), (C) DMBA+ 300 mg/kgBW EGP; (D) DMBA+750 mg/kgbw EGP. At autopsy, liver organ were removed and fixed in 10% buffered formalin. 3-5 µm tissue slices were embedded in paraffin, and stained with $AgNO_3$. Argyrophilic nucleolar organiser regions (AgNORs) are visible as dark dots within the plasma cell nuclei (pointed by black arrow). Magnification x1000.

DMBA needs to be metabolized to become a reactive metabolite. DMBA is a substrate of the enzyme cytochrome P450 (CYP), CYP1A1 and CYP1B1.[14] In the phase I metabolism, DMBA is changed to 8.9-; 5.6-; 3,4-epoxide DMBA by CYP1A1 [15] and 3,4-epoxide DMBA by CYP1B1.[15,16] DMBA 3,4-epoxide compounds can undergo several reaction such as hydration and oxidation to form ultimate carcinogens that are highly mutagenic.[17] The epoxide metabolite also can interact with glutathione S-transferase (GST) to generate glutathione conjugates that are readily metabolized to the mercapturic acid and will be eliminated from the body .[18]

Expression of CYP and GST are inducible. CYP expression is regulated by transcription factor named Aryl hydrocarbon Receptor (AhR).[19] Some compound are CYP inducer.[19] DMBA is an autoinducer of CYP 1A1 expression.[20]Induction of CYP 1A1 leads to increasing of DMBA reactive metabolite. Expression of GST is also regulated by transcription factor such as Antioxidant-Responsive Element (ARE), Xenobiotik-Responsive Element (XRE), GST-P Enhancer 1 (GPE) or glucocorticoid-Rensonsive Element (GRE).[21] Induction of GST expression is important to eliminate DMBA reactive metabolite from the body.

A previous study [20] reported that treatment of DMBA induced high CYP1A1 expression, but low expression of GSTμ on female rat liver. Treatment of EGP 300 mg/kgbw significantly inhibit CYP1A1 and induced expression of GSTμ on female rat liver induced by DMBA. We proposed that the mechanism of EGP antiproliferative activity on male rat liver is via inhibition of CYP1A1 and induction of GST, but the mechanism nedds to be explored further. Our present study showed that the higher concentration of EGP, the lower proliferative activity on rat liver induced by DMBA. This phenomena is similar to the previous study on female rats.[8,20,22] The phenomenon is probably due to saturation of enzymatic receptor, but the mechanism need to be clarified more details.

In the present study, EGP inhibited proliferation of rat liver induced by DMBA. We conclude that EGP inhibited carcinogenesis of DMBA on male rats liver. Ethanolic extract of *Gynura procumbens* is potential to be developed as anticancer.

Conclusion

Ethanolic extract of *G. procumbens* leaves showed antiproliferative activity on male rats liver induced by DMBA.

Acknowledgements

We would like to Sitarina Widyarini, DVM, PhD. (Faculty of Veterinary Medicine, Universitas Gadjah Mada, Yogyakarta) for helping on analysis of histopathology.

Conflict of interest

Authors declare no conflict of interest.

Abbreviations

Ethanolic extract of *G. procumbens* leaves (EGP)

References

1. Jemal A, Bray F, Center MM, Ferlay J, Ward E, Forman D. Global Cancer Statistics. *CA Cancer J Clin* 2011;61:69-90.
2. Li S, Zhou Y, Wang R, Zhang H, Dong Y, Ip C. Selenium Sensitizes MCF-7 Breast Cancer Cells to Doxorubicin-Induced Apoptosis Through Modulation of Phospho-Akt and Its Downstream Substrates. *Mol Cancer Ther* 2007;6:1031-1038.
3. Walaszek Z, Hanausek M, Slaga TJ. Mechanisms of Chemopreventiion. *Suppl. Am. Coll. Phys* 2004;125, 128-133.
4. Sugiyanto, Sudarto B, Meiyanto E, Nugroho AE, Jenie UA. Anticarcinogenic Activity of Plant Isolate. *Indo J Pharm* 2003;14(4):216-225.
5. Meiyanto E, Septisetyani EP. Antiproliferative Activity and Apoptosis Induction of Phenolic Fraction *Gynura procumbens* (Lour.) Merr. Leaves Ethanolic Extract on HeLa Cells. *Artocarpus* 2005;5(2):74 – 80.
6. Jenie RI, Meiyanto E. Antiangiogenic Effect of Sambung Nyawa (*Gynura procumbens* (Lour.) Merr.) Leaves Ethanolic Extract on Chick Chorio Allantois Membrane. *Indo J Pharm* 2006;17(1): 50-55.
7. Jenie RI, Meiyanto E. Co-chemotherapy of Sambung Nyawa (*Gynura procumbens* (Lour.) Merr.) Leaves Ethanolic Extract and Doxorubicin on Breast Cancer Cells. *Indo J Pharm 2007;*18(2):81– 87.
8. Meiyanto E, Susilowati S, Tasminatun S, Murwanti R, Sugiyanto Dan. Chemopreventive Effect of Ethanolic Extract of *Gynura procumbens* (Lour), Merr on the Carcinogenesis of Rat Breast Cancer Development. *Indo J Pharm* 2007;18(3):154 – 161.
9. Meiyanto E, Tasminatun S, Susilowati S, Murwanti R, Sugiyanto Dan. Suppression of DMBA-induced Carcinogenesis of Breast Cancer in Post Initition Stage by Ethanolic Extract of *Gynura procumbens* (Lour), Merr leaves. *Indo J Pharm* 2007;18(4):169 – 175.
10. Pich A, Margaria E, Chiusa L, Bortolin P, Palestro G. Relationship Between AgNORs, MIB-1 and OncogeneExpression in Male Breast Carcinoma and Papillary Superficial Bladder Neoplasm. *Oncology Reports* 2003;10:1329-1335.
11. Bánkfalvi A, Giuffré G, Őfner D, Diallo R, Poremba C, Buchwalow IB, Barresi V, Bőcker W, Tuccari G. Relationship Between HER2 Status and Proliferation Rate in Breast Cancer Assesed by Immunohistochemistry, Fluorescence in Situ Hybridisation and Standardised AgNOR Analysis. *International Journal of Oncology* 2003; 23:1285-1292.
12. Rizali E, Auerkari EI. Teknik Pewarnaan *Silver* (AgNOR) Sebagai Salah Satu Cara Menentukan Aktivitas Proliferasi Sel Tumor dan Apoptosis. *Jurnal Kedokteran Gigi Indonesia* 2003;10(3):41-45 (In Indonesia).

13. Hamid IS. Proliferation Activity of Gland Mammae After Treated with Gynura procumbens Leaves Extract and DMBA Initiation on Sprague Dawley Rats. *Veterinaria Medika.* 2009;2:1979-1305.
14. Shimada T, Guengerich FP. Inhibition of Human Cytochrome P450 1A1-, 1A2-, and 1B1-Mediated Activation of Procarcinogens to Genotoxic Metabolites by Polycyclic Aromatic Hydrocarbons. *Chem Res Toxicol* 2006, 19:288-294.
15. Weimer TL, Ashok PR, Ulrich H, David AS, Craig S, Michael RM, William B, Jerry H, Bailey G. Influence of ß-Naphthoflavone on 7,12-Dimethylbenz(a)anthracene Metabolism, DNA Adduction, and Tumorigenicity in Rainbow Trout. *Toxicological Sci* 2000;57, 217-228.
16. Heidel SM, Holston K, Jeroen T, Buters M, Gonzales FG, Jefcoate CR, Czupyrynski CJ. Bone Marrow Stromal Cell Cytochrome P4501B1 is Required for Pre-B Cell Apoptosis Induced by 7,12-Dimethylbenz(*a*)antracene. *Molecular Pharmacology* 1999;56(6):1317-1323.
17. Kleiner HE, Vulimiri SV, Uberecken MJRA, DiGiovanni J. Role of Cytochrome P450 1A1 and 1B1 in the Metabolic Activation of 7,12-Dimethylbenz[*a*]anthracene and the Effects of Naturally Occurring Furanocoumarins on Skin Tumor Initiation, *Chem. Res. Toxicol* 2002;15 :226-235.
18. Yanaida Y, Kohno H, Yoshida K, Hirose Y, Yamada Y, Mori H, Tanaka T. Dietary Silymarin Supresses 4-Nitroquinoline 1-Oxide-Induced Tongue Carcinogenesis in Male F344 Rats. *Carcinogenesis* 2002;23(5):787-794.
19. Rodriguez-Antona C, Ingelman-Sundberg M. Cytochrome P450 Pharmacogenetics and Cancer. *Oncogene* 2006;25:1679–1691.
20. Hamid IS, Sugiyanto, Meiyanto E, Widyarini S. CYP1A1 and GSTμ expression of hepatocytes induced by 7,12-dimethylbenz(a)anthracene and the influence of Ethanolic Extract of *Gynura procumbens. Indo J Pharm* 2009;20(4) : 198-206.
21. Hayes JD, Pulford DJ. The Glutathione S-transferase Supergene Family: Regulation of GST and the Contribution of The Isoenzymes to Cancer Chemoprotection and Drug Resistance. *Chem Mol Biol* 1995, *30*:445-600.
22. Hamid IS, Sugiyanto, Meiyanto E, Widyarini S. p53 Expression in Sprague Dawley Rat Mammary After Initiation of 7,12-dimethylbenz[a]anthracene (DMBA) and Give Chemoprevention of *Gynura procumbens. Media Ked Hewan* 2008;24(3): 171-176.

13

On the mechanism of agglomeration in suspension

Maryam Maghsoodi[1*], Katayoun Derakhshandeh[2], Zahra Yari[2]

[1] *Drug applied Research Center and School of Pharmacy, Tabriz University of Medical Sciences, Tabriz, Iran.*

[2] *School of Pharmacy, Kermanshah University of Medical Sciences, Kermanshah, Iran.*

ARTICLE INFO

Keywords:
Agglomeration
Carbamazepine
Binding liquid

ABSTRACT

Purpose**:** Agglomeration in suspension is a size enlargement method that facilitates operation of solid processing and preserves the solubilization properties of fine particles. A small quantity of binder liquid is added into a suspension of microparticles, directly in the stirred vessel where the precipitation or crystallization took place. This study deals with the evaluation of the effect of agitation time before and after addition of binder liquid on agglomerates properties in order to give some insights into the mechanism of the formation of the agglomerates. ***Methods*****:** Carbamazepine is used as a model drug and isopropyl acetate is used as binder liquid. The agglomerates characterization includes the particle size, morphology and density. ***Results*****:** The results showed that, by increasing the agitation time before addition of binder liquid, smaller agglomerates with less density and irregular forms composed of larger crystals were obtained. However, with increasing agitation time after addition of binder liquid the agglomerates size and density increases and morphology improves. Indeed, by continuing agitation along the course of agglomeration the properties of the particles change gradually but substantially. ***Conclusion*****:** With optimized agitation time before and after addition of binder liquid, spherical and dense agglomerates can be obtained.

Introduction

Agglomeration in liquid systems with a wide range of objectives including separation of colloidal particles from a liquid, spherical granulation, removal and recovery of fine solids from liquid wastes, and selective separation of some components in a mixture of particles has gained increasing attention in recent years due to its relative simplicity and ease of operation. [1]
The further finding of spherical agglomeration of crystals during crystallization processes, named spherical crystallization by Kawashima et al. [2], has offered a promising approach to particulate design for engineering pharmaceuticals and chemicals. [3] The possibility of agglomerating the microcrystals directly inside the reactor presents many advantages for the processing of these particles.

Agglomeration is capable of modifying the micromeritic properties of pharmaceutical powders, such as flowability, packability, and solubility. It can also reduce the dust-releasing properties of an intermediate or the final product, and avoid segregation caused by vibration during handling and processing. All of these advantages ensure reliable and efficient powder handling and processing (e.g., mixing, granulation) as well as improvement in the bioavailability of the product. [4]

While a significant number of studies have been conducted on spherical agglomeration, the mechanisms of this technique have not been fully elucidated. As a result, there exist very few general guidelines for the application of this technique. The reasons for the preparation of agglomerates in liquid phase in particular conditions in the literature concerned were often not stated. Therefore it would appear that further application of the technique to other compounds could only be based on experience and /or trial and error.

Therefore, this technique is still not extensively used in industry due to the problems in understanding and controlling the process parameters that allow production of agglomerates with the reproducible desired properties. In particular the aim of the present work is to bring further insight into how the agglomerates are formed and evolve during the process, and into the mechanisms behind the agglomeration in suspension. For this purpose the effect of the agitation time before and after addition of binder liquid on the agglomerates properties was investigated. Carbamazepine was used as model compound in the present work. Carbamazepine normally crystallizes as needles or flake that can be difficult to handle in downstream processing and are unsuitable for direct compression into tablets. Carbamazepine was crystallized from ethanol by drowning out with water and agglomerated using Isopropyl acetate as binder liquid according to our previous study. [5]

***Corresponding author:** Maryam Maghsoodi (PhD), E-mail: maghsoodim@tbzmed.ac.ir

Materials and Methods

Materials

In this work carbamazepine was supplied by Arasto Pharmaceutical Chemical Inc, Iran and solvents (ethanol and isopropyl acetate) were purchased from Merck, Germany.

Agglomeration experiments

The crystallization process used in this study was similar to method which was introduced in previous study as the spherical crystallization technique. [5] A solution of 0.5 g of carbamazepine in 10 ml of ethanol was poured into 84 ml of water at 25°C under stirring with a propeller-type agitator with four blades at 400 rpm in a cylindrical vessel. After different agitation time including 5,10 and 15 min for A_1, A_2 and A_3 samples respectively, 6 ml of isopropyl acetate as a binder liquid was introduced into the crystallization medium in a dropwise manner and agitation continued for 40 min. The agglomerates obtained were filtered, washed with water, and dried in an oven at 80 °C for 12 h.

In series B, the purpose is to be able to track how the properties of the agglomerates gradually change during the corresponding series A experiment. Because of that in series B the conditions correspond to A_1 experiment but agitation continued for different times (5,10, 20 and 40 min for B_1, B_2, B_3 and B_4 samples respectively) after addition of binder liquid.

The analysis of the product includes particle morphology, size and density.

Characterization of the agglomerates

Pictures of at least 60 particles of each powder were taken using a CCD camera (Canon digital, Japan) connected to a light microscope (Leitz, Portugal). Digital images were acquired at 5× magnification. For each particle the heywood diameter and the aspect ratio (AR) were determined by using the scion image software. According to the software specification the aspect ratio as a shape factor was calculated using the following equation

$$AR = dmax/dmin$$

where dmax and dmin were the longest and shortest Feret diameters measured, respectively.

To determine the primary particle size, the agglomerates were disintegrated in an aqueous solution of tween 80 (0.05%) using Ultrasonicator (Model starsonic 18-35, liarre casal flumanese, Italy) for 30s at 100 W before determining the particle size. Then the particle size of the primary crystals, which composed the agglomerates, was measured using a laser diffraction and scattering particle sizer (SALD_2101, shimadzu, Japan).

Apparent particle density

Apparent particle density was determined by the projective image count method as follows. Particles were placed on a glass plate. Heywood diameter and particle number were measured by using the scion image software. Subsequently, the apparent particle density was calculated according to following equation

$$\text{Apparent particle density} = \frac{W}{V} = \frac{W}{\sum(\pi d^3 n/6)}$$

where W = weight of particles, V = volume of particles, d = Heywood diameter, and n = number of particles. [6]

Statistical evaluation of data

Quantitative data were reported as mean ± standard deviation (SD). Statistical analysis was performed using the analysis of variance (ANOVA). Comparison between the two means was determined using the Tukey's test with statistical significance evaluated at $P< 0.05$.

Results

In this study, a three-solvent system was utilized to produce the agglomerates of carbamazepine. The drug was first dissolved in ethanol and the resultant solution was poured into water then isopropyl acetate was added as binder liquid. Before binding liquid injection, the suspension produced by precipitation is totally opaque. Immediately after injection and dispersion of binder liquid, the suspension becomes clearer and particles gather into flocs of all shapes and all sizes which can be measured less than 1 min after injection.

The agglomerates disintegrated easily into primary crystals under ultrasonic agitation of the aqueous suspension of agglomerates. A size analysis was carried out on the constituent crystals of the agglomerates. It can be seen in Table 1 that with increasing agitation time before addition of binder liquid (series A) the obtained agglomerates composed of bigger and more elongated crystals. According to Figure 1 and Table 1 for the bigger primary crystals the obtained agglomerates are smaller, less spherical with rough surface and less density. The morphology of the particles from series B experiments is shown in the Figure 2. This Figure shows that there appears to be a gradual improvement of the shape of the particles as stirring time continues. The particles obtained after 5 min are dominated by irregularly shaped agglomerates, which adhere together as a big clusters and when agitation is continued for up to 20 min the agglomerates were found separately and their surface seems to be much smoother and the overall shape is clearly more regular.

After 40 min agitation the agglomerates starts to look spherical. However, in reality some of the agglomerates are somewhat tabular and not completely spherical. Figure 3 shows the spherical agglomerates prepared after 40min agitation were closely compacted with fine primary crystals, while after 5 min agitation, the agglomerates composed with loosely compacted fine primary crystals were observed. Table 1 also confirmed this fact and shows that in series B with continuing agitation the particle density significantly increases ($p<0.05$).

Table 1. micromeritic properties of the samples

samples	Aspect ratio	Crystal size (μ) (Length)	Median ±σ (μ)	Particle density (g/cm^3)	Yield (%)
A_1	1.23±0.20	6.0±0.8	1237.4+148.5	0.59±0.09	84.0±0.9
A_2	2.01±0.19	8±0.9	1147.5+188.7	0.40±0.08	84.4±0.8
A_3	2.3 8±0.21	15±0.9	1096.5+222.7	0.34±0.08	76.3±0.8
B_1	1.70±0.23	15±0.8	1456±346	0.66±0.07	86.1±0.9
B_2	1.83±0.20	15±0.9	1118±230	0.65±0.06	86.4±0.7
B_3	2.17±0.19	15±0.7	1136±193	0.75±0.09	84.3±0.8
B_4	1.2 3±0.20	15±0.8	1237.4+148.5	0.97±0.06	84.0±0.9

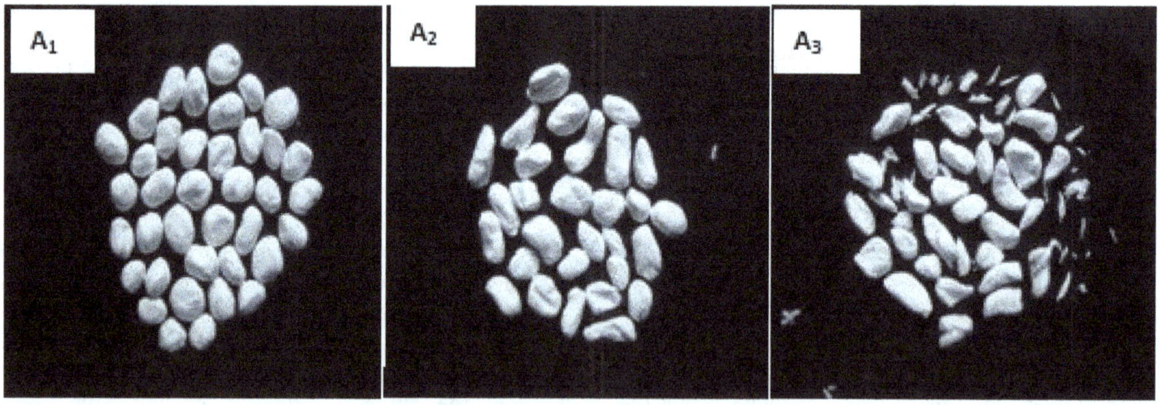

Figure 1. Particle morphology of series A (× 10).

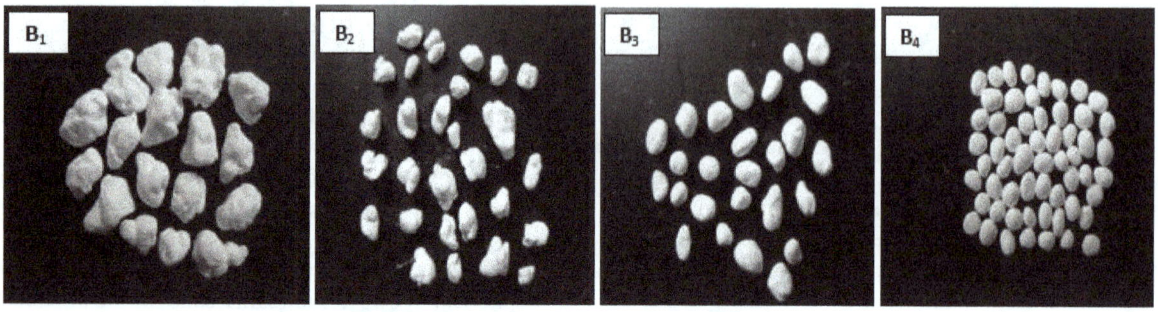

Figure 2. Particle morphology of series B(× 10).

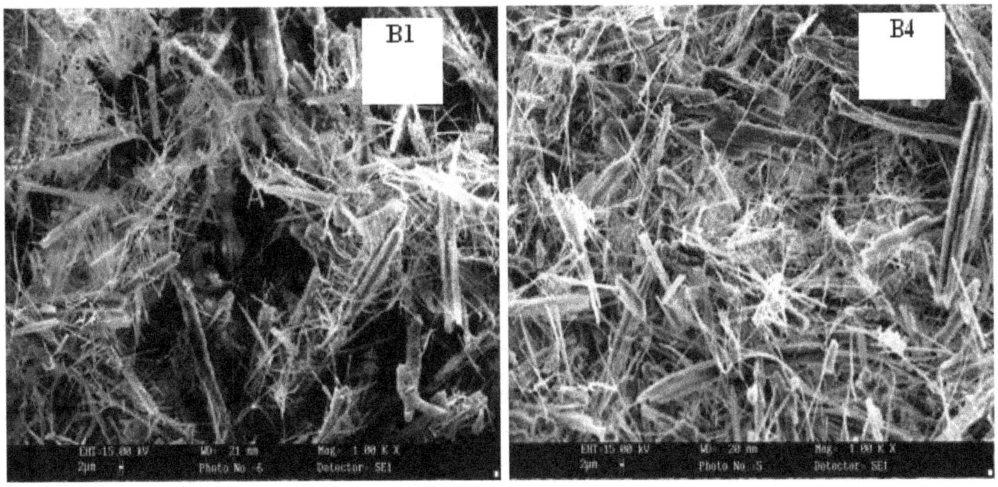

Figure 3. Surface of the particles from series B_1 and B_4.

Discussion

Results of series A showed that agglomeration of large crystals is more difficult especially if they are more elongated, while, smaller crystals give rise to more spherical and larger agglomerates with smoother surface and denser structure. Indeed, the agglomeration process was less efficient for bigger primary crystals and some fines were not incorporated in to the agglomerates (A_3) which consequently results in decreasing agglomeration yield. This fact might be interpreted by considering the other investigation [7] which showed fine crystals required less amount of binder liquid for agglomeration, since the adhesive force of fine crystals with binder liquid was stronger than those coarse crystals as a consequence of higher surface area. Therefore, higher amount of available binder liquid on the outer surface of the agglomerates of fine crystals making the surface more deformable and might promote further agglomeration. Increasing agglomerates size with an increase in the amount of available binder liquid for agglomeration has been shown in the numerous studies. [8-10] On the other hand, smoother surface of the agglomerates composed of finer crystals is expectable since smaller particles will cause smaller surface asperities. Denser structure of the agglomerates obtained at lower agitation time in series A might be attributed to this fact that, the fine and isotropic particles was compacted during agglomeration more closely than that of coarse and needle-like particles. [11] These results can also be interpreted by considering the mechanism of agglomeration.

The process of agglomeration in suspension can be described as a two-step process. [12] The first step is the nucleation period, where the particles come into contact with the liquid binder droplets and form agglomerate nuclei. Several mechanisms of the nucleation period are proposed, which depend on the diameter ratio of the crystals to the binder droplet. [13,14]

When the crystals are bigger than the binder droplet, the nucleation takes place by a distribution mechanism, i.e. the liquid droplets are coating the solid particles. This leads to the formation of agglomerates with an irregular shape and a looser structure. When the crystals are smaller than the binder droplet, nucleation occurs by an immersion mechanism. The particles impact against the surface of the droplet and enter the droplet until the droplet internal volume is saturated with solid particles. This leads to the formation of agglomerates with a narrower particle size distribution and a more spherical shape with a denser structure.

The results of series A can also be described according to above explanation about the nucleation mechanism of agglomeration, because finer crystals offer a greater potential for nucleation by immersion than larger ones, and that immersion leads to the formation of agglomerates with a narrower particle size distribution, a more spherical shape and with a denser structure than distribution.

In other part of this study, in order to bring insight into the mechanism of the agglomeration, agglomerate size, shape and density evaluation was carried out after binder liquid injection and continuing stirring for different time (5,10, 20 and 40 min) which allowed to follow the change in the agglomerate properties during the agglomeration process (series B). Firstly it is notable that, by measuring primary crystal size of agglomerates produced in series B, it was found that the particle size of the primary crystals during agglomeration remained unchanged ($p>0.05$), which was in agreement with some other investigations. [3, 15-17] Results revealed a marked change from irregularly shaped agglomerates to more regular with smoother surface agglomerates throughout agitation in series B. According to Table 1, aspect ratio of these samples decreases ($p<0.05$) with agitation time which confirmed the rounding effect of further agitation. Also, by continuing agitation in series B, particle density markedly increases ($p<0.05$). Results of series B can be interpreted by considering the second step of the agglomeration process. [12] The second step of agglomeration is the growth and consolidation period by a mechanism of collision and coalescence of the agglomerates in the stirred reactor. According to Figure 2 in initial stage of the agglomeration the particles were adhered together, which indicate the coalescence of the particles. In this stage the coalescence is easier because the agglomerates can be deformed and compacted and the elementary particles can move to be piled up in a more compact way.

By continuing agitation the agglomerates become more and more compact (increasing particle density) and regular (decreasing AR), thanks to the numerous shocks between agglomerates (which are also responsible for the agglomerates enlargement when they induce an efficient coalescence) or between the agglomerates and different parts of the vessel.

This growth period ends when the agglomerates become too compact to be deformed and arranged during the collision.

Conclusion

Results showed that the influence of agitation is of great importance for the creation of the regular shape of the particles by agglomeration in suspension method. With increasing agitation time before addition of binder liquid obtained agglomerates composed of bigger and more elongated crystals. Needle-like particles are more difficult to pack than isotropic particles. Moreover, the particle surface area available is decreased when the particle size is increased for an equivalent solid concentration. These two phenomena have an effect on the deformability of the agglomerates and reduce the agglomeration efficiency when bigger crystals are used. Therefore, in order to control the size of the agglomerates produced, it seems important to control the size of the crystals to be agglomerated. In second part of this study by varying the stirring time after addition of binder liquid, it was shown that the spherical shape of the agglomerates does not appear immediately but develops gradually. The spherical shape is due to the mechanical forces of the agitation exerted on the particles over a long period of time, similar to the consolidation in granulation process.

Acknowledgments

The financial support from Kermanshah University of Medical Sciences is greatly acknowledged.

Conflict of interest

The authors report no conflicts of interest. The authors alone are responsible for the content and writing of the paper.

References

1. Capes C, Fouda A. Agglomeration in liquid systems. in: Fayed M.E, Otten(Eds.) L.P.Handbook of Powder Science and Technology. New York; Van Nostrand Reinhold Com, 1984; pp: 331–344.
2. Kawashima Y, Okumura M, Takenaka H. Spherical crystallization: direct spherical agglomeration of salicylic acid crystals during crystallization. *Science* 1982; 216: 1127–1128.
3. Kawashima Y. New process-application of spherical crystallization to particulate design of pharmaceuticals for direct tabletting and coating. and new drug delivery systems. in: Chulia D, Deleuil M, Pourcelot (Eds.) Y.Powder Technology and Pharmaceutical Processes. New York: Elsevier, 1994; pp: 493–512.
4. Kawashima Y. Spherical crystallization: direct spherical agglomeration of salicylic acid crystals by the wet spherical agglomeration technique. *Science* 1982; 219:1127–1128.
5. Nokhodchi A, Maghsoodi M, Hassan-Zadeh D, Barzegar-Jalali M. Preparation of agglomerated crystals for improving flowability and compactibility of poorly flowable and compactible drugs and excipients. *Powder Technology* 2007;175: 73–81.
6. Sato Y, Kawashima Y, Takeuchi H, Yamamoto H. In vitro evaluation of floating and drug releasing behaviors of hollow microspheres (microballoons) prepared by the emulsion solvent diffusion method. *European Journal of Pharmaceutics and Biopharmaceutics* 2004; 57: 235–243.
7. Kawashima Y, OkumuraM, Takenaka H. The effects of temperature on the spherical crystallization of salicylic acid. *Powder technolog* 1984; 39: 41-47.
8. Bos AS. Agglomeration in suspension. PhD thesis. University of Technologie of Delft. The Netherland,1983.
9. Blandin AF, Mangin D, Rivoire A, Klein JP, Bossoutrot JM. Agglomeration in suspension of salicylic acid fine particles: influence of some process parameters on kinetics and agglomerate final size. *Powder Technol* 2003; 130: 316–323.
10. Maghsoodi M, Barghi L. Design of Agglomerated Crystals of Ibuprofen During Crystallization: Influence of Surfactant. Iran J Basic Med Sci 2011;14(1):57-66.
11. Kawashima Y, Okumura M, Takenaka H. The effects of temperature on the spherical crystallization of salicylic acid. *Powder technolog* 1984; 39: 41-47.
12. Blandin AF, Mangin D, Subero-Couroyer C, Rivoire A, Klein JP, Bossoutrot JM. Modelling of agglomeration in suspension: Application to salicylic acid microparticles. *Powder Technol* 2005; 156: 19–33.
13. Amaro-Gonza´lez D, Biscans B. Spherical agglomeration during crystallization of an active pharmaceutical ingredient. *Powder Technol* 2002; 128: 188–194.
14. Abberger T, Seo A, Schæfe T. The effect of droplet size and powder particle size on the mechanisms of nucleation and growth in fluid melt agglomeration. *Int J Pharm* 2002; 249: 185–197.

14

Preparation and In vitro Investigation of Chitosan Compressed Tablets for Colon Targeting

Negar Bashardoust[1,2], **Josephine Leno Jenita**[1], **Parvin Zakeri-Milani**[3,4*]

[1]*Department of Pharmaceutics, Dayananda Sagar College of Pharmacy, Kumaraswamy Layout, Bangalore – 560078, Karnataka, India*

[2]*Student Research Committee, Tabriz University of Medical Sciences, Tabriz, Iran*

[3]*Faculty of Pharmacy, Tabriz University of Medical Sciences, Tabriz, Iran*

[4]*Drug Applied Research Center, Tabriz University of Medical Sciences, Tabriz, Iran*

ARTICLE INFO

Keywords:
Colon targeting
Polysaccharide
Chitosan
Ibuprofen
Compressed coated
Tablet

ABSTRACT

Purpose: The aim of the present study was minimizing the drug release in upper gastro intestinal tract and targeting to colon by using the principles of compression coat. ***Methods:*** Compression coated tablets of Ibuprofen were prepared by direct compression method using chitosan (300, 250, 200 & 175 mg). Tablets were evaluated for their physicochemical properties and in vitro drug release studies. In vitro drug release studies were performed with and without rat caecal contents. ***Results:*** In the rat caecal contents tablets showed enhanced drug release due to degradation of chitosan coat by colonic colonic enzymes. The *in vitro release* studies in pH-6.8 phosphate buffer containing 2% w/v of rat caecal contents showed the cumulative percentage release of Ibuprofen after 26h as 31.94% ±0.59, 67.89% ± 0.45 and 55.87 % ± 0.45 and 82.52 % ± 0.92 respectively. Coat thickness and amount of chitosan controls the release rate. Formulations are best fitted with Korsmeyer-Peppas kinetics and mechanism of drug release was non-Fickian. FTIR studies reveals there is no drug-polysaccharide interaction. F_1 formulation was a promising system for drug targeting to colon. ***Conclusion:*** Based on the obtained results chitosan as a press coat could target ibuprofen to the colon.

Introduction

Among all the routes of drug administration that have been explored for the development of controlled release systems the oral route has by far achieved the most attention and success. This is due, in part to the ease of administration as well as to the fact that gastrointestinal physiology offers more flexibility in dosage form design than most other routes. On the other hand the most direct route for delivery of drugs into the colon is by rectal administration. Since there are problems in both patient acceptability and accessing the proximal colon using rectally administered dosage forms, orally administered colon specific delivery systems have been developed. There are three practical mechanisms by which a delivery system can be targeted into the colon following oral administration[1]: Coating with pH dependent polymers, Time release dosage forms, and Delivery systems based on the metabolic activity of colonic bacteria. Colonic bacteria degraded the prodrugs and polysaccharides enzymatically and then the drug releases into the colon. Previously several polysaccharides have been reported as carriers to colon-specific drug delivery.[2-5]For example amylase, cross linked guar gum, chondrotinsulphate, chitosan for peptides, pectin and its salts. Oral compression coated tablets (CCT) compose of an inner solid core that contains an active pharmaceutical ingredient and any other pharmaceutically acceptable carriers or excipients which is substantially covered with an outer layer that dissolves or disintegrates slowly to produce the pre-determined lag time.[6] The advantage of this manufacturing technique is that it is simple, inexpensive and it is not hazardous to the environment since it doesnot require the use of high amounts of organic solvents. Ibuprofen was used as model drug because it is absorbed at different sites in the human gastrointestinal tract and also well absorbed throughout the colon.[1] It is a non-steroidal anti-inflammatory agent, which is widely used in treatment of mild to moderated

***Corresponding author:** Parvin Zakeri-Milani (PhD), E-mail: pzakeri@tbzmed.ac.ir

pain and fever. This study selected ibuprofen as a drug for formulating colonic drug delivery system to avoid gastrointestinal discomfort associated with ibuprofen therapy.In the present study, chitosan in the form of compression coat was evaluated as a suitable carrier for colonic targeting of ibuprofen. Chitosan is a non-acetylated or partially acetylated chitin derivative which is tough, bio-degradable and non-toxic.[7] In vitro drug release studies were carried out on ibuprofen core tablets compression coated with different amounts of chitosan in simulated gastro intestinal fluids in the presence and absence of rat caecal contents.

Material and methods

Materials

Ibupeofen was obtained from Strides Acro Labs, Bangalore, India. Chitosan was purchased from Alembic Pharma, Baroda, India. Microcrystalline cellulose, Sodium starch glycholate, Potassium dihydrogen Phosphate and Magnesium stearate were obtained from Spectrochem Pvt. Ltd. Mumbai. Sodium hydroxide pellets were received from Sd fine chem. Ltd., Mumbai, India. Talk was obtained from Leo chem. Bangalore, India. Potassium chloride and Potassium bromide (IR grade) were from Thomas Baker , Mumbai, India and Merck specialities Pvt. Ltd., Germany respectively. Hydrochloride (HCl) was provided from Swastik Pharmaceuticals, Mumbai, India. The instruments used were as follows: Dissolution test apparatus (Lab India, India), Disintegration test apparatus (Serweal Instrument Inc., Bangalore, India), FT-IR Spectrometer (Shimadzu, Japan), UV- Visible Spectrophotometer (Shimadzu, Japan), Hot Air Oven (Serwell Instrument Inc., Bangalore, India), Digital weighing balance (Acculab Sartorius Group, Bangalore, India), Tablet compression machine (I.P/B.P/U.S.P. standard) 12 Station (Karnavati Engineering, Ahmedabad, India), Hardness tester (Scientific Engineering Corp., Delhi, India), Friability tester (Dutta Scientific Works., Madras, India), Humidity cabinet (Remi Laboratories Ltd., India), Hydraulic pellet press (S.V.Scientific), pH meter (Serwell Instrument Inc., Bangalore, India).

FT-Infrared spectroscopy

To find out the compatibility between the ibuprofen and the chitosan, 10 mg of the sample and 400 mg of KBr were taken in a mortar and triturated. A small amount of the triturated sample was taken into a pellet maker and was compressed at 10 kg/cm^2 using a hydraulic press. The pellet was kept onto the sample holder and scanned from 4000 cm^{-1} to 400 cm^{-1} in Shimadzu FT-IR spectrophotometer. Samples were prepared for drug ibuprofen, polymer chitosan, and physical mixture of drug and polymer. The spectra obtained were compared and interpreted for the functional group peaks.

Preparation of ibuprofen core tablets

Each core tablet (average weight 150 mg) for invitro drug release studies consisted of ibuprofen(100 mg), microcrystalline cellulose (MCC, 46 mg) , dried starch (4mg). The materials were weighed, mixed and passed through a mesh(250 µm) to ensure complete mixing. The tablets were prepared by compressing the thoroughly mixed materials using 7 mm round, flat and plain punches on a single station tablet machine (Cadmach, India). The thickness of the core tablet was 0.2 mm and their crushing strength was checked. It was about 3 Kg/cm^2.

Compression coating of ibuprofen core tablets

The Ibuprofen core tablets were compression coated with different concentrations of chitosan. Since the coating material alone gave very soft coats. Microcrystalline cellulose was included in the coat formulations to impart enough hardness. Half the quantity of the coating material was placed in the die cavity, the core was carefully positioned in the center of the die cavity and was filled with other half of the coating material. The coating material was compressed around the core at an applied force of 5,000 kg using 10 mm round, flat and plain punches. The strength of the compression coat tablet was 5 kg/cm^2 (Table 1).

Table 1. Composition of chitosan coats used to cover ibuprofen core tablets

Batch code	Coat Weight (mg)	Composition (mg)			
		Chitosan	MCC	MgStearate	Talc
F_1	300	270	25	2	3
F_2	250	220	25	2	3
F_3	200	170	25	2	3
F_4	175	145	25	2	3
F_5	150	120	25	2	3

Characterization of ibuprofen compression coated tablets

Hardness test

The prepared tablets were subjected to hardness test. It was carried out using hardness tester and expressed in Kg/cm^2.

Friability test

The friability was determined using Roche friabilator and expressed in percentage (%). 10 tablets from each batch were weighed separately and placed in the friabilator, which was then operated for 100 revolutions at 25 rpm. The tablets were reweighed and the percentage friability was calculated for each batch using the following formula:

$$F(\%) = \frac{(W_{initial}) - (W_{final})}{(W_{initial})} X\,100$$

Weight variation test

Twenty tablets were selected at random from the lot, weighed individually and the average weight was determined. The percent deviation of each tablets weight against the average weight was calculated. The test requirements are met, if not more than two of the individual weights deviate from the average weight by more than 5% and none deviates more than 10%.

Uniformity of drug content

The prepared ibuprofen tablets were tested for their drug content. Five tablets of each formulation were weighed and finely powdered. About 0.1 g equivalent of ibuprofen was accurately weighed and completely dissolved in pH 6.8 phosphate buffer and the solution was filtered. One ml of the filterate was further diluted to 100 ml with pH 6.8 buffer. Absorbance of the resulting solution was measured by UV- visible spectrophotometer at 223 nm and the amount of drug in the solution were calculated using the standard curve (r^2=0.999).

In vitro drug release studies

USP dissolution apparatus type I was employed to study the in vitro drug release from various formulations prepared. The dissolution medium used was 900 ml of acidic buffer of pH 1.2 for 2 h and phosphate buffer of pH 7.4 for 3 h. Temperature was maintained at 37°C ± 0.5°C and the stirring rate was 100 rpm. Two samples each of 1 ml were taken, suitably diluted and analyzed spectrometrically.

Preparation of rat caecal content medium

To induce bacterial enzymes postulated to be in the caecum, five Wister rats, weighing 200-300 g were intubated with Teflon tubing for 7 days before the release experiments were initiated.Each day 1 ml of 2% w/v of chitosan dispersion was directly administered to the rat stomach through the Teflon tubing. This process provides the best conditions for in vitro evaluation 30min before the commencement of drug release studies, rats were killed by spinal traction. The abdomen was opened, the caecum was isolated, ligated at both ends, dissected and immediately transferred into pH 6.8 phosphate buffer previously bubbled with CO_2.[7,8] The caecal bags were opened, their contents were individually weighed, pooled and then suspended in PBS, to give a final caecal dilution of 2% w/v. As the caecum is naturally anaerobic, all these operations were carried out under CO_2. The studies simulating the drug release in colon were carried out using USP dissolution rate test apparatus (apparatus I, 100 rpm. 37°C) with slight modification.[7] A beaker containing 200 ml of dissolution medium immersed in water containing 1000 ml vessel, which was placed in the water bath of the apparatus. The tablets were placed in the baskets of the apparatus and immersed in the dissolution medium containing rat caecal contents. The drug release studies were carried out for 21 h. (asuming colonic transit time of 20-30 h) and 1 ml samples were taken at different time intervals and replaced with 1 ml of fresh 6.8 pH PBS to maintain a constant volume and pH. The samples were diluted and analyzed spectrometrically. This part of the study was approved by Institutional Animal Ethics Committee.

Release kinetics

Data obtained from the in vitro release studies of compression coated tablet of ibuprofen formulations were fitted to various kinetic equations such as zero order, first order, Higuchi model and Korsmeyer-Pappas model using following equations: $Q = Q_0 - K_0t$ (For Zero order model), $\ln Q = \ln Q_0 - K_1t$ (for First order model), $Q = K_2t_{1/2}$ (for Higuchi model), and $Q/Q_0 = K\ t_n$ (for Korsmeyer - Pappas model). Where, K_0 to K_2 were release rate constants, Q/Q_0 was fraction of drug released at time t, K was a constant and n was diffusion constant that indicates general operating release mechanism.[9] For Fickian (diffusion controlled), $n \leq 0.5$; for non- Fickian (anomalous/ zero order) release, 'n' value is in between 0.5 to 1.0; for zero order release, n=1.0; for super case transport II, n > 1.0.

Results and Discussion

Drug-polymer interaction study by FTIR spectrophotometer

The spectra obtained from FTIR studies at wavelength from 4000 cm^{-1} to 400 cm^{-1} are shown in Figure 1. Comparing the IR spectrum of ibuprofen, chitosan and their mixtures confirm that the drug and polymer in the formulation are compatible with each other. From the figures, it is clear that, there is no appreciable change in the positions of the characteristic bands of the drug along with the IR spectrum of the drug/polymer physical mixture during the present investigation. Since there is no change in the nature and position of the bands in the physical mixture, it can be concluded that the drug maintains it's identity without going any chemical interaction with the chitosan.

Characterization of Ibuprofen core tablets

The results of physicochemical evaluation of prepared core tablets are shown in Table 2. The tablets were evaluated for weight variation, drug content, hardness and friability and disintegration. The drug content was found to be 97.84 ± 0.15%. The hardness was found to be 4.58 ± 0.42 (kg/cm^2) and in all cases the friability was less than 1%.

The results of physicochemical evaluation of compression coated tablet of ibuprofen are shown in Table 3. The tablets were evaluated for weight variation, hardness and friability. The hardness was found to be from 4.58 ± 0.42 to 5.06±0.18 (kg/cm^2) and in all the cases the friability was less than 1%.

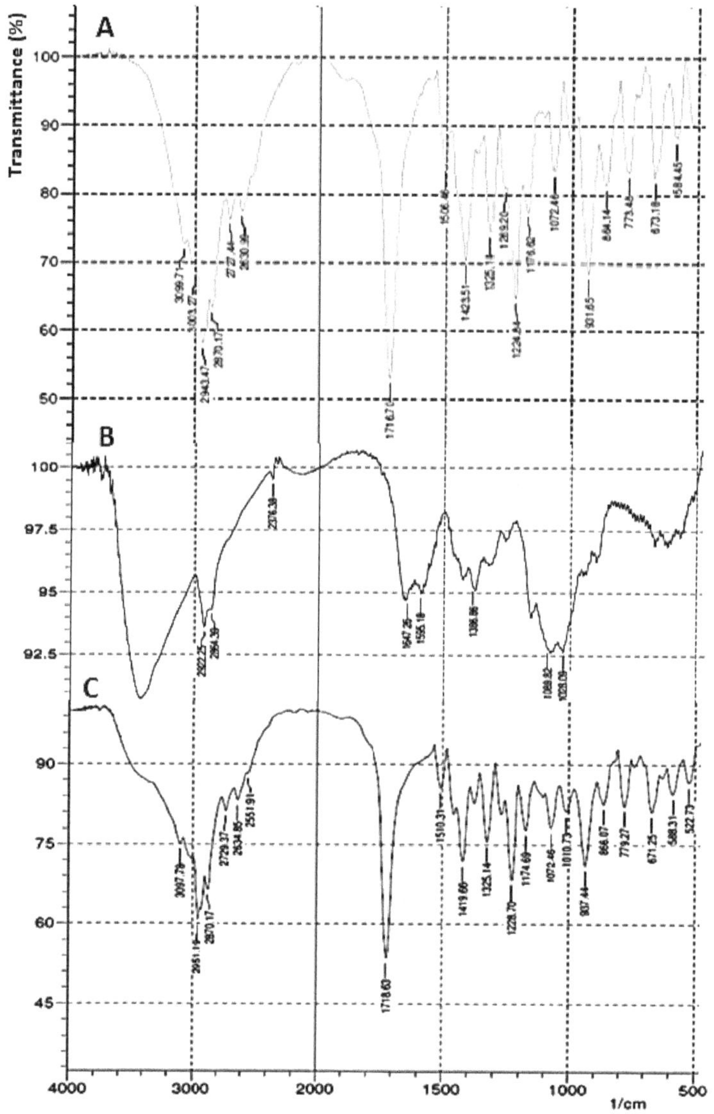

Figure 1. IR Spectrum of (A), Chitosan (B), and their physical mixture (C)

Table 2. Physicochemical evaluations of Ibuprofen core tablets.

Hardness(kg/cm^2)(±S.D)	Friability(%)(±S.D)	Weight variation(%)(±S.D)	Drug content (%)(±S.D)	Disintegration(sec)
4.58±0.42	0.20±0.021	1.403±0.012	97±0.15	60

Table 3. Physicochemical evaluations of Compression Coated Tablet of Ibuprofen

Batch Code	Parameter		
	Hardness (kg/cm^2)(± S.D)	Friability (%) (± S.D)	Weight variation (%)(± S.D)
F_1	5.06±0.18	0.065±0.014	0.51±0.016
F_2	4.8±0.09	0.14±0.034	0.67±0.038
F_3	4.7±0.12	0.11±0.017	0.96±0.052
F_4	4.6±0.35	0.13±0.015	0.57±0.034
F_5	4.82±0.12	0.062±0.029	0.73±0.056

In vitro drug release studies

Drug release studies from compression coated tablets with different coat weight, are presented in figure 2. For colon targeting, it is desirable that the system remains intact and shows minimal drug release in the stomach and the small intestine and starts drug release in the tracts of the colon. Therefore in this investigation an attempt was made to formulate a dosage form, which showed minimal drug release in conditions mimicking mouth-to-colon transit and ensured maximum drug release in the environments of the colon. The compression coat was designed to undergo bacterial degradation in the colon, exposing the rapidly disintegrating drug containing core in the colon.

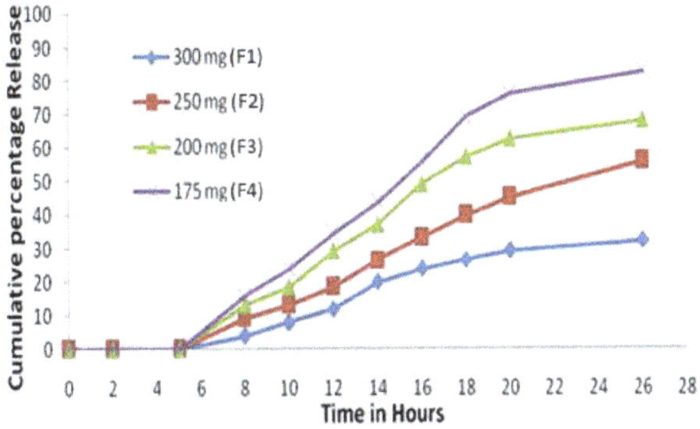

Figure 2. Cumulative percentage release profile of ibuprofen in formulations F_1 to F_4 with rat caecal content.

Formulation F_1 containing 300 mg of Chitosan released 31.94% of drug, Formulation F_2 containing 250mg of Chitosan released 67.89% of drug, Formulation F_4 containing 175 mg of Chitosan released 82.52% of drug, Formulation F_5 containing 150 mg of Chitosan was not able to cover the core tablet,From the above results, it was found that the rate of drug release, from the ibuprofen tablets decreased with increasing concentration of coating polymer. At the end of the 26 h of testing, ibuprofen tablet coated with coat formulation F_1 was found to be intact. Tablets with coat formulation F_3 found broken at one point indicating commencement of the disintegration of the coat, whereas the coat formulation F_4 was completely disintegrated.

Dissolution studies without rat caecal content

The percentage drug released at different time periods from ibuprofen tablets compression coated with coat formulations F1-F4 in 0.1N HCl (2 h), pH 7.4 phosphate buffer (3 h) and pH 6.8 phosphate buffer are shown in figure 3. At the end of the experiment, all these formulations were found to be intact retaining their coats and slight swelling of coats due to water sorption were observed. The results were found to be F_1:10.37%, F_2: 16.63%, F_3: 30.25%, F_4: 32%. From these results, it was found that the percent drug released from ibuprofen tablets were less in 6.8 phosphate buffer than the percent drug released in 6.8 phosphate buffer containing 2% w/v of rat caecal contents.

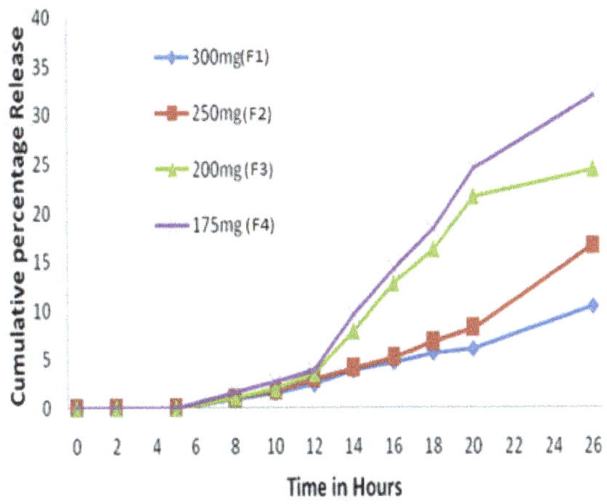

Figure 3. Cumulative percentage release profile of ibuprofen in formulations F_1 to F_4 without rat caecal content.

Successful delivery of drugs specifically to the colon requires the protection of drug from being released in stomach and small intestine. In this study polymer in the form of compression coat was applied over ibuprofen core tablets and drug release studies were carried out under conditions mimicking mouth to colon transit. The drug delivery systems targeted to the colon should not only protect the drug from being released on the physiological environment of stomach and small intestine, but also release the drug in colon after enzymatic degradation by colonic bacteria. Hence in vitro drug release studies were carried out in pH 6.8 phosphate buffer containing 2% w/v of rat caecal contents. At the end of 26 h of testing which includes testing simulated gastric and intestinal fluid, the percent drug released from ibuprofen tablets coated with coat formulation F_1 was found to be 39.91% and the coat remained intact. The presence of higher amount of polymer might not have allowed the disintegration of the coat during the time period of testing. This also indicates that the drug will not be released unless the coat is broken. The percent drug release from tablets coated with coat formulation F_3 were found to increase from 18 h on wards indicating the commencement of breaking of gum coats. The percent drug released after 26 h of testing was 67.89% and the tablet coat was found to be broken at one point making way for the release of the drug. In the case of tablet coated with coat formulation F_4 a significant increase in percent drug released was observed from 16 h on wards and at the end of the experiment and 94.46% of ibuprofen was released. The coat was completely degraded by the rat caecal thereby releasing the drug into the dissolution medium. Since the polymer content and thickness of coat formulation F4 was lesser compared to others, the coat might have been completely hydrated and subsequently degraded by the caecal enzymes at a faster rate resulting in the release of about 94.46%. On the other hand, drug release studies in the absence of rat caecal contents showed that at the end of 26 h of testing which includes testing simulated gastric and intestinal fluid, the percent drug released from the coated tablets are lesser when compared to the results of study with rat caecal contents. Moreover at the end of 26 h of testing, the coat for all the tablets remained intact which proved that the drug release were found to be dependent on bacterially triggered delivery system. In a study by A.V. Bhosale et al., tablet systems coated with films composed of guar gum and HPMC offered potential as colonic drug delivery systems for ibuprofen.[1] In another study by Kalyani Chithaluru and co-workers combination of guargum/metalose 90 SH polymers were used to prepare compression coated ketorolac tablets.[10] As it was seen in the present study, in the rat caecal contents formulations showed enhanced ketorolac release due to degradation of guar gum coat by colonic galactomannanase enzyme. Stability study were carried out at room temperature and 40°C / 75% RH over a period of 1 month for tablets prepared using coat F_4. Samples were evaluated at 0, 10, 20 and 30 days for different parameters such as physical appearance, hardness, weight variation, drug content and dissolution. The results of the stability studies are given in Table 4.

Table 4. Stability studies of compression coated tablet of ibuprofen using chitosan polymer coat 175 mg (F_4)

Evaluationparameter	Initial	Observation in Day					
		Room temperature			45± 1°C / 75% RH		
		10	20	30	10	20	30
Physicalappearance	Coated tablets	No change	No change	No change	No change	No change	No change
Averageweight (mg)	176	178	179	177	179	180	184
Hardness (kg/cm^2)	4.6	4.6	4.8	4.8	4.7	4.7	4.9
Drug content* (%w/w)	100	98.87±0.23	98.65±0.11	98.73±0.05	98.89±0.32	98.54±0.14	98.23±0.21
% CDR*	82.52±0.92	82.31±0.21	82.62±0.19	81.07±0.43	85.64±0.35	82.44±0.29	82.23±0.35

*(n=3 ± SD), Initial Drug content as 100% w/w

Invitro release of Ibuprofen from formulation F_4 as a sample was best explained by Korsmeyer-Peppas equation indicated a good linearity (r^2=0.997). The respected values for first-order, zero-order and Higuchian release models were 0.609, 0.934 and 0.838 respectively. The release exponent n was between 0.5 and 1, which indicates a coupling of the diffusion and erosion mechanism so called anomalous diffusion and may indicate that the drug release is controlled by more than one process.[10]

Conclusion

The result from this study clearly shows chitosan in the form of compression coat, is a potential carrier for drug targeting to the colon. This polymer is capable of retarding the release of core materials until they reach the colon, an environment rich in bacterial enzymes, which degrade the chitosan allowing the drug release.

Acknowledgement

The authors would like to thank the authority of Dayananda Sagar College of Pharmacy, Karnataka, India, for their support.

Conflict of interest

The authors report no conflicts of interest in this work.

References

1. Bhosale AV, Hardikar SR, Patil N, Patel U, Sumbe Y, Jagtap R. Formulation and in-vitro evaluation of microbially triggered ibuprofen delivery for colon targetting. *Int J Pharm Tech Res* 2009;1:328-333.
2. Chithaluru K, Tadikonda RR. Formulation and evaluation of microbially triggered compression coated tablets of ketorolac tromethiamine. *Der Pharmacia Lettre* 2011;3:485-495.
3. Hovgaard L, Brøndsted H. Current applications of polysaccharides in colon targeting. *Crit Rev Ther Drug Carrier Syst* 1996;13:185-223.
4. Esseku F, Adeyeye MC. Bacteria and pH-sensitive polysaccharide-polymer films for colon targeted delivery. *Crit Rev Ther Drug Carrier Syst* 2011;28:395-445.
5. Krishnaiah YS, Muzib YI, Rao GS, Bhaskar P, Satyanarayana V. Studies on the development of colon targeted oral drug delivery systems for ornidazole in the treatment of amoebiasis. *Drug Deliv* 2003;10:111-117.
6. Shah R, Patel S, Patel H, Pandey S, Shah S, Shah D. Formulation development of Carvedilol compression coated tablet. *Pharm dev Technol* 2011 Jul 28. [Epub ahead of print]
7. Raghavan CV, Muthulingam C, Jenita JA, Ravi TK. An in vitro and in vivo investigation into the suitability of bacterially triggered delivery system for colon targeting. *Chem Pharm Bull* 2002;50:892-895.
8. Sinha VR, Mittal BR, Bhutani KK, Kumria R. Colonic drug delivery of 5-fluorouracil: an in vitro evaluation. *Int J Pharm* 2004;269:101-108.
9. Dash V, Mishra SK, Singh M, Goyal AK, Rath G. Release kinetic studies of aspirin microcapsules from ethyl cellulose, cellulose acetate phthalate and their mixtures by emulsion solvent evaporation method. *Sci Pharm* 2010; 78; 93–101.
10. Chithaluru K, Tadikonda RR. Formulation and evaluation of microbially triggered compression coated tablets of ketorolac tromethiamine. *Der Pharmacia Lettre* 2011;3:29-39.

15

Socio-demographic characteristics of the addicted inmates of Qom and Tabriz prisons in Iran

Sattari Mohammadreza[1,5], Islambulchilar Mina[2,5], Toluyi Mohsen[3], Mashayekhi Siminozar[4,5]*

[1] *Neurosciences Research Centre, Tabriz University of Medical Sciences, Tabriz, Iran.*

[2] *Infectious and Tropical Diseases Research Centre, Tabriz, Iran.*

[3] *Students Research Committee, Tabriz University of Medical Sciences, Tabriz 51664-14766, Iran.*

[4] *NPMC, Tabriz University of Medical Sciences, Tabriz 51664-14766, Iran.*

[5] *Faculty of Pharmacy, Tabriz University of Medical Sciences, Tabriz, Iran.*

ARTICLE INFO

Keywords:
Addiction
Inmates
Opiates

ABSTRACT

Purpose: The aim of this investigation was to study the factors responsible for drug addiction amongst the inmates of Tabriz and Qom prisons, to further understand the reasons for drug abuse particularly in the young and find improved methods for combating these widespread problems. ***Methods:*** A multi-choice questionnaire was provided to inmates to potentially assess the reasons for their drug addiction psychiatric, personal, social, economical, and political factors were thought to be implicated. Two hundred drug addicted prisoners were individually interviewed randomly in both Tabriz and Qom prisons. A questionnaire including questions about the inmates' demographic characteristics and 49 multiple answers questions, was provided to identify the effects of different reasons for drug addiction for instance: psychiatric, personal, social, economical, and political factors. The collected data were analyzed by Student t-test and chi-squared test using SPSS software. ***Results:*** The results showed that the following factors could lead to drug addiction e.g. company with addicted friends and offenders, curiosity, imitation, illiteracy, family problems, crowded family, poverty, unemployment, and lack of self confidence. There were significant differences between Tabriz and Qom prisoners in relation to age, starting age of addiction, job, income, education, class of addiction, marital status, and hobbies. Mean age, mean starting age of addiction, poverty, alcohol drinking before addiction, marital status, heroin addiction, codeine and benzodiazepines abuse were significantly greater for Tabriz prisoners than those of Qom. ***Conclusion:*** It is clear that the governmental programs for reducing unemployment, creation of safe hobbies, proper control on drug dispensing in the pharmacies, proper birth control programs, and encouragement to higher education could alleviate addiction problem in Iran.

Introduction

Besides the improvement in technology and science, and in spite of the benefits on socioeconomics and amelioration of life facilities new problems such as new diseases have arisen. Nowadays, we have been able to overcome many problems including eradicating many diseases such as smallpox and polio. However, there are many other obstacles in the way of reaching a healthy lifestyle eg drug addiction and subsequently some incurable diseases like HIV and hepatitis C.

A report has indicated that 87% of Asian countries have had increasing numbers of prisoners over the past twenty years.[1] In Iran, the prison population has increased from about 100,000 in 1993 to 160,000 in 2002, with a rate of 229 inmates per 100,000 of general population.[1] The recent boom in Afghan opium production, propelled by a resurgent Taliban, has had an increasing impact on Iranians, both young and old, across the border. Although, the police of Iran have been tackling the drug problem for many years, Iran has an estimated 3 million drug users and by many accounts, the world's worst heroin problem.[2]

Addiction is a psychological and behavioral syndrome characterized by an intense desire for the drug and overwhelming concern about its continued availability. Addiction or substance dependence unlike tolerance and physical dependence is not a predictable response to exposure for reward-producing drugs but may occur in biologically and psychologically susceptible

***Corresponding author:** Siminozar Mashayekhi (PHD), Faculty of Pharmacy, Tabriz University of Medical Sciences, Tabriz, Iran.
E-mail: mashayekhis@yahoo.co.uk

individuals.[3] There is a significant increase in the production and use of illicit drugs throughout the world.[4,5] Dependence on heroin continues to rise for example from one-half million in the 1980s to approximately 750,000 in the 1990s, the numbers now appear to have markedly increased to about 1 million.[6] Opiate use continues to spread and is an increasing burden especially in developing countries like Iran [4]. Few reports have shown that the pattern of drug abuse has started to change from opium to other drugs. However, some other studies have shown opium to be the most frequent substance abused in Iran.[7,8] Less is known about the epidemiology of substance abuse, addiction and therefore its complications in Iran.[8,9] The cultivation of opium in Iran has been banned since 1979 and since that time, the law has recognized addiction as a social problem. Despite this legislation, the use of illegal substances has continued as a hidden activity associated with social disapproval and stigma. On the other hand a consequence of drug trafficking from the opium producing areas of Afghanistan and Central Asia to Europe through Iran, may be increasing the availability of opium which could influence the prevalence of opium usage in Iran.[4]

The United Nations Office on Drugs and Crime (UNODC) estimates 60 percent of Afghanistan's opium is trafficked across Iran's border (much of it in transit to Europe). A report indicated that Iran had at least 1,200,000–2,000,000 cases of drug dependency or abuse, constituting 1–2% of the general population in 2002.[10] According to the report for 2005, Iran has the highest proportion of opiate addicts in the world, 2.8 percent of the population over age 15.[11] The majority of previous studies have demonstrated unemployment, illegal income, drug use by family members, and pleasure/enjoyment as the main reasons for substance abuse in Iran.[12] In a study in the north of Iran, there was a significant correlation between opium use and male sex, unemployment and cigarette smoking.[13] In another study on 920 professional drivers of Iran, 434 cases (46.8%) and 256 cases (27.6%) were using opium and crack respectively.[14] Of the 3840 participants who were studied in the Fars province of Iran, 689 (17.9%) admitted use of opium once or more times during their lives (28.4% of men and 7.4% of women). Three hundred thirty-nine (8.8%) were current opium users (14.3% of men and 3.3% of women).[15] Of the 153 women, 47.4% had a lifetime history of drug treatment.[16] Heroin is the most frequent cause of fatal intoxication in most countries.[17] Heroin use predominates among urban residents, whilst villagers are more likely to be opium users.[18] Unemployment in Iran is somewhere between 11 percent (the official level) and 25 percent (the estimate given by some outside economists).[2] One in four Iranians lives in poverty. Experts say because of these dire economic conditions, particularly among those under thirty, who comprise 70 percent of Iran's population; people turn to drugs.[2]

In a study on the self-admitted illicit drug users in police custody within the Metropolitan Police Service in London, UK in 2003, heroin and crack cocaine were the most frequently used drugs (93% and 87% respectively).[5] A number of studies have suggested that there are risk factors which can lead adolescents to the abuse of alcohol and other drugs.[19-25] Labouvie et al.[26] described three basic categories of risk factors: demographic, social, and behavioural. Bragger et al[27] suggested that individual characteristics of adolescents are also involved in the onset of substance abuse. The objective of this study was to show the differences between the two main cities of Iran regarding demographic, social, and behavioral risk factors.

Materials and Methods

Two hundred drug addicted prisoners (23 females and 177 males), aged between 18 and 65 years (median 30) were individually interviewed at random in both Tabriz and Qom prisons (100 each prison) . *Tabriz* is the fourth largest and the second industrial city in Iran and the capital of East Azerbaijan Province in the north-west of Iran, with a population of about 1,400,000 (http://en.wikipedia.org/wiki/Tabriz). Qom is a religious city of Iran, the capital of Qom Province, in the south of Tehran, with an estimated population of 1,042,309 in 2005.The city is the largest center for Shi'a scholarship in the world, and is a significant destination of pilgrimage (http://en.wikipedia.org/wiki/Qom). Tabriz and Qom prisons comprise of 625 (562 males and 87 females) and 463 (403 males and 60 females) addicted inmates respectively. The majority of the inmates recruited for the study chose not to participate. A questionnaire including questions about the inmates' demographic characteristics and 49 multiple answers questions, was provided to identify the effects of different reasons for drug addiction for instance: psychiatric, personal, social, economical, and political factors. The inmates were selected for participation in the study from May to September, 2007. They were free to choose to attend the survey or not. Demographic and background characteristics of the sample are described in Table 1. The collected data were analyzed by Student t-test and Pearson chi-squared test using SPSS (ver. 17) software.

Results

Demographic characteristics

The majority of addicts were men in Tabriz (90%) and Qom (87%). The proportions of men to women in Tabriz and Qom were 9:1 and 6.7:1 respectively. There was no significant difference between gender in the two cities ($P>0.05$). The average ages of subjects were 34.52 ± 10.68 (SD) and 30.71 ± 7.69 respectively ($P<0.001$). The most common age group in Tabriz was 21-25 years (21%), while, it was 26-30 years (40%) in Qom ($P<0.001$). About 23% of the addicts of Tabriz were illiterate compared to 4% of the addicts of Qom.

26 and 49% had primary school, 13 and 15% middle school, 20 and 15% high school, and 7 and 1% of the addicts of Tabriz and Qom had university education respectively (P<0.001). There were more single addicts in Tabriz (70%) than in Qom (40%) (P<0.05). Only 4% of the addicts of Tabriz and 3% of Qom were employed, while 94% in Tabriz and 79% in Qom were unemployed or false-employed. Most of the addicts (72% in Tabriz and 53% in Qom) in both cities earned less than US$300 in a month before onset of drug addiction. Low income addicts in Tabriz were significantly more than Qom (P<0.05) (Table 1).

Age at drug addiction commencement

The majority of addicts stated that they commenced drug abuse between 16 and 20 years of age (38% in Tabriz and 34% in Qom). The mean age of drug abuse commencement in Qom (20.03±6.25) was significantly lower than Tabriz (23.72±7.71) (P<0.01) (Table 2).

Table 1. Results of demographic characteristics of the inmates of Tabriz and Qom

Demographic Characteristics of the Addicts		Tabriz (%)	Qom (%)
Mean Age (± SD)		34.52±10.68	30.71±7.69
Sex	Male	90	87
	Female	10	13
Education	Illiterate	23	4
	Primary school	26	49
	Middle school	13	15
	High school	20	15
	Higher education	7	1
	NA*	11	16
Employment status	Employed	4	3
	Unemployed or false-employed	94	79
	NA	2	18
Marital status	Single	70	40
	Married	29	58
	NA	1	2
Monthly income	<$300	42	29
	$300 to 600$	30	24
	$600 to $900	8	12
	$900 to $1200	3	11
	$1200 to $1500	3	10
	$1500 to $1800	3	6
	>$1800	6	8

*Not Acquired

Smoking and drinking alcohol before onset of drug addiction

Smoking and drinking alcohol has already been shown to encourage drug addiction.[28-32] In Tabriz and Qom 70% and 73% confessed to smoking cigarette respectively and 58% in Tabriz and 49% in Qom confirmed they were drinking alcohol prior to the onset of drug addiction, although drinking alcohol is illegal in Iran after the Islamic revolution in 1978. There were no significant differences between the two cities regarding smoking and drinking alcohol before commencement of drug addiction (P>0.05) (Table 2).

Hobbies and friendship before drug addiction

Hobbies and the role of close friends are very important in the development of smoking, alcohol and drug abuse among teenagers.[33-38] Twenty seven percent of Tabriz's and 56% of Qom's addicts suggested that they used to spend their spare times with their close friends (P<0.001) and 22% of the addicts' hobbies in Tabriz and 12% in Qom were sport (P<0.001). Other hobbies e.g. reading, cinema, and doing second job were less important and similar in both cities (Table 2). Most of the addicts in both cities confirmed that they were usually abusing their drugs with friends (39% in Tabriz and 27% in Qom) or alone out of their families' sight (21% in Tabriz and 30% in Qom). In both cities

(Tabriz: 69% and Qom: 64%) the majority of addicts confirmed the importance of the role of close friends in starting their drug addiction, while family members and relatives were less important in both cities (Table 3).

Table 2. Other information acquired from the inmates of Tabriz and Qom

Other Characteristics of the Addicts		Tabriz (%)	Qom (%)
Age at drug addiction commencement	<15	7	26
	16-20	38	34
	21-25	14	15
	26-30	13	14
	31-35	11	4
	36-40	7	1
	>41	2	0
	Mean	23.72±7.71	20.03±6.25
	NA	8	6
Smoking before drug addiction	Positive	70	73
	Negative	26	25
	NA	4	2
Drinking alcohol before drug addiction	Positive	58	49
	Negative	37	47
	NA	5	4
Hobbies before drug addiction	Reading	4	7
	Sport	22	12
	Being with friends	27	56
	Cinema	6	5
	Second job	9	7
	Others	23	9
	NA	9	4
Causes of returning to drug addiction	Humiliation by others	11	6
	Unemployment	30	30
	Intolerability to physical and psychiatric problems	24	44
	Intolerability to social problems	15	8
	NA	20	12
Usual time for drug abuse	At home near family	16	18
	At home out of sight of family	21	30
	Work place	3	11
	After work	16	7
	With friends	39	27
	NA	0	1
Awareness about drug adverse events	None	12	14
	Little	29	23
	Much	18	27
	Very much	37	32
	NA	4	4

Causes of returning to drug addiction

All of the inmates who were interviewed had given up their addiction at least once. The majority of them said they could not find any proper job (30% in both cities) or they were intolerable to physical and psychiatric problems (24% in Tabriz and 44% in Qom) after giving up their addiction and leaving jail (Table 2). Therefore, they found drugs the "best friend" again, although, most of them (77.1%) said they had decided to stop abusing drugs (Table 3).

Table 3. Other information acquired from the inmates of Tabriz and Qom

Other Characteristics of the Addicts		Tabriz (%)	Qom (%)
Decision to give up drugs	Positive	73	82
	Negative	17	14
	NA	8	4
First drug abuse offered by:	Family member	9	4
	Relatives	7	11
	Friends	69	64
	Others	10	16
	NA	5	5
The first motivation to addiction	Curiosity	26	28
	Pleasure	17	20
	Analgesic effects	19	9
	Missing a dear one	5	10
	Treatment of a psychological disease	16	16
	Family problem	7	11
	Other	6	4
	NA	4	2
Causes of arrest	Robbery	10	12
	Trafficking drugs	30	35
	Fighting	1	1
	Drug addiction	42	43
	Smuggling illegal materials	5	0
	Other	4	5
	NA	8	4

Usual time for drug abuse

Addicts usually like to enjoy abusing drugs in private or with friends. The majority of our subjects declared that they were regularly using their drugs with friends (30%) or at home in private (25.5%) (Table 2).

Awareness about drug adverse events

Only 12% in Tabriz and 14% in Qom were aware of adverse drug events, whereas, 29% in Tabriz and 23% in Qom had little information and 55% in Tabriz and 59% in Qom were approximately aware of such adverse events. The question remains "Why abuse drugs knowing what is likely to occur?"

Influence of people and reason for commencement of drug addiction

Addicts are not encouraged by television or radio programs nor by magazines advertisements but often their friends are involved in offering the first drug to them. Many of our subjects believed that their friends had offered them drugs for the first time (66.5%). They said they started drug abuse because they were curious about them (27%), wanted to be delighted (18.5%), to treat a psychological disease (16%) or pain (14%), to remove sadness about missing a dear person (7.5%) or a family problem (9%), and/or some other reasons (Table 3).

Reasons of arrest

A large proportion of addicts have no employment or income, so they earn money from illegal or criminal acts such as robbery, smuggling, and shoplifting. According to Iranian law and our subjects' beliefs, the majority of them (42.5%) were in jail because of their addiction. Despite that, 30% and 11% of them were arrested in relation to smuggling and robbery respectively.

Replaced drugs

Though most abused drugs can cause some degree of physiologic dependence, the severity of withdrawal varies considerably among these drugs. Some of these symptoms are; nausea, vomiting, diarrhoea, yawning, restlessness, rhinorrhea, lacrimation, tachycardia, and hypertension. Addicts regularly replace some other drugs to eliminate the above symptoms [39]. The majority of addicts in Tabriz and Qom said that they used codeine (36% and 19%) or alcohol (14% and 26% respectively) to eliminate the withdrawal symptoms of the main abused drug. Other drugs used for this purpose included: diphenoxylate, barbiturates, benzodiazepines, phenothiazines, and amphetamines. There was not any significant difference in the variety of substituted drugs between the two cities (P>0.05) (Table 4).

Table 4. Other information acquired from the inmates of Tabriz and Qom

Information about Drugs Abused by the Addicts		Tabriz (%)	Qom (%)
The first experience in drug abuse	Heroin	19	16
	Opium	44	62
	Hashish or Marihuana	32	15
	LSD	0	2
	Ecstasy	0	1
	Amphetamine	5	4
	NA	19	16
Effects following the first abuse of drugs	Drowsiness	13	14
	Pleasure	48	43
	Hyperthermia	4	1
	Analgesia	12	8
	Amnesia	5	10
	Physical effects	1	6
	Psychological effects	0	2
	Headache	5	1
	Dizziness	8	7
	NA	0	5
Type of addiction	Heroin	43	29
	Opium	40	58
	Hashish or Marihuana	11	29
	LSD	0	1
	Ecstasy	0	2
	Amphetamine	1	1
	NA	5	5
Replaced drugs	Alcohol	14	26
	Barbiturates	1	1
	Amphetamines	1	0
	Diphenoxylate	3	2
	Codeine	36	19
	Phenothiazines	3	0
	Benzodiazepines	9	0
	Other drugs	9	0

Discussion

The influence of demographic characteristics on drug addiction has already been demonstrated in different societies.[19,22,25,40-44] We showed in this study that men are usually at higher risk of getting addiction to drugs compared to women probably because they are more curious, bolder, more interested in variety, and less tolerable under social or familial stresses compared to women. We also showed that the addicted inmates of Tabriz were significantly older than those of Qom. Possibly, according to our data (Tab. II), the prison inmates of Tabriz commenced their drug abuse when older in age compared to those Qom. Research has indicated that certain younger people are more prone to drug abuse[45] and lifetime prevalence of abuse is higher between the ages of 18 and 29 than other cohorts for both men and women.[46] We showed that around 64% in both cities had started their drug abuse between 16 and 30 years of age that confirms Young et al's findings. Younger people have inadequate knowledge on illicit drugs and their attitudes become more liberal as age increases. They are also more curious, bolder, and less timorous than other ages. Like other countries,[47-49] unemployment and low income, singleness, low education, looking for fun, being trained in a violent area with rough families or friends are other reasons for the high prevalence of addiction commencing at a young age in Iran.The effect of families, relatives and friends on drug abuse has already been demonstrated in previous studies.[50-55] In the present study, the majority of subjects (66.5%) said that they have been offered their drugs by their friends for the first time. These addicts usually had less control from their parents during their childhood. Single addicts of Tabriz (70%) were significantly more than those of Qom (40%). This difference might be because of the low age of marriage in villages and small cities compared to the large cities in Iran. We revealed that only 17.5% of inmates had high school education or above, and the rest were illiterate or had primary or middle school education. We also showed that the most of our subjects (62.5% in both cities) had under $300 income in a month and 86% in total were unemployed or false-employed. Therefore, organization of job opportunities, encouragement of singles to get married, establishment of leisure centres, and raise in knowledge of teenagers about the adverse effects of drugs will help the drug abuse prevalence among teenagers in Iran to be diminished.

In this study we found that most of the addicts, who had given up drug abuse and left the prison, were arrested again after a short term. Unemployment, humiliation, intolerability to social problems, and hopelessness for their future were the most important reasons for their returning to the drugs. There is easy access to drugs in Iran because of the many dealers who are looking for customers among these people and encourage them with exciting offers. Therefore, rehabilitation programs should coincide with combating drug dealers. Accepting that opioid use and crime are associated and develop together, amongst opioid-using criminals the need for opioids may cause crime on a day-to-day basis or both may tend to be determined by some other set of factors. A study showed that heavy opioid users committed crimes significantly more frequently than did moderate opioid users, non-opioid polydrug users, cannabis users or alcohol users.[56] There is a correlation between imprisonment and problematic drug use. Many people are imprisoned for possession or distribution offences, many commit crimes while under the influence of drugs and commit astounding amounts of property crime to pay for their regular supply.[57] The majority of our subjects were in jail because of addiction or related crimes e.g. drug trafficking and smuggling.

Some of our subjects (15%) mentioned the role of pain-killer drugs in their addiction to drugs. Previous studies have shown that the increasing prescription of opioids is associated with a rise in aberrant drug-related behaviour. The causes of this behaviour are multifactorial. Some pharmacotherapeutic, but in particular psychosocial risk and etiologic pain factors have been identified. The indication for the prescription of opioids must be very carefully evaluated in the presence of any risk factor. In the absence of successful opioid therapy, the treatment must be discontinued to avoid iatrogenic damage, substance abuse and illegal diversion.[58] Furthermore, strategies to help identify the early signs of addiction and the best clinical practices for use of these agents will help minimize the likelihood of addiction.[59]

Acknowledgments

We wish to thank to Dr. Derek Buss (Cardiff University) for his collaboration in writing this paper and the personnel of the prisons of Tabriz and Qom for their cooperation.

Conflict of interest

The authors report no conflicts of interest in this work.

References

1. Assadi SM, Noroozian M, Pakravannejad M, et al. Psychiatric morbidity among sentenced prisoners: prevalence study in Iran. *Br J Psychiatry* 2006;188:159-64.
2. Afghanistan's Role in Iran's Drug Problem Council on Foreign Relations; 2006. http://www.cfr.org/publication/11457/afghanistans_role_in_irans_drug_problem.html. Accessed January 28, 2011.
3. Hojsted J, Sjogren P. Addiction to opioids in chronic pain patients: a literature review. *Eur J Pain* 2007;11(5):490-518.
4. Karbakhsh M, Salehian Zandi N. Acute opiate overdose in Tehran: the forgotten role of opium. *Addict Behav* 2007;32(9):1835-42.
5. Payne-James JJ, Wall IJ, Bailey C. Patterns of illicit drug use of prisoners in police custody in London, UK. *J Clin Forensic Med* 2005;12(4):196-8.
6. Kelber HD. Future advances in addiction treatment. *Clinical Neuroscience Research* 2005;5(2):201-5.
7. Rajabizade G, Ramezani MA, Shakibi MR. Prevalence of opium addiction in Iranian drivers 2001–2003. *Journal of Medical Sciences* 2004;4:210-3.
8. Ziaaddini H, Ziaaddini MR. The household survey of drug abuse in Kerman. *Journal of Applied Sciences* 2005;5:380–2.
9. Ahmadi J, Arabi H, Mansouri Y. Prevalence of substance use among offspring of opioid addicts. *Addict Behav* 2003;28(3):591-5.
10. Mokri A. Brief overviewof the status of drug abuse in Iran. *Archives of Iranian Medicine* 2002;5:184-90.
11. Vick K. Opiates of the Iranian People. *Despair Drives World's Highest Addiction Rate* 2005; http://www.washingtonpost.com/wpdyn/content/article/2005/09/22/AR2005092202287.html. Accessed October, 2010.
12. Rafiey H, Narenjiha H, Shirinbayan P, et al. Needle and syringe sharing among Iranian drug injectors. *Harm Reduct J* 2009;6:21.

13. Meysamie A, Sedaghat M, Mahmoodi M, Ghodsi SM, Eftekhar B. Opium use in a rural area of the Islamic Republic of Iran. *East Mediterr Health J* 2009;15(2):425-31.
14. Narenjiha H, Rafiey H, Jahani MR, Assari S, Moharamzad Y, Roshanpazooh M. Substance-dependent professional drivers in Iran: a descriptive study. *Traffic Inj Prev* 2009;10(3):227-30.
15. Ahmadi J, Pridmore S, Alimi A, et al. Epidemiology of opium use in the general population. *Am J Drug Alcohol Abuse* 2007;33(3):483-91.
16. Walton-Moss B, McCaul ME. Factors associated with lifetime history of drug treatment among substance dependent women. *Addict Behav* 2006;31(2):246-53.
17. Preti A, Miotto P, De Coppi M. Deaths by unintentional illicit drug overdose in Italy, 1984-2000. *Drug Alcohol Depend* 2002;66(3):275-82.
18. Dalvand S, Agahi C, Spencer C. Drug addicts seeking treatment after the Iranian Revolution: a clinic-based study. *Drug Alcohol Depend* 1984;14(1):87-92.
19. Beman DS. Risk factors leading to adolescent substance abuse. *Adolescence* 1995;30(117):201-8.
20. Bennett EM, Kemper KJ. Is abuse during childhood a risk factor for developing substance abuse problems as an adult? *J Dev Behav Pediatr* 1994;15(6):426-9.
21. Brown SA. Life events of adolescents in relation to personal and parental substance abuse. *Am J Psychiatry* 1989;146(4):484-9.
22. Danielson CK, Amstadter AB, Dangelmaier RE, Resnick HS, Saunders BE, Kilpatrick DG. Trauma-related risk factors for substance abuse among male versus female young adults. *Addict Behav* 2009;34(4):395-9.
23. Hernandez JT. Substance abuse among sexually abused adolescents and their families. *J Adolesc Health* 1992;13(8):658-62.
24. Maltzman I, Schweiger A. Individual and family characteristics of middle class adolescents hospitalized for alcohol and other drug abuse. *Br J Addict* 1991;86(11):1435-47.
25. Newcomb MD, Maddahian E, Skager R, Bentler PM. Substance abuse and psychosocial risk factors among teenagers: associations with sex, age, ethnicity, and type of school. *Am J Drug Alcohol Abuse* 1987;13(4):413-33.
26. Labouvie EW, Pandina RJ, White HR, Johnson V. Risk factors of adolescent drug use: an affect-based interpretation. *J Subst Abuse* 1990;2(3):265-85.
27. Bragger U, Schurch EJr, Gusberti FA, Lang NP. Periodontal conditions in adolescents with cleft lip, alveolus and palate following treatment in a co-ordinated team approach. *J Clin Periodontol* 1985;12(6):494-502.
28. Biener K. Problems of smoking, alcohol and drug addiction in prisoners (author's transl). *Offentl Gesundheitswes* 1980;42(2):55-8.
29. Butters JE, Smart RG, Mann RE, Asbridge M. Illicit drug use, alcohol use and problem drinking among infrequent and frequent road ragers. *Drug Alcohol Depend* 2005;80(2):169-75.
30. Hafner H. Epidemiology of alcohol and drug addiction. Report on a WHO conference. *Fortschr Med* 1973;91(14):617-21.
31. Kryspin-Exner K. Relationship between alcohol and drug addiction. *Offentl Gesundheitswes* 1971;33(9):548-55.
32. Schmidt L. Relation between smoking, alcoholism, and drug addiction. *Rehabilitation (Bonn)* 1972;25(1):53-4.
33. Ghanizadeh A. Shiraz University students' attitude towards drugs: an exploratory study. *East Mediterr Health J* 2001;7(3):452-60.
34. Mohammad Poorasl A, Vahidi R, Fakhari A, Rostami F, Dastghiri S. Substance abuse in Iranian high school students. *Addict Behav* 2007;32(3):622-7.
35. Urberg KA, Degirmencioglu SM, Pilgrim C. Close friend and group influence on adolescent cigarette smoking and alcohol use. *Dev Psychol* 1997;33(5):834-44.
36. Miller P, Plant M. Truancy and perceived school performance: an alcohol and drug study of UK teenagers. *Alcohol Alcohol* 1999;34(6):886-93.
37. Miller P. Family structure, personality, drinking, smoking and illicit drug use: a study of UK teenagers. *Drug Alcohol Depend* 1997;45(1-2):121-9.
38. Chanin A. Toward an understanding of teenagers. Alternatives to drug abuse. *Clin Pediatr (Phila)* 1969;8(1):6-10.
39. Guthrie SK, Brower KJ, Karam-Hage M. Substance-Related Disorders. In: Chisholm-Burns MA, Wells BG, Schwinghammer TL, et al., eds. *Pharmacotherapy, Principles & Practice*. New York: McGraw-Hill, 2008:525-48.
40. Aytaclar S, Erkiran M, Kirisci L, Tarter R. Substance abuse and associated psychosocial risk factors among Turkish male adolescents. *Addict Behav* 2003;28(8):1419-29.
41. Bandason T, Rusakaniko S. Prevalence and associated factors of smoking among secondary school students in Harare Zimbabwe. *Tob Induc Dis 2010;*8:12.
42. Christensen H, Low LF, Anstey KJ. Prevalence, risk factors and treatment for substance abuse in older adults. *Curr Opin Psychiatry* 2006;19(6):587-92.
43. Gil AG, Vega WA, Turner RJ. Early and mid-adolescence risk factors for later substance abuse by African Americans and European Americans. *Public Health Rep* 2002;117 Suppl 1:S15-29.
44. Weinberg NZ. Risk factors for adolescent substance abuse. *J Learn Disabil* 2001;34(4):343-51.
45. Royo-Bordonada MA, Cid-Ruzafa J, Martin-Moreno JM, Guallar E. Drug and alcohol use in

Spain: consumption habits, attitudes and opinions. *Public Health* 1997;111(5):277-84.
46. Young SE, Corley RP, Stallings MC, Rhee SH, Crowley TJ, Hewitt JK. Substance use, abuse and dependence in adolescence: prevalence, symptom profiles and correlates. *Drug Alcohol Depend* 2002;68(3):309-22.
47. Iliev Y, Akabaliev V, Doychinov I. Characteristics of adult acute poisoning mortality in a large industrial-agrarian region of Bulgaria during socioeconomic transition and crisis (1990-1998). *Vet Hum Toxicol* 2000;42(6):366-9.
48. Lamontagne Y, Garceau-Durand Y, Elie R, Blais S. [The young homeless of Montreal: a longitudinal study]. *Can J Psychiatry* 1988;33(8):716-22.
49. Ruiz-Perez I, Olry de Labry-Lima A. [Suicide in Spain today]. *Gac Sanit* 2006;20 Suppl 1:25-31.
50. Beauvais F. Drug use of friends: a comparison of reservation and non-reservation Indian youth. *Am Indian Alsk Native Ment Health Res* 1992;5(1):43-50.
51. Diaz CJ, Brands B, Adlaf E, Giesbrecht N, Simich L, Wright Mda G. [Drug consumption and treatment from a family and friends perspectives: Guatemala]. *Rev Lat Am Enfermagem* 2009;17 -:824-30.
52. Knight DK, Simpson DD. Influences of family and friends on client progress during drug abuse treatment. *J Subst Abuse* 1996;8(4):417-429.
53. Lacy WB. The influence of attitudes and current friends on drug use intentions. *J Soc Psychol* 1981;113(First Half):65-76.
54. Lagu T, Anderson BJ, Stein M. Overdoses among friends: drug users are willing to administer naloxone to others. *J Subst Abuse Treat* 2006;30(2):129-33.
55. Smart RG, Stoduto G. Interventions by students in friends' alcohol, tobacco, and drug use. *J Drug Educ* 1997;27(3):213-22.
56. Hammersley R. Drug addiction and crime. *Br J Addict* 1988;83(4):445-6.
57. Trace M. Tackling drug use in prison: a success story. *Drug Policy* 1998;9(4):277-82.
58. Jage J, Willweber-Strumpf A, Maier C. [Risk factors for substance abuse and dependence in opioid therapy for chronic noncancer-related pain]. *Schmerz* 2005;19(5):434-436, 437-40.
59. Compton WM, Volkow ND. Major increases in opioid analgesic abuse in the United States: concerns and strategies. *Drug Alcohol Depend* 2006;81(2):103-7.

16

Formulation of cefuroxime axetil oral suspension and investigation of its pharmaceutical properties

Hadi Valizadeh[1,2], Aynoor Farajnia[3,4], Parvin Zakeri-Milani[1,5*]

[1]*Faculty of Pharmacy, Tabriz University of Medical Sciences, Tabriz, Iran*

[2]*Research Center for Pharmaceutical Nanotechnology, Tabriz University of Medical Sciences, Tabriz, Iran*

[3]*Student Research Committee, Tabriz University of Medical Sciences, Tabriz, Iran*

[4]*Drug Applied Research Center, Tabriz University of Medical Sciences, Tabriz, Iran*

[5]*Liver and Gastrointestinal Diseases Research Center, Tabriz University of Medical Sciences, Tabriz, Iran*

ARTICLE INFO

Keywords:
Cefuroxime axetil
oral suspension
viscosity
zeta potential
sedimentation volume
degree of flocculation

ABSTRACT

Purpose: Cefuroxime is the second generation cephalosporin, which its intravenous and oral dosage forms are available. Oral route is the selective method for administration of most of the drugs. The aim of this study was formulating 'for oral' cefuroxime axetil suspensions. ***Methods:*** Minitab (ver.15) was used to design the formulations containing 125 mg of cefuroxime in 5 ml vehicle. After selecting the acceptable preparations, physical stability tests and other tests such as dissolution rate, pH, zeta potential and viscosity measurement of formulations were performed. ***Results:*** From all 33 formulations, only 9 were selected to further investigation. Considering no sedimentation, the sedimentation volume was determined to be 1. The degrees of flocculation were also equal to 1. All selected formulations released the drug between 81-100% in 30 minutes which was acceptable according to the USP32 criteria. The results of assay test also proved that all formulations contain the drug in acceptable range (91-106%). The viscosity curves showed that the systems were pseudo plastic and thixotrop. ***Conclusion:*** Designed cefuroxime axetil formulations had good qualities and could be added as a new product to Iran drug marketing.

Introduction

Cefuroxime is1-acetoxyethyl ester of a β-lactamase-stable cephalosporin.[1] This second generation-cephalosporin is active against a wide range of Gram-positive and Gram-negative organisms[2] which makes it useful in treating a variety of infections caused by b-lactam-producing strains of *Haemophilus influenzae*, *Moraxella catarrhalis* and *Staphylococcus aureus.* An advantage of cefuroxime over other second-generation cephalosporins is that it is effective in the treatment of *Neisseria gonorrhea* and *H influenzae*. It is characterized by being the only second-generation cephalosporin which adequately penetratesinto the cerebrospinal fluid (CSF).[3] The use of Cefuroxime by the oral route requires its administration in the form of prodrug, cefuroxime axetil. Since cefuroxime is not absorbed orally, the 1-acetyloxyethyl (axetil) ester of cefuroxime was used to improve its gastrointestinal absorption.[4] Oral route is the selective method for administration of most of the drugs because of its ease and patient compliance.[5] Because of the advantages of using a suspension and high bioavailability in comparison to other dosage forms (except solutions), in this investigation the aim was formulating oral cefuroxime axetil suspensions.

Materials and Methods

Materials

Cefuroxime axetil was purchased from Dana Pharmaceutical Company, Tabriz, Iran. Avicel, Colloidal silicon dioxide, Silloidal silicon dioxide were purchased from Exir Pharmacrutical Company, Boroujerd, Iran. Xanthan, Ploxamer were purchased from Sigma-Aldrich, Basal, Switzerland. All other chemicals were purchased fromMerck, Darmstadt, Germany.

***Corresponding author:** Parvin Zakeri-Milani (PhD), E-mail: pzakeri@tbzmed.ac.ir

Formulation of suspensions

One of the methods for making the suspension, is the dispersion of a particle in a vehicle that can be done by mechanical instruments or by the use of surfactants that contains three steps: a) wetting of particles, b) disintegration of aggregated particles, and c) prevention of re-aggregation of particles in the vehicle.[6]

For suspension formulation equivalent to 125 mg of cefuroxime was suspended in 5 ml vehicle, after selecting the type and concentration of wetting agent, other ingredients such as flocculating agents, suspending agents, preservatives and flavors were added.[6] Minitab (ver.15) software was used to design the formulations.

Evaluation of physical stability

Made formulations are then evaluated for physical stability tests in which the sedimentation volume (the ratio of the final volume of the sediment to the original volume of the suspension) and degree of flocculation (the ratio of the ultimate sediment volume of flocculated suspension to the ultimate sediment volume of deflocculated suspension) were conducted.[7]

Assay test

Prepared formulations were evaluated by UV system in 281 wavelengths, for the standard solution 20 mg of the drug was dissolved in 50 ml methanol and 10.61 concentration of it was made by dilution and the absorbance was read. For the assay solution 5 ml of suspension was dissolved in 50 ml methanol and after shaking for 5 minutes 200 ml of medium was added and after achieving 10.61 concentrations the absorbance was read.

Dissolution test

For 3 of each formulation, dissolution test was performed with USP 2 apparatus (Paddle) in 50 rpm for 30 minutes. 900 ml of medium (3.7 g of monobasic sodium phosphate and 5.7 g of anhydrous dibasic sodium phosphate) was transferred to each vessel and the absorbances of the samples were read in maximum absorption wavelength of 281. Then using equation derived from calibration curve ($y = 0.0344x + 0.0233$ و $R^2 = 0.9991$) the percentage of drug release was calculated.[8]

Other tests, including measurement of pH, viscosity and zeta potential measurements were performed and finally the best formulations were selected.

Results

From all 33 formulations designed in Minitab software, only 9 was selected to further investigation that are listed in the Table 1. The sedimentation volume was calculated to be 1 in all the suspensions, therefore there was no need to re-dispersion test and the degree of flocculation value was also 1. All selected formulations released more than 60% of the drug (81-100%) that was acceptable according to the USP32 criteria. In Figure 1 the percentage of release in all the formulations are presented. Assay tests also show that the amount of drug in all formulations are in the range of 91-106% and all are acceptable (Table 2). After calculating the viscosity, the curves of viscosity against shear rate were plotted. A sample of these curves is shown in Figure 2.

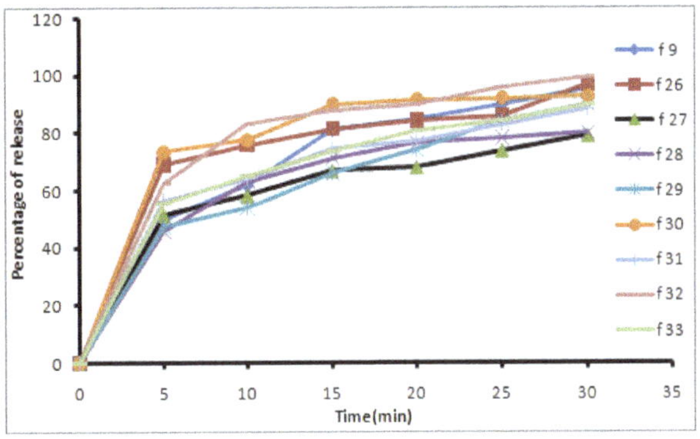

Figure 1. Percentage of release for all selected formulations

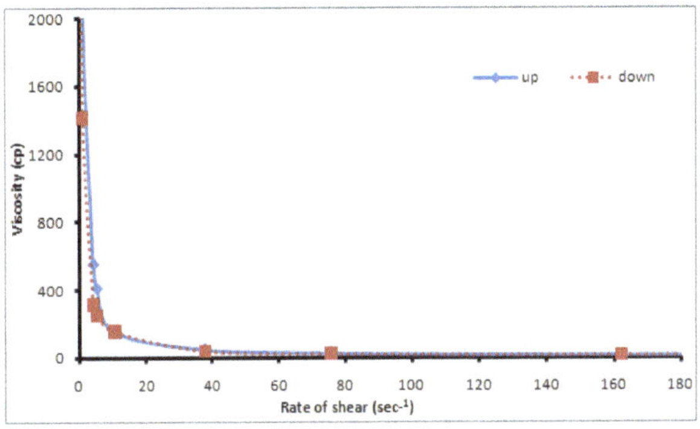

Figure 2. A sample viscosity curve for formulated suspension

Table 1. Composition of selected formulations designed in Minitab (ver.15)

Formulations	Drug%	Glucose%	Avicel%	Polaxamer%	Silloidal silicon dioxide%	Xanthan%	Colloidal silicon dioxide%
9	20	50	12.5	0.55	0.275	0.175	16.5
26	20	50	5	1	0.05	0.05	23.9
27	20	50	5	1	0.5	0.3	23.2
28	20	50	5	0.1	0.05	0.05	24.35
29	20	50	5	0.1	0.05	0.3	24.55
30	20	50	5	1	0.05	0.3	23.65
31	20	50	5	0.1	0.05	0.05	24.8
32	20	50	5	1	0.5	0.05	23.45
33	20	50	5	0.1	0.5	0.3	24.1

Table 2. Results of assay test

Formulations	concentration (µg/ml) sample 1	concentration (µg/ml) sample 2	concentration (µg/ml) sample 3	Percent of labeled amount
9	9.97	11.05	10.29	98.36
26	13.26	9.77	10.29	104.66
27	10.03	9.53	9.68	91.87
28	9.26	10.11	10.48	93.78
29	10.35	10.93	10.46	99.73
30	10.48	10.44	10.67	100.37
31	11.08	10.7	10.81	102.37
32	11.54	11.19	11.25	106.76
33	11.1	10.58	10.76	101.92

Discussion

General criteria for selecting a suitable suspension can be considered as proper appearance of uniformity and homogeneity, the number of low-frequency shaking for the complete distribution, the high volume of sediment, no crystal growth and appropriate pour ability. According to these properties a general discussion is presented. 33 formulations were designed with Minitab (ver.15) software and only 9 were pourable and had ideal characteristics to continue more other tests. There was no sediment in selected formulations and the sediment volume was 1 for all of them so there was no need for re-dispersion test and the degree of the flocculation was also 1 that was probably because of the high viscosity of the system. pH measurement indicated that all the suspensions' pH were between 5 - 6 that was acceptable according to the pharmacopeia. Release test approved that all the formulations released drug more than 60% in 30 minutes. According to the curve each formulation released 95.44, 96.82, 79.10, 81.10, 89.69, 92.62, 88.14, 99.28, and 89.69 in 30 minutes. The assay test showed that all the formulations contain drug in acceptable range according to the pharmacopeia and all contains between 91-106%.

According to the viscosity curves, the suspensions were pseudo plastic, i.e., the viscosity decreases as the shear rate increases. This is probably because of xanthan and sodium carboxymethyl cellulose (exists in the avicel RC-591 in the amount between 8-13%)[9] which give pseudo plastic property to the vehicle. Considering the differences of the viscosity in up and down curves the thixotropy of the system is obvious so the vehicle was pseudo plastic and thixotrop. Also the system was found to be time-depended. That means after a while takes the stress off, the initial viscosity of the suspension is achieved and that's a good chance to pour the suspension after each re-dispersion which is one of the most important characteristics in suspensions, also because of the high viscosity of the system despite of having flocculated particles in the vehicle according to Stokes's law the sedimentation rate was low.[4]

The charge of the particles effects their distribution in the environment and increases the concentration of opposite charge on the surface close to them which produces electric double layer. The potential of the moving layer around each particle is called zeta potential. Quantity of zeta potential can indicate the potential stability of the colloidal system, if the particles have a large positive or negative zeta potential they will have a tendency to repel each other and in too low zeta potentials particles will accumulate and attract each other. Overall, the borderline between stable and unstable suspensions is usually considered zeta potentials between + 30 mv or - 30 mv means those particles which have zeta potential more than +30 or lower than -30 mv considered stable.[10,11] In this investigation all the formulations had zeta potential lower than -30 mv but all of them were stable so it seems that mechanisms other than the zeta potential of the particles is involved in the formulation of stable formulations In other words, polymer bridging was the main mechanism for controlled flocculation in the present work.

Conclusion

According to the obtained results and considering the ideal characteristics of prepared suspension formulations, this product can be added to drug market.

Acknowledgement

The authors would like to thank Dana Pharmaceutical Co. Tabriz, Iran for the supply of cefuroxime axetil. This article is based on a thesis submitted for Pharm Dr degree (No.3541) in Faculty of Pharmacy, Tabriz University of Medical Sciences, Tabriz, Iran.

Conflict of interest

The authors report no conflicts of interest.

References

1. Dhumal R, Biradar V, Yamamura SH, Paradkar R, York P. Preparation of amorphous cefuroxime axetil nanoparticles by sonoprecipitation for enhancement of bioavailability. *Eur J Pharm Biopharm* 2008; 70: 109-115.
2. Jelinska A, Dudzinska I, Zajac M, Oszczpowiez I. The stability of the amorphous form of cefuroxime axetil in solid state. *J Pharm Biomed Anal* 2006; 41: 1075-1081.
3. Al-Said MS, Al-Khamis KI, Niazy EM, El-Sayed YM, Al-Rashood KA, Al-Bella S, Al-Yamani MA,

Al-Najjar TA, Alam SM, Dham R. Bioequivalence evaluation of two brands of cefuroxime 500 mg tablets (cefuzime and zinnat) in healthy volunteers. *Biopharm Drug Dispos* 2000; 21: 205-210.
4. Ruiz-Carretero P, Merino-Sonjuan M, Casabo VG. Pharmacokinetic models for the saturable absorption of cefuroxime axetil and saturable elimination of cefuroxime axetil. *Eur J Pharm Sci* 2004; 21: 217-223.
5. Kulshreshtha AL, Singh ON, Wall GM. Pharmaceutical suspensions from formulation to manufacturing. New York: Springer; 2010.1-38.
6. Sinko JP, Singh YA. *Martin's Physical Pharmacy and Pharmaceutical Sciences*. USA: Wolters Kluwer/ Lippincott Williams & Wilkins; 2011.
7. Bowman JB, Mofner C, Schott H. Colloidal dispersion. In: Troy DB, Hauber MJ, Brien MA. *Remington the science and practice of Pharmacy.* USA: Lippincott Williams & Wilkins; 2006. 293-337.
8. Tabibi S, Rhodes CH. Disperse system. In:Banker SG, Rhodes TC. Modern Pharmaceutics. New York: Marcel Dekker; 1996. 365-436.
9. *The United States Pharmacopeia (USP)*. Port City Press; 2009.1864-1865.
10. Epshtein NA. A new approach to HPLC analysis of medicinal suspensions. *Pharm Chem J* 2001; 35: 686-689.
11. Benitez EI, Lozano JE. Influence of the soluble solids on the zeta potential of the cloudy apple juice. *Lat Am Appl* 2006; 36: 163-168.

Antioxidant Activity of Rhizoma Cibotii *in vitro*

Wenqiong Mai[1], Dongfeng Chen[2], Xican Li[1]*

[1] *School of Chinese Herbal Medicine, Guangzhou University of Chinese Medicine, Guangzhou, China.*

[2] *School of Basic Medicine, Guangzhou University of Chinese Medicine, Guangzhou, China.*

ARTICLE INFO

Keywords:
Rhizoma Cibotii
Antioxidant activity
Radical scavenging
Total phenolics
HPLC
Caffeic acid

ABSTRACT

Purpose: The paper tried to systematically investigate the *in vitro* antioxidant activity of Rhizoma Cibotii (RC) for the first time. ***Method***: The methanol extract from RC (MERC) was prepared then systematically investigated by various antioxidant assays, including: DPPH• (1, 1-diphenyl-2-picrylhydrazyl radical), ABTS•$^+$ (3-ethylbenzthiazoline-6- sulfonic acid diammonium salt radical), •O_2^- (superoxide anion radical), •OH (hydroxyl radical) scavenging assays, Fe^{3+} reducing power, Cu^{2+} reducing power assays, compared with positive controls Trolox (± -6 -hydroxyl -2,5, 7, 8-tetramethlychromane-2-carboxylic acid) and BHA (butylated hydroxyanisole). Its total phenolics and caffeic acid content were also measured by Folin-Ciocalteu method and HPLC, respectively. ***Result***: MERC exhibited effective antioxidant activity in dose-dependent manners and its IC_{50} values were calculated as 44.2 ± 0.62, 19.84 ± 0.31, 137.66 ± 2.90, 22.94 ± 0.90, 289.73 ± 46.17, 53.52 ± 1.51 μg /mL, for DPPH•, ABTS•$^+$, •O_2^-, •OH scavenging assays, Fe^{3+} reducing power, Cu^{2+} reducing power assays, respectively. Its total phenolics content was 50.88 ± 1.24 mg CAE /g and the caffeic acid content was 1.82 ± 0.19 mg/g. ***Conclusion***: Rhizoma Cibotii has effective *in vitro* antioxidant activity which may attribute to its total phenolics, among which caffeic acid can be considered as one of the active components. The pharmacological effects or healthcare functions of whole RC may result from the synergistic effects caused by the combination of its components and its antioxidant effect plays an important role in the synergistic effects.

Introduction

Rhizoma Cibotii (RC), the root of *Cibotium barometz* (L.) J. Sm. in Dicksoniaceae, is a commonly used Chinese herbal medicine. From the viewpoint of traditional Chinese medicine (TCM), RC has the efficacies of tonifying the liver and the kidney, strengthening bones and tendons, relaxing the meridian, dispelling wind-dampness.[1] Hence, it is usually used as the main ingredient with other Chinese herbal medicine to pickle wine for drinking for body building and disease treatment like waist sour, rheumatism and so on. In modern clinical applications, RC is used to treat lumbar and leg pain, numbness, hemiplegia, leucorrhea spermatorrhea, women bleeding and kinds of tumors such as osteoma, osteosarcoma, brain tumors, and multiple myeloma.[2,3]

Phytochemical study on RC indicated that RC mainly contained fatty acid (e.g. oleic acid, palmitic acid, and octadecaonic acid),[4,5] phenolic acids (e.g. caffeic acid, protocatechuic acid),[6,7] flavonoids (e.g. kaempferol, onychin)[8,9] and so on. Pharmacological investigations revealed that palmitic acid has anti-inflammatory effect and octadecaonic acid can lower blood lipid[4], water-soluble phenolic acids such as caffeic acid and protocatechuic acid are the active constituents for rheumatoid arthritis and osteoarthritis [10], flavonoids like kaempferol and onychin possess antioxidant activity and anticancer effects.[11-13]

Despite that the components in RC possess various pharmacological effects, according to the free radical biology & medical, the pharmacological effects or healthcare functions of Chinese medicine of whole RC may closely related to it antioxidant activity.[14] However, to our knowledge, the comprehensive evaluation of antioxidant activity of RC has not been reported yet. Therefore, this paper tries to evaluate its *in vitro* antioxidant activity for the first time by various methods, including DPPH•, ABTS•$^+$, •O_2^- and •OH radical-scavenging, Fe^{3+} reducing power and Cu^{2+} reducing power assays. Its total phenolics and caffeic acid content were also measured by chemical methods.

Obviously, the study is helpful to explain the mechanism of pharmacological effects or healthcare functions of RC.

***Corresponding author:** Xican Li, School of Chinese Herbal Medicine, Guangzhou University of Chinese Medicine, Guangzhou, China.
E-mail: lixican@126.com

Materials and Methods

Plant material

Rhizoma Cibotii was purchased from Guangzhou University of TCM Yanghe Interlink Limited Company and identified by Prof. Tang Shuhui.

Chemicals and reagents

DPPH• (1,1-Diphenyl-2-picrylhydrazyl radical), pyrogallol, Trolox (± -6 -hydroxyl -2,5, 7, 8-tetramethlychromane-2-carboxylic acid), BHA (butylated hydroxyanisole) and neocuproine (2,9-dimethyl-1,10-phenanthroline) were purchased from Sigma Co.; ABTS diammonium salt [2,2′-Azino-bis (3-ethylbenzothiazoline-6-sulfonic acid diammonium salt)] , and D-2-deoxyribose were obtained from Amresco Co.; HPLC-grade acetonitrile was purchased from Kermel Co. (Tianjin, China); Caffeic acid was purchased from NICPBP; All other chemicals were of analytical grade.

Preparation of plant extract

The plant was powdered then extracted with methanol by Soxhlet extractor for 12 hours. The extract was concentrated under reduced pressure to a constant weight then stored at 4°C.

DPPH• scavenging assay

DPPH• radical-scavenging activity was determined as previously described by Li.[15] Briefly, 1 mL of DPPH• solution (0.1 mol/L) was mixed with 0.5 mL of various concentrations of samples dissolved in 95% ethanol. The mixture was kept at room temperature for 30 min, and then the absorbance at 519 nm was measured on a spectrophotometer (Unico 2100, Shanghai, China), using 95% ethanol as the blank. Trolox and BHA were used as the positive controls and the percentage DPPH• inhibition of the test samples was calculated: Inhibition % = $(1 - A_S/A_0) \times 100$. Where A_S is the absorbance in the presence of RC or positive controls, while A_0 is the absorbance in the absence of RC and positive controls.

ABTS•$^+$ scavenging assay

The scavenging activity of ABTS•$^+$ was measured by a previously described method.[15]The ABTS•$^+$ was produced by mixing 0.35 mL of ABTS diammonium salt (7.4 mmol/L) with 0.35 mL of potassium persulfate (2.6 mmol/L). The mixture was kept in the dark at room temperature for 12 h to allow completion of radical generation, and then diluted with 95% ethanol (about 1:50) so that its absorbance at 734 nm was 0.70 ± 0.02 measured on a spectrophotometer (Unico 2100, Shanghai, China). To determine the scavenging activity, 1.2 mL of ABTS•$^+$ reagent was mixed with 0.3 mL of sample or negative control (95% ethanol), and the absorbance at 734 nm was measured 6 min after the initial mixing, using 95% ethanol as the blank. The percentage inhibition of the samples was calculated as: Inhibition % = $(1 - A/A_0) \times 100\%$. Where A_0 is the absorbance at 734 nm of the negative control, A is the absorbance at 734 nm of the mixture with sample or positive controls.

Superoxide anion (•O_2^-) radical-scavenging assay

Measurement of superoxide anion scavenging activity of RC was based on the pyrogallol autoxidation method of Marklund S and Marklund G,[16] as described by Li *et al.*[15] Briefly, a sample solution (1 mg/m L, x μL, where x = 0, 50, 100, 150, 200, 250 μL) was mixed with Tris-HCl buffer (2920 - x μL, 0.05 mol/L, pH 8.2) containing EDTA (1 mmol/L) and pyrogallol (80 μL, 6 mmol/L), then shaken rapidly at room temperature. The absorbance at 325 nm of the mixture was measured (Unico 2100, Shanghai, China) against the Tris-HCl buffer as blank per 30 s for 5 min. Trolox and BHA were used as the positive controls. The slope of the correlation of absorbance with time was calculated. The reaction mixture without sample was used as the control. The •O_2^- scavenging ability was calculated as: (1 - Slope of sample/ Slope of control) × 100 %.

Hydroxyl (•OH) radical-scavenging assay

The scavenging activity on the hydroxyl radical was investigated by the deoxyribose method [17], with some modification. Our preliminary experiments demonstrated that most organic solvents especially alcohol can promote the inhibition percentage value. Hence, the inhibition of the hydroxyl radical was evaluated as follows: all test samples (2 mg/mL) were first dissolved in methanol and 10-110 μL sample solution was taken into mini tubes, and the methanol then removed at 80 °C to eliminate its interference. The reactions were performed in 0.2 M phosphate buffer (pH 7.4), containing 2.8 mmol/L deoxyribose, 2.8 mmol/L H_2O_2, 25 μM $FeCl_3$, 80 μM Na_2EDTA, and the test sample (20-220 μg). The reaction was started by adding ascorbic acid to a final concentration of 100 μM, and the reaction mixture (800 μL in total) was incubated for 20 min at 50°C in a water bath. After incubation, the color was developed by addition of 0.5 mL 2-thiobarbituric acid (1 g/100 mL) followed by 0.5 mL trichloroacetic acid (5 g/100 mL) and heating in an oven at 105°C for 15 min. The sample was cooled and its absorbance was measured at 532 nm against buffer (as blank). The reaction mixture without test sample was used as control. The scavenging activity on hydroxyl radicals was expressed as: Inhibition % = $(1 - A/A_c) \times 100\%$. Where A_c is the absorbance at 532 nm of control (without sample), and A is the absorbance at 532 nm of the reaction mixture containing sample.

Reducing power assay

Ferric ions (Fe^{3+}) reducing power

Ferric cyanide (Fe^{3+}) reducing power was determined by the method of Oyaizu [18], as described by Li *et al.* [15]. Sample solutions (1 mg/mL, x mL, x = 20, 40, 60, 80, 100, 120 μL) were mixed with Na_2HPO_4 / KH_2PO_4 buffer (350-x μL, 0.2 M, pH 6.6) and $K_3Fe(CN)_6$ (250 μL, 1 g/100 mL). The mixture was incubated at 50°C for 20 min, before 250 μL of trichloroacetic acid (10 g/100 mL) was added, and the mixture centrifuged at 3000 *g* for 10 min. The supernatant (400 μL) was recovered, mixed with distilled water (400 μL) and $FeCl_3$ (400 μL, 0.1 g/100 mL) and placed immediately into the spectrophotometer (Unico 2100, Shanghai, China), and the timer started. The absorbance at 700 nm was measured at 90 s. Samples were analyzed in groups of three samples, and when the analysis of one group was finished, the next group of three samples were mixed with $FeCl_3$ to avoid oxidization by air. Trolox and BHA were used as the positive controls, and an increased absorbance indicated increased reducing power. The percentage reducing power of the sample as compared with the maximum absorbance tested, which appeared in BHA at 83.3 μg/mL, was calculated by using the formula: $(A_s / A_m) \times 100$. Here, A_m =maximum absorbance tested , A_s = absorbance of sample.

Cupric ions (Cu^{2+}) reducing power

The cupric ions (Cu^{2+}) reducing power capacity was measured by Gülçin [19], with slight modification. Briefly, 125 μL $CuSO_4$ aqueous solution (10 mmol/L), 125 μL neocuproine ethanolic solution (7.5 mmol/L) and 500 μL CH_3COONH_4 buffer solution (100 mmol/L, pH 7.0) were added to test tubes with different volumes of MERC(1 mg/mL, 20-100 μL). Then, the total volume was adjusted with the buffer to 1 mL and mixed vigorously. Absorbance against a buffer blank was measured at 450 nm after 30 min. Increased absorbance of the reaction mixture indicates an increase of reduction capability. Trolox and BHA were used as the positive controls. The percentage reducing power of the sample as compared with the maximum absorbance tested, which appeared in BHA at 100 μg/mL, was calculated by using the formula: $(A_s /A_m) \times 100$. Here, A_m = maximum absorbance tested, A_s = absorbance of sample.

Determination of total phenolics

The total phenolics content of MERC was determined using a modified Folin-Ciocalteu colorimetric method [20], with CA (caffeic acid) as a standard. The MERC (5 mg/mL, 500μL) was mixed with the Folin-Ciocalteu reagent (0.25 mmol/L, 500 μL) and 15% sodium carbonate solution (Na_2CO_3 ,1.0 mL). The mixture was centrifuged at 3500 ***g*** for 3 min after incubation for 30 minutes at room temperature. The absorbance of supernatant was determined at 760nm and the total phenolics content was expressed as caffeic acid equivalent (CAE) in milligram per gram dry extract.

Caffeic acid determination using HPLC

HPLC analysis was performed using Techcomp LC2000, Dikma Diamonsil C_{18} (250 mm×4.6 mm, 5 μm particle size). The mobile phase consisted of solvent A (acetonitrile) and solvent B (0.1 % acetic acid in water), the flow rate was 0.5 mL/min, injection volume was 10 μL and absorption was measured at 323 nm. The content of caffeic acid in the MERC was obtained on the basis of the standard calibration curve.

Statistical analysis

Results were reported as the mean ± standard error of three measurements and analyzed by SPSS (Version 10.0). The IC_{50} values were calculated by linear regression analysis and all linear regression in this paper was analyzed by Origin 6.0 professional software. One-way analysis of variance (ANOVA) and multiple comparisons were carried out to test any significant difference between the means. A *P* value of less than 0.05 was considered to be significant.

Results

Scavenging ability on DPPH•

As DPPH• is a stable free radical, it is widely used for radical scavenging assay.[19] The radical can dissolve in methanol or ethanol, and their colors show characteristic absorption at 519 nm. When an antioxidant scavenges the free radical by hydrogen donation, the colors in the DPPH• assay solutions become lighter.[14] As presented in Figure 1, the radical-scavenging effect of MERC on DPPH• was in a concentration-dependent manner and had an effective capacity at high concentration. The scavenging effect of MERC and the positive controls on the DPPH radical decreased in the order of Trolox(96.8%) ≈ BHA(93.1.5%) > RC (79.6%), at the concentration of 80 μg/mL. The IC_{50} values of RC, Trolox and BHA were 44.26 ± 0.62, 4.02 ± 0.71, and 2.03 ± 0.28 μg /mL, respectively (Table 1).

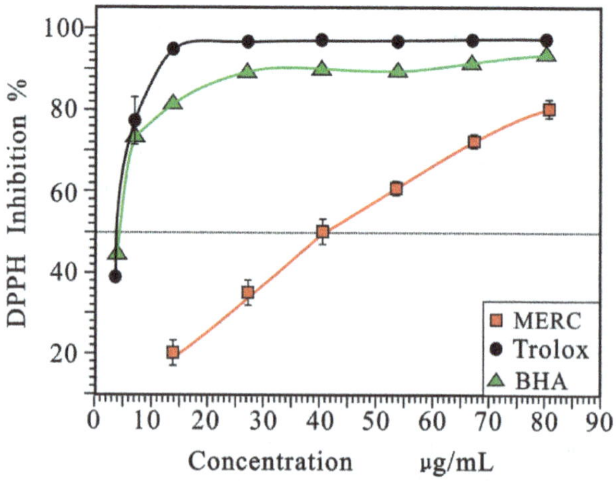

Figure 1. Radical-scavenging activity on DPPH• of MERC and positive controls.
(Each value is expressed as mean ± standard deviation, n =3. MERC, methanolic extract from Rhizoma Cibotii.)

Scavenging ability on $ABTS^{•+}$

Unlike the reactions with DPPH•, which involve H-atom transfer, the reactions with $ABTS^+$ involve an electron-transfer process. Generation of the $ABTS^{+}$• cation forms the basis of one of the spectrophotometric methods that have been applied to the measurement of the total antioxidant activity of pure substances, aqueous mixtures.[21] As presented in Figure 2, the scavenging ability of MERC on $ABTS^{+}$• was enhancing along with its concentration and was similar to the positive controls at high concentration. As listed in Table 1, the IC_{50} of MERC, BHA and Trolox were 19.84 ± 0.31, 2.03 ± 0.28 and 1.49 ± 0.00 μg/mL, respectively. Although the IC_{50} of RC was higher than BHA and Trolox, it still showed an effective antioxidant capacity.

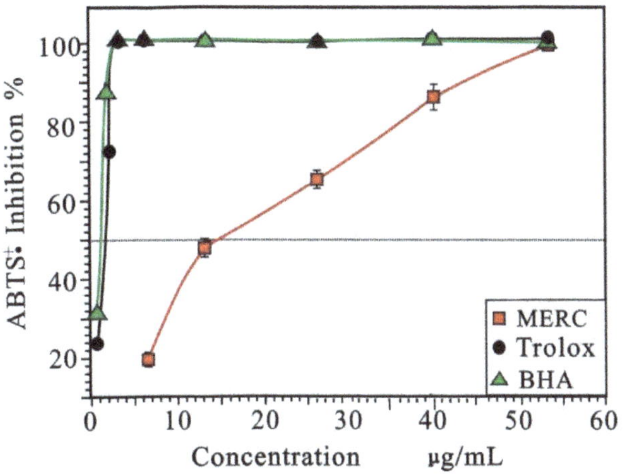

Figure 2. Radical-scavenging activity on •$ABTS^{+}$ of MERC and positive controls.
(Each value is expressed as mean ± standard deviation, n =3. MERC, methanolic extract from Rhizoma Cibotii.)

Scavenging ability on •O_2^-

Superoxide anion (•O_2^-) is one of the most important free radicals in living cells. As Figure 3 shown, the •O_2^- radical-scavenging effect of MERC was in a dose-response manner. As listed in Table 1, the IC_{50} of MERC, BHA and Trolox were 137.66±2.90, 2568.62±11.78, 799.11±72.30 μg/mL, respectively. So, MERC exhibited stronger •O_2^--scavenging activity than the positive controls.

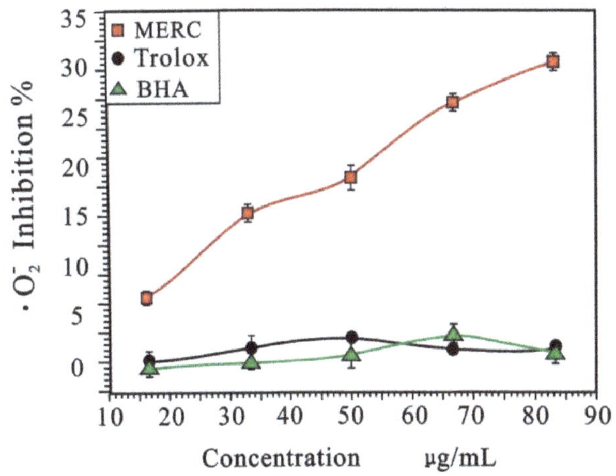

Figure 3. Radical-scavenging activity on O_2^-• of MERC and positive controls.
(Each value is expressed as mean ± standard deviation, n =3. MERC, methanolic extract from Rhizoma Cibotii.)

Scavenging ability on •OH

Hydroxyl radical (•OH) is also one of the most important free radicals in living cells. However, as the most dangerous form of ROS, it has a high reactivity with a very half-life of approx. 10^{-9} s *in vivo*.[22] In the study, the •OH scavenging activity was evaluated by the Fenton reaction using the deoxyribose assay. A mixture of Fe^{3+}-EDTA, hydrogen peroxide (H_2O_2), and ascorbic acid were used to generate hydroxyl radicals (•OH). The response degrades D-2-deoxyribose into fragments which under heating with 2-thiobarbituric acid at acidic solution, are detected at 540 nm because they generate a pink chromogen. Figure 4 revealed that the percentage •OH scavenging effect of MERC and the positive controls (Trolox and BHA) were in concentration-dependent manners. Their relative scavenging activity on •OH decreased in the order of BHA ≈ RC > Trolox. Their IC_{50} (showed in Table 1) were 22.94 ± 0.90, 26.39 ± 0.28 and 41.84 ± 3.79 μg/mL, respectively.

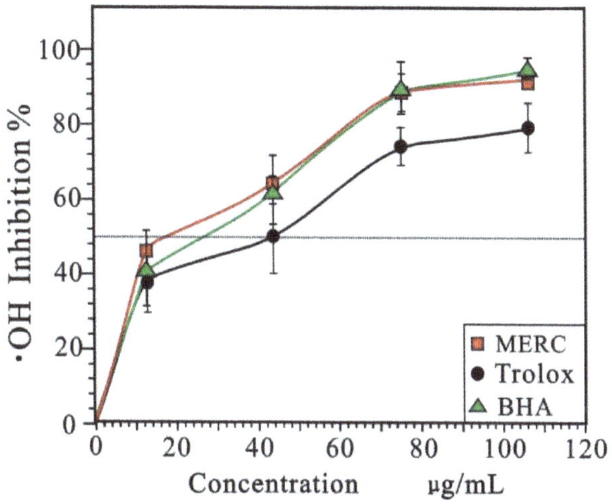

Figure 4. Radical-scavenging activity on •OH of MERC and positive controls.
(Each value is expressed as mean ± standard deviation, n =3. MERC, methanolic extract from Rhizoma Cibotii.)

Reducing power

Many reports have revealed that there is a direct correlation between antioxidant activities and reducing power.[23] Hence, reducing capacity may serve as a significant indicator of its potential antioxidant activity. As shown in Figure 5, it can be seen that the reducing power percentage values of MERC and the positive controls (BHA and Trolox) increased with the increasing of sample concentration in the range of the tested concentration. Their relative reducing powers on Cu^{2+} were as follows: BHA >Trolox > MERC. Their IC_{50} were 34.14 ± 0.26, 44.96 ± 0.60, 289.73 ± 46.17 μg/mL, respectively. The similar result could be also observed in Cu^{2+} reducing power assay as presented in Figure 6. The IC_{50} of MERC, BHA and Trolox were 523.52 ± 1.51, 5.74 ± 0.23 and 11.32 ± 0.09 μg/mL, respectively.

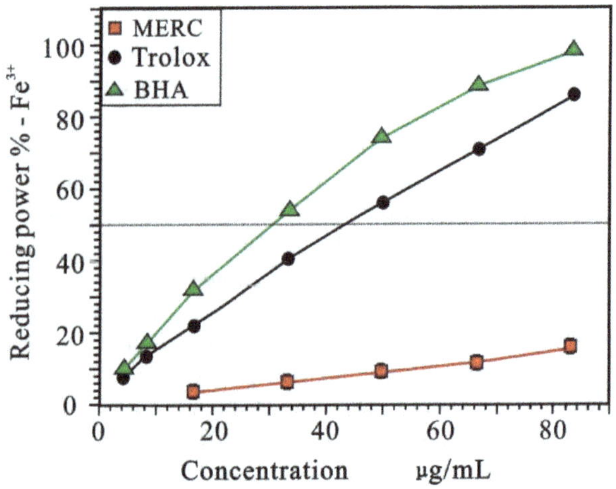

Figure 5. Reducing activity on Fe^{3+} of MERC and positive controls.
(Each value is expressed as mean ± standard deviation, n =3. MERC, methanolic extract from Rhizoma Cibotii.)

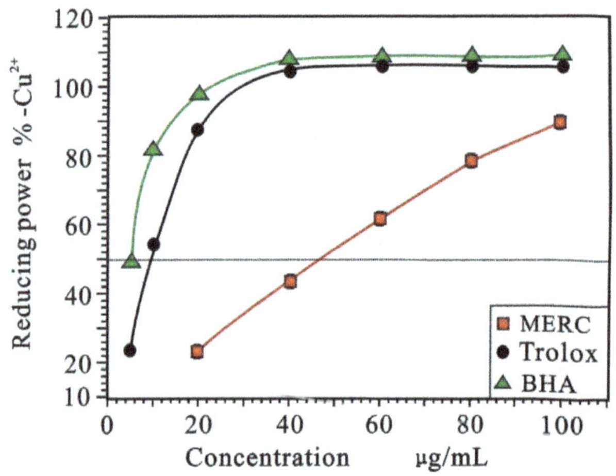

Figure 6. Reducing activity on Cu^{2+} of MERC and positive controls.
(Each value is expressed as mean ± standard deviation, n =3. MERC, methanolic extract from Rhizoma Cibotii.)

Table 1. The IC_{50} values of MERC and positive controls (µg/mL)

Assays	Rhizoma Cibotii	BHA	Trolox
DPPH	44.26 ± 0.62 [a,b]	2.03 ± 0.28	4.02 ± 0.71
ABTS	19.84 ± 0.31 [a,b]	2.03 ± 0.28	1.49 ± 0.00
• O_2^-	137.66 ± 2.90 [a,b]	2568.62 ± 11.78	799.11 ± 72.30
• OH	22.94 ± 0.90 [a,b]	26.39 ± 0.28	41.84 ± 3.79
Reducing power (Fe^{3+})	289.73 ± 46.17 [a,b]	34.14 ± 0.26	44.96 ± 0.60
Reducing power (Cu^{2+})	53.52 ± 1.51 [a,b]	5.74 ± 0.23	11.32 ± 0.09

All values were mean ± SD (n=3). Results were analyzed by ANOVA. Value with [a] significantly different from Trolox ($P < 0.05$); Value with [b] significantly different from BHA ($P < 0.05$). MERC, methanolic extract from Rhizoma Cibotii.

Total phenolics content

In this study, Folin-Ciocalteu method was used for determining total phenol content. The principle of the assay is described as follows: Folin-Ciocalteu reagent can oxidate the total phenols compounds quantificationally and is reduced to a blue compound and the color depth is positively related with the total phenols content. In the assay, caffeic acid was used as the standard and the result showed a good liner relationship, according to the linear regression equation: $y = 0.0653x + 0.102$ (R=0.994, x for sample amount, y for absorbance). The total phenolics content of MERC was 50.88 ± 1.24 mg CAE/ g.

Identification and quantification of caffeic acid by HPLC

Sample was identified by the peck symmetry and retention time, by comparison with reference substance at the same conditions. Chromatograms of caffeic acid and MERC were shown in Figure 7 & 8. According to the linear regression equation $y = 51374.17x - 197426.85$ (R=0.9992, x for sample amount, y for peak area), caffeic acid contents in MERC was calculated as 1.82 ± 0.19 mg/g.

Discussions

Our results showed that MERC and the standards dose-dependently increased the radical inhibition (or reducing power) values in all antioxidant assays, including DPPH•, ABTS•$^+$, •O_2^-, •OH, Fe^{3+} & Cu^{2+} reducing power assays, suggesting that RC had effective radical-scavenging activity or reducing powers.

On the other hand, a great deal of studies proved that the antioxidant activity of plants may likely be attributed to the phenolic content in it. Our data suggested that RC contained relatively high levels of total phenolics (50.88 ± 1.24 mg CAE/g). As previously mentioned, phytochemical study on RC had indicated the presence of phenolic compounds, including caffeic acid, protocatechuic acid, kaempferol, and onychin (Figure 9).

Since caffeic acid has been proved to be extremely versatile in pharmacological activity,[24] it was analyzed by HPLC method in the present study. The results revealed that the caffeic acid contents in MERC was calculated as 1.82 ± 0.19 mg/g and a higher ratio (1.82: 50.88) of caffeic acid *vs.* total phenolics content suggested that caffeic acid was one of main phenolic compounds in MERC.

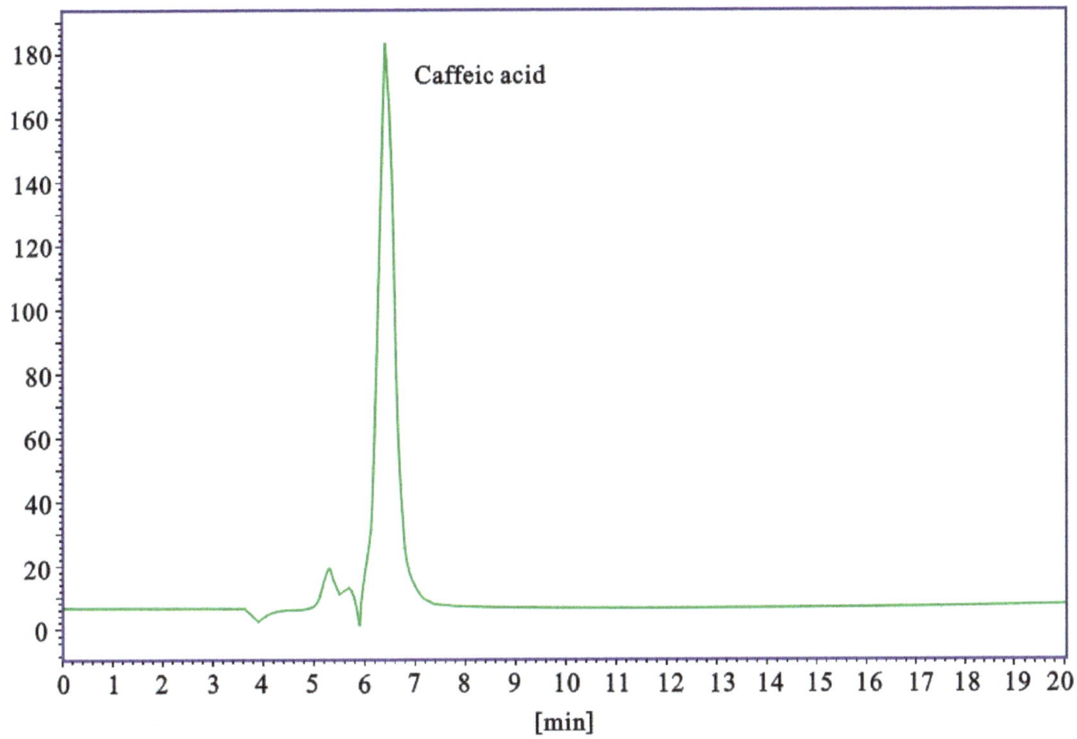

Figure 7. HPLC chromatogram of caffeic acid

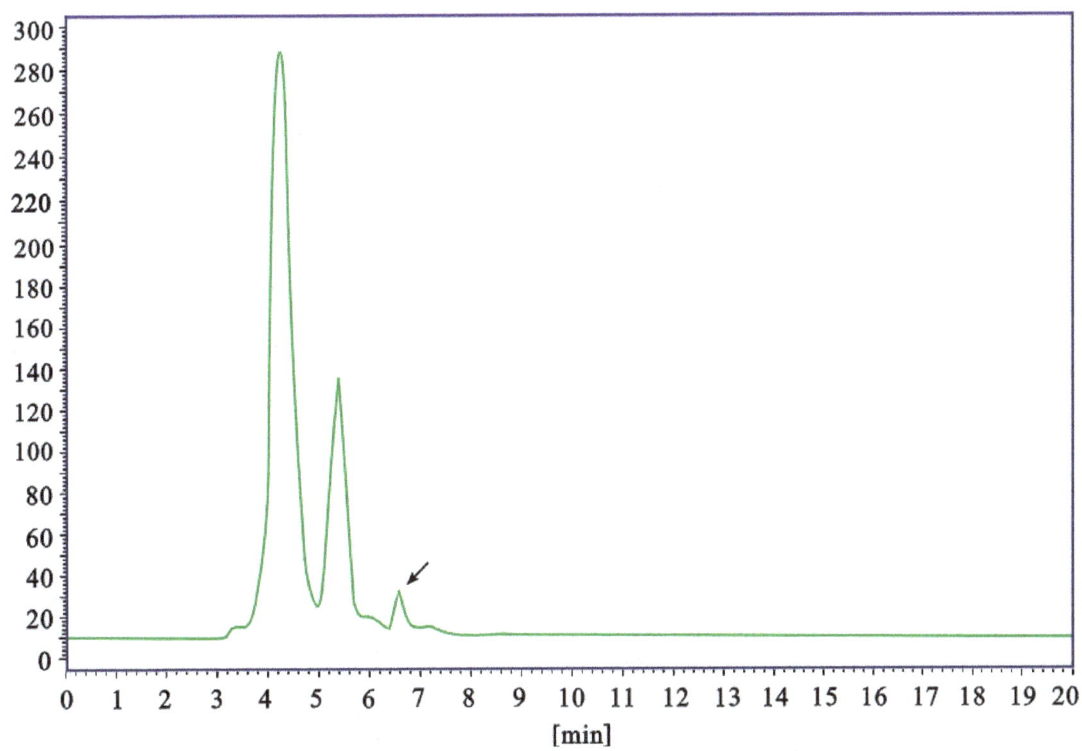

Figure 8. HPLC chromatogram of MERC (methanolic extract from Rhizoma Cibotii)

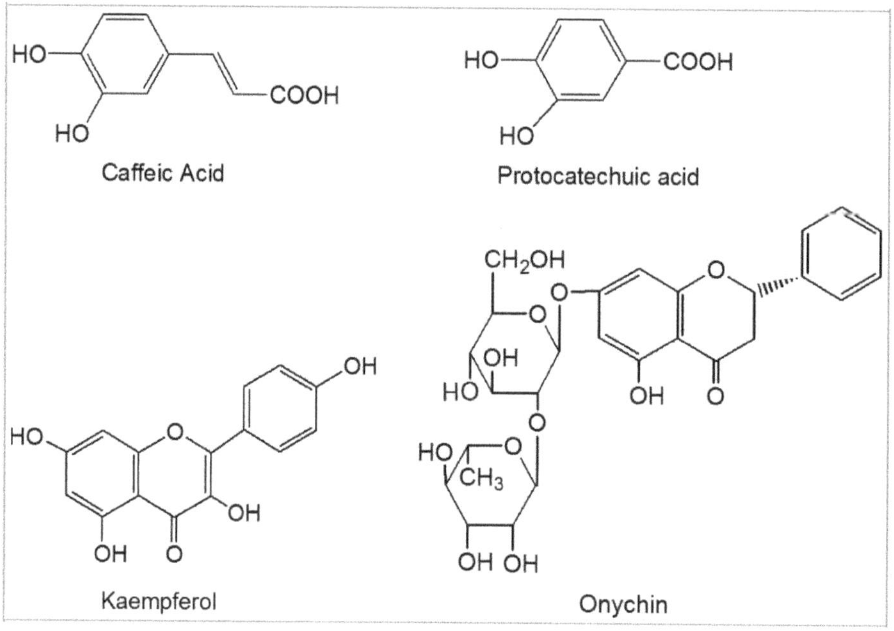

Figure 9. Chemical structure of caffeic acid, protocatechuic acid, kaempferol, and onychin

As described previously, besides phenolic compounds, other compounds were also found in RC and pharmacological investigations revealed that those compounds possessed different pharmacological effects, therefore, we assumed that the pharmacological effects or healthcare functions of whole RC is likely due to the synergistic effects caused by the combination of its components. Undoubtedly, antioxidant effect plays an important role in the synergistic effects.

Conclusion

As a traditional Chinese medicine herb, Rhizoma Cibotii possesses an effective *in vitro* antioxidant activity which can contribute to its medicinal or health-care effects. Its antioxidant activity may result from the radical-scavenging & reducing power, and can attribute to the total phenolics, among which caffeic acid is regarded as one of bioactive compounds.

Conflict of interests

The authors declare that they have no competing interests.

References

1. China Pharmacopoeia Committee: *Chinese Pharmacopoeia (Volume I)*. Beijing: Chemical Industry Press; 2010.
2. Xu ZY, Chen ZD, Chen ZL, Hou LB. The progress in research of *Cibotium barometz. Journal of Chinese Medicine Materials (Chinese)* 2000; 23: 160-161.
3. Zhao Y, Zhu JY, Zhang GJ. *Chinese Medicine (Basis and application of TCM)*. Beijing: People's Medical Publishing House; 2007.
4. Jia TZ, Zhang JP. Comparative Study on essential oil in Rhizoma Cibotii and processed product. *China Journal of Chinese Material Medica* 1996; 21:216-217.
5. Xu ZY, Chen ZD, Chen ZL, Hou LB, Zhang K. Studies on the Chemical Constituents of *Cibotium Barometz*(Ⅱ). *Pharmaceutical Journal of Chinese People's Liberation Army* 2000; 16:65-68.
6. Zhang CL, Wang ZX. Studies on the Constituents of *Cibotium barometz* (L) J. Sm. Rhizome. *Chinese Journal of Medicinal Chemistry*. 2001; 11:279-280.
7. Cheng QH, Yang ZL, Hu YM. Studies on the chemical constituents of Rhizoma Cibotii. *Progress in Pharmaceutical Sciences* 2003; 27:298-299.
8. Xu ZY, Yan Y, Chen ZD, Chen ZL, Zhang K. Studies on the Chemical Constituents of *Cibotium Barometz* (Ⅱ). *Pharmaceutical Journal of Chinese People's Liberation Army* 2004; 20:337-339.
9. Hu YW, Yu JL. Advances in Study on Chemical Constituents and Pharmacological effects of Rhizoma Cibotii. *LiShiZhen Medicine and Medica Medica Research* 2006; 17:275-276.
10. Yuan Z, Yu JT, Su SW. Determination of Protocatechuic Acid and Caffeic Acid in Rhizoma Cibotii and Rhizoma Pteris by TLCs. *Journal of Shenyang Pharmaceutical University* 2000; 17:338-340.
11. Yang FX, Zhu BY, Zheng X, Hu JF, Ge XL, Huang HL, Liao DF. Protective Effect of Onychin on Lipid Peroxidation in Experimental Liver Damage of Mice. *Journal of Nanhua University (Medical Edition)* 2002; 30:4-6.
12. Kim J K, Choi S J, Cho H Y. Protective effects of kaempferol(3,4′,5,7-tetrahydroxyflavone) against amyloid beta peptide (Abeta)-induced neurotoxicity in ICR mice. *Biosci Biotechnol Biochem*. 2010;

74(2):397-401.

13. Zhang J, Zhao CC, Han WN, Liu FZ. Effects of Flavonoids on Myocardial Apoptosis. Chinese Pharmacological Bulletin 2008, 24:635-639.Xu ZY, Chen ZD, Chen ZL, Hou LB. The progress in research of *Cibotium barometz*. *Journal of Chinese Medicine Materials (Chinese)* 2000; 23:160-161.
14. Ling GT: *Antioxidant food and health (Chinese)*. Beijing: Chemical Industry Press; 2004.
15. Li XC, Wu XT, Huang L. Correlation between antioxidant activities and phenolic contents of Radix Angelica Sinensis (Danggui) *Molecules.* 2009; 14: 5349-5361.
16. Marklund S, Marklund G. Involvement of the superoxide anion radical in the autoxidation of pyrogallol and convenient assay for superoxide dismutase. *European Journal of Biochemistry* 1974; 47: 469-474.
17. Kitts DD, Arosha, N W, Chun H. Antioxidant properties of a North American ginseng extract. *Molecular and Cellular Biochemistry* 2000; 203: 1-10.
18. Oyaizu M. Studies on product of browning reaction prepared from glucose amine. *Japanese Journal of Nutrition* 1986; 44: 307-315.
19. Gülçin İ. Antioxidant properties of resveratrol: A structure-activity insight. *Innovative Food Science and Emerging Technologies* 2010; 11: 210-218.
20. Lacikova L, Muselik J, Msterova I, Grancai D. Antioxidant Activity and Total Phenols in Different Extracts of Four *Staphylea* L. Species. *Molecules*2007; 12: 98-102.
21. Re R, Pellegrini N, Proteggente A, Pannala A, Yang M, Rice-Evans C. Antioxidant activity applying an improved $ABTS^{+}$ radical cation decolorization assay. *Free Radical Biology and Medicine* 1999; 26: 1231-1237.
22. Valko M, Leibfritz D, Moncol J, Cronin MTD, Mazur M, Telser J. Free radicals and antioxidants in normal physiological functions and human disease. *The International Journal of Biochemistry & Cell Biology* 2007; 39: 44-84.
23. Yildirim A, Mavi A, Kara AA. Determination of antioxidant and antimicrobial activities of *Rumex crispus* L. extracts. *Journal of Agricultural and Food Chemistry* 2001; 49:4083-4089.
24. Touaibia M, Jean-Francois, Doiron J. Caffeic Acid, a Versatile Pharmacophore: An Overview. *Mini Reviews in Medicinal Chemistry* 2011; 11(8):695-713.

Synthesis and Pharmacological Evaluation of Some New Pyrimidine Derivatives Containing 1,2,4-Triazole

Shantaram Gajanan Khanage[1]*, S. Appala Raju[2], Popat Baban Mohite[3], Ramdas Bhanudas Pandhare[3]

[1] *Research scholar, Department of Pharmacy, Vinayaka Missions University, Salem, Sankari main road, NH-47, Tamilnadu, India.*

[2] *Department of Pharmaceutical chemistry, H.K.E.'S College of Pharmacy, Sedam road, Gulbarga, Karnataka, India.*

[3] *Department of Pharmaceutical chemistry, M.E.S. College of Pharmacy, Sonai, Tq-Newasa, Dist.-Ahmednagar, Maharashtra, India.*

ARTICLE INFO

Keywords:
Chalcones
Condensation
Dihydropyrimidine
Antimicrobial activity
MES activity
Antitumor agent

ABSTRACT

Purpose: An efficient method has been described for synthesis of 6-(substituted aryl)-4-(3,5-diphenyl-1H-1,2,4-triazol-1-yl)-1, 6-dihydropyrimidine-2-thiol, as a beneficial antimicrobial, anticonvulsant and anticancer agents. ***Methods:*** The clalcones of title compounds were synthesized in three steps and subsequently these chalcones were further reacted with thiourea in the presence of KOH in ethanol, which led to the formation of dihydropyrimidine derivatives (4a-j). Compounds 4a-j were screened for their *in vitro* antimicrobial activity by agar well method and their anticonvulsant activity by the MES model. Anticancer activity of two newly synthesized heterocycles were evaluated at National Cancer Institute (NCI) Maryland, USA against 60 cell lines of different human tumor at a single dose of 10^{-5}M. ***Results:*** Compound 4b, 4c, 4d, 4i and 4j were exhibited significant antimicrobial potential against tested strains at 50µg/ml and 100µg/ml concentrations. Out of the ten compounds studied 4a, 4b, 4c, 4h and 4j showed comparable MES activity to Phenytoin and Carbamazepine after 0.5h. Tested compounds did not showed to be more potent than standard drugs after 4h. Compound 4a and 4d were found active on Non-Small Cell Lung Cancer (HOP-92). ***Conclusion:*** Ten noveldihydropyrimidine analogues has been synthesized, characterized and found to bepromising antibacterial, anticonvulsant and antitumor agents.

Introduction

Heterocycles bearing a symmetrical triazole moiety were reported to show a broad spectrum of pharmacological properties like anticancer,[1,2] antimicrobial,[3-6]anticonvulsant,[7] antiinflammatory, analgesic[8,9] antidepressant,[10] antitubercular,[11,12] antimalarial[13] and hypoglycemic[14] activities. The pyrimidine ring system is a six membered heterocyclic ring structure composed of two nitrogen atoms and used in the synthesis of pharmaceuticals. The pyrimidine moiety is a versatile lead molecule in pharmaceutical development and has a wide range of biological activities. In the past few years, the therapeutic interest of pyrimidine derivatives in pharmaceutical and medicinal field has been given a great attention to the medicinal chemist. Literature survey reveals that pyrimidine derivatives are well known to have antimicrobial,[15-17] antimalarial,[18] anticonvulsant,[19] anticancer,[20] antiinflammatory, analgesic,[21,22] antitubercular[23] activities. In recent years, the extensive studies have been focused on pyrimidine derivatives because of their diverse chemical reactivity, accessibility and wide range of biological activities. We have recently reported the *in vitro* antimicrobial potential of 1-(3,5-diphenyl-1H-1,2,4-triazol-1-yl)-3-(substituted aryl) prop-2-en-1-one (chalcones) and MIC values of different derivatives were determined by liquid broth method.[24]

The widespread properties of 1,2,4-triazoles and pyrimidines have prompted us to synthesize them in single molecular framework in order to study their pharmacological activity. Hence, the present investigation was undertaken to study the antimicrobial, anticonvulsant and antitumorpotential ofpyrimidine derivatives containing 1,2,4-triazole moiety. In this dissertation, we achieved the successful synthesis and significant antimicrobial, anticonvulsant and anticancer potential of a series of 6-(substituted aryl)-4-(3,5-diphenyl-1*H*-1,2,4-triazol-1-yl)-1,6-dihydropyrimidine-2-thiol (4a-j).

Materials and methods

The chemicals and solvents used for the experimental work were commercially procured from E. Merck India and Qualigens India. The melting points of all synthesized compounds were determined by open tube capillary using Thermonik precision apparatus in

***Corresponding author:** Shantaram Gajanan Khanage, M.E.S. College of Pharmacy, Sonai, At post-Sonai, Tq-Newasa, Dist.-Ahmednagar, Maharashtra-414105, India. Email: shantaram1982@gmail.com

Celsius scale and uncorrected. IR spectra were recorded using KBr pellets on PERKIN ELMER 8201 PC IR spectrophotometer, ^{1}H-NMR spectra of the final compounds 4a-j were recorded on BRUKER DRX NMR spectrometer (400 MHz). All spectra were obtained in DMSO. Mass spectra (FAB-MS) of compounds 4a-j were recorded on 70V on JEOL D-300 spectrophotometer (Jeol Ltd., Tokyo, Japan). Elemental analysis for C, H and N were performed on a PERKIN ELMER 240 elemental analyzer.

Synthesis protocol

Compounds 1, 2, and 3a-j were synthesized according to the reported method.[24]

Synthesis of 3,5-diphenyl-1H-1,2,4-triazole (1)

Benzohydrazide (0.1 mole) was dissolved in methanol, to this solution benzamide (0.1 mole) was added and stirred to get clear solution, then the resulting reaction mixture was refluxed for two hours on water bath. Therafter the reaction mixture was cooled at room temperature and poured in ice cold water to get precipitated 3,5-diphenyl-1*H*-1,2,4-triazole. Then obtained product was recrystallized by dioxane:ethanol mixture with an yield 83 %, m.p. 196-198°C.

Synthesis of 1-(3,5-diphenyl-1H-1, 2, 4-triazol-1-yl) ethanone (2)

To a solution of compound 1 (0.05 mole) dissolved in methanol, acetic anhydride (0.05 mole) and 2-3 drops of concentrated sulfuric acid were added, then the resulting reaction mixture was warmed on a water bath for 20 min. The reaction mixture was cooled at room temperature and poured in to ice cold water to get precipitate of compound 2. The precipitate of compound 2 was purified by dioxane:ethanol mixture with an yield 76 %, m.p. 176-178°C.

General procedure for synthesis of 1-(3,5-diphenyl-1H-1,2,4-triazol-1-yl)-3-(substituted aryl) prop-2-en-1-one(Chalcones) 3a-j

Compound 2 (0.05 mole) in methanol was treated with substituted aromatic aldehydes (0.05 mole) and 20% 10 ml NaOH, afterward stirred the reaction mixture for 7-8 hours at room temperature. The mixture was poured in ice cold water to get precipitate of compounds 3a-j, subsequently recrystallized by dioxane:ethanol mixture.

General procedure for synthesis of 6-(substituted aryl)-4-(3,5-diphenyl-1H-1,2,4-triazol-1-yl)-1,6-dihydropyrimidine-2-thiol (4a-j)

A mixture of 0.01 mole of the required chalcones (3a-j), 0.01 mole thiourea and KOH (1gm) in 20 ml ethanol was heated under reflux for 6 hours, then cooled and poured on to crushed ice. The solid product obtained was filtered and recrystallized from dioxane:ethanol mixture.

Physical and spectral data of the compounds 4a-j are mentioned bellow.

Physical and spectral data of compounds 4a-j.

***6-(4-chlorophenyl)-4-(3,5-diphenyl-1H-1,2,4-triazol-1-yl)-1,6-dihydropyrimidine-2-thiol* (4a).**

Yield 67 %, m.p. 120-122°C. Elemental analysisFound C 64.89; H 4.02; N 15.70, Calculated for ($C_{24}H_{18}ClN_5S$), C 64.93; H 4.09; N 15.78.IR(KBr, cm^{-1}): 2940, 3075, 3151 (Ar-CH), 1629 (C=N, triazole), 1415 (C=C, pyrimidine), 787 (-Cl), 2626 (-SH). MS m/z: 443(M^+). ^{1}H NMR (400 MHZ, DMSO) δ: 7.69-8.40 (14H, m, Ar-H), 4.46 (d, 1H, NH-C<u>H</u>), 5.92 (d, 1H, CH), 13.39 (S, 1H, Ar-SH), 5.27 (s, 1H, NH).

***6-(2-chlorophenyl)-4-(3,5-diphenyl-1H-1,2,4-triazol-1-yl)-1,6-dihydropyrimidine-2-thiol*(4b).**

Yield 71 %, m.p. 125-127°C. Elemental analysisFound C 64.84; H 4.12; N 15.72, Calculated for ($C_{24}H_{18}ClN_5S$), C 64.93; H 4.09; N 15.78.IR(KBr, cm^{-1}): 2939, 3073, 3175 (Ar-CH), 1624 (C=N, triazole), 1419 (C=C, pyrimidine), 779 (-Cl), 2616 (-SH). MS m/z: 443(M^+). ^{1}H NMR (400 MHZ, DMSO) δ: 7.65-8.47(14H, m, Ar-H), 4.48 (d, 1H, NH-C<u>H</u>), 5.94 (d, 1H, CH), 13.41 (S, 1H, Ar-SH), 5.25 (s, 1H, NH).

***6-(3-nitrophenyl)-4-(3,5-diphenyl-1H-1,2,4-triazol-1-yl)-1,6-dihydropyrimidine-2-thiol*(4c).**

Yield 65 %, m.p. 107-109°C. Elemental analysisFound C 63.44; H 4.06; N 18.40, Calculated for ($C_{24}H_{18}N_6O_2S$), C 63.42; H 3.99; N 18.49.IR(KBr, cm^{-1}): 2942, 3078, 3180 (Ar-CH), 1628 (C=N, triazole), 1417 (C=C, pyrimidine), 1551 (-NO_2), 2619 (-SH). MS m/z: 454(M^+). ^{1}H NMR (400 MHZ, DMSO) δ: 7.64-8.38 (14H, m, Ar-H), 4.45 (d, 1H, NH-C<u>H</u>), 5.96 (d, 1H, CH), 13.44 (S, 1H, Ar-SH), 5.26 (s, 1H, NH).

***6-(4-methoxyphenyl)-4-(3,5-diphenyl-1H-1,2,4-triazol-1-yl)-1,6-dihydropyrimidine-2-thiol*(4d).**

Yield 68 %, m.p. 130-132°C. Elemental analysisFound C 68.33; H 4.82; N 15.83, Calculated for ($C_{25}H_{21}N_5OS$), C 68.32; H 4.82; N 15.93.IR(KBr, cm^{-1}): 2947, 3075, 3181 (Ar-CH), 1625 (C=N, triazole), 1415 (C=C, pyrimidine), 1159 (-OCH_3), 2618 (-SH). MS m/z: 439(M^+). ^{1}H NMR (400 MHZ, DMSO) δ: 7.64-8.38 (14H, m, Ar-H), 4.44(d, 1H, NH-C<u>H</u>), 5.96 (d, 1H, CH), 13.55 (S, 1H, Ar-SH), 3.82 (3H, s, OCH_3),5.27 (s, 1H, NH).

***6-(4-dimethylaminophenyl)-4-(3,5-diphenyl-1H-1,2,4-triazol-1-yl)-1,6-dihydropyrimidine-2-thiol*(4e).**

Yield 74 %, m.p. 140-142°C. Elemental analysisFound C 69.06; H 5.33; N 18.57, Calculated for ($C_{26}H_{24}N_6S$), C 69.00; H 5.35; N 18.57.IR(KBr, cm^{-1}): 2939, 3076, 3174 (Ar-CH), 1623 (C=N, triazole), 1412 (C=C, pyrimidine), 3159, 3146 (-NCH_3), 2606 (-SH). MS m/z: 452(M^+). ^{1}H NMR (400 MHZ, DMSO) δ: 7.61-8. 56 (14H, m, Ar-H), 4.47(d, 1H, NH-C<u>H</u>), 5.90 (d, 1H, CH), 13.49 (S, 1H, Ar-SH), 3.19 (6H, s, -$N(CH_3)2$), 5.23 (s, 1H, NH).

***6-(phenyl)-4-(3,5-diphenyl-1H-1,2,4-triazol-1-yl)-1,6-dihydropyrimidine-2-thiol* (4f).**
Yield 72 %, m.p. 115-117°C. Elemental analysisFound C 70.36; H 4.60; N 17.19, Calculated for ($C_{24}H_{19}N_5S$), C 70.39; H 4.68; N 17.10.IR(KBr, cm^{-1}): 2946, 3072, 3182 (Ar-CH), 1621 (C=N, triazole), 1411 (C=C, pyrimidine), 2609 (-SH). MS m/z: 409(M^+). ^1H NMR (400 MHZ, DMSO) δ: 7.56-8.39 (15H, m, Ar-H), 4.45 (d, 1H, NH-C<u>H</u>), 5.93 (d, 1H, CH), 13.61 (S, 1H, Ar-SH), 5.29 (s, 1H, NH).

***6-(2-furul)-4-(3,5-diphenyl-1H-1,2,4-triazol-1-yl)-1,6-dihydropyrimidine-2-thiol*(4g).**
Yield 68 %, m.p. 111-123°C. Elemental analysisFoundC 66.12; H 4.34; N 17.44, Calculated for ($C_{22}H_{17}N_5OS$), C 66.15; H 4.29; N 17.53.IR(KBr, cm^{-1}): 2942, 3079, 3178 (Ar-CH), 1628 (C=N, triazole), 1416 (C=C, pyrimidine), 1224 (C-O-C), 2611 (-SH). MS m/z: 399(M^+). ^1H NMR (400 MHZ, DMSO) δ: 7.06-8. 37 (13H, m, Ar-H), 4.46 (d, 1H, NH-C<u>H</u>), 5.97(d, 1H, CH), 13.47 (S, 1H, Ar-SH), 5.28 (s, 1H, NH).

***6-(4-bromophenyl)-4-(3,5-diphenyl-1H-1,2,4-triazol-1-yl)-1,6-dihydropyrimidine-2-thiol*(4h).**
Yield 58 %, m.p. 117-119°C. Elemental analysisFound C 59.04; H 3.67; N 14.39, Calculated for ($C_{24}H_{18}BrN_5S$), C 59.02; H 3.71; N 14.34.IR(KBr, cm^{-1}): 2936, 3066, 3173 (Ar-CH), 1625 (C=N, triazole), 1413 (C=C, pyrimidine), 698 (-Br), 2615 (-SH). MS m/z: 488(M^+). ^1H NMR (400 MHZ, DMSO) δ: 7.55-8.48 (14H, m, Ar-H), 4.47 (d, 1H, NH-C<u>H</u>), 5.94 (d, 1H, CH), 13.38 (S, 1H, Ar-SH), 5.27 (s, 1H, NH).

***6-(4-hydroxyphenyl)-4-(3,5-diphenyl-1H-1,2,4-triazol-1-yl)-1,6-dihydropyrimidine-2-thiol*(4i).**
Yield 72 %, m.p. 127-129°C. Elemental analysisFoundC 67.79; H 4.49; N 16.42, Calculated for ($C_{24}H_{19}N_5OS$), C 67.74; H 4.50; N 16.46.IR(KBr, cm^{-1}): 2946, 3073, 3175 (Ar-CH), 1622 (C=N, triazole), 1412 (C=C, pyrimidine), 3357 (-OH), 2616 (-SH). MS m/z: 425(M^+). ^1H NMR (400 MHZ, DMSO) δ: 7.48-8.59 (14H, m, Ar-H), 4.49 (d, 1H, NH-C<u>H</u>), 5.96 (d, 1H, CH), 13.41 (S, 1H, Ar-SH), 10.16 (s, 1H, Ar-OH), 5.26 (s, 1H, NH).

***6-(2,4-dimethoxyphenyl)-4-(3,5-diphenyl-1H-1,2,4-triazol-1-yl)-1,6-dihydropyrimidine-2-thiol*(4j).**
Yield 65 %, m.p. 133-135°C. Elemental analysisFound C 66.59; H 4.89; N 14.92, Calculated for ($C_{26}H_{23}N_5O_2S$), C 66.50; H 4.94; N 14.91.IR(KBr, cm^{-1}): 2941, 3079, 3186 (Ar-CH), 1624 (C=N, triazole), 1416 (C=C, pyrimidine) 1155 ($-OCH_3$), 2626 (-SH). MS m/z: 469(M^+). ^1H NMR (400 MHZ, DMSO) δ: 7.31-8.44 (13H, m, Ar-H), 4.45 (d, 1H, NH-CH), 5.95 (d, 1H, CH), 13.39 (S, 1H, Ar-SH), 3.89 (6H, s, OCH_3), 5.28 (s, 1H, NH).

Pharmacological assessment

Antimicrobial Activity

The *in vitro* antimicrobial activity of the target compounds 4a-j was performed by agar well method (diffusion technique) against *S. aureus* NCIM 2079, *E. coli* NCIM 2065, *C. albicans* NCIM 3471 and *A. niger* NCIM 1196. The antibiotic Ampicillin and the antifungal agent Fluconazole were used as standard drugs for the study. The fresh bacterial culture was obtained by inoculating bacteria into peptone water liquid media and incubating at 37± 2 °C for 18-24 hours. This culture was mixed with nutrient agar media and poured in to Petri dishes. After culture media solidification four wells were made at equal distance by using a sterile steel cork borer (8mm diameter). In to these wells different concentrations of standard drug and synthesized compounds were introduced. Dimethyl Formamide (DMF) was used as a control. After introduction of standard drug and synthesized compounds, the plates were placed in a refrigerator at 8-10 °C for proper diffusion of drugs into the media. After two hours of cold incubation, the Petri plates were transferred to incubator and maintained at 37±2 °C for 18-24 hours. After the incubation period, the petri plates were observed for growth inhibition zone by using vernier scale. The results were evaluated by comparing the growth inhibition zone shown by the synthesized compounds with standard drugs. The results were presented as the mean value of growth inhibition zone measured in millimeters of three sets (Table 1). The standard drugs and synthesized compounds were dissolved in a minimum quantity of Dimethyl Formamide (DMF) and adjusted, to made up the volume with distilled water to get 50μg/ml and 100μg/ml concentrations.

Anticonvulsant Activity: Maximal Electroshock Seizure Test (MES)

The compounds 4a-j were screened for their anticonvulsant activity by Maximal electroshock seizure method. Study protocol was approved by the Institutional Animal Ethics Committee for the purpose of control and supervision on experiments on animals (IAEC, Approval No.1211/ac/08/CPCSEA) before experiment. Initial anticonvulsant evaluations of the test compounds were undertaken by following the anticonvulsant drug development (ADD) program protocol.[25] The animals Albino mice (20-25 g) of either sex were stimulated through corneal electrodes to 50 mA current at a pulse of 60 Hz applied for 0.2 s. Animals were previously given the test drug intraperitoneally. Abolition of the hind limb tonic extension spasm was recorded as the anticonvulsant activity. The test compounds were suspended in a 0.5% methyl cellulose-water mixture. In preliminary screening, each compound was administered through an intraperitoneally injection at three dose levels (30, 100 and 300 mg/kg) and the anticonvulsant activity was assessed after 0.5 h and 4 h intervals of administration. The anticonvulsant efficacy was evaluated by the maximal electroshock-induced seizure (MES) and screening data of compounds 4a-j are presented in Table 2.

Table 1. Antimicrobial activity of compounds 4a-j.

Compound	Zone of inhibition (in mm)							
	S. aureus		*E. coli*		*C. albicans*		*A. niger*	
	50μg	100μg	50μg	100μg	50 μg	100μg	50 μg	100μg
4a	19	21	18	23	20	23	18	21
4b	18	21	19	23	22	25	23	22
4c	21	24	24	24	19	22	18	23
4d	19	22	19	22	23	22	22	21
4e	18	19	17	20	20	21	19	20
4f	15	17	14	17	18	19	16	18
4g	16	19	17	20	15	19	17	21
4h	19	21	21	19	19	22	21	19
4i	21	19	22	20	21	18	22	22
4j	22	21	20	20	19	18	16	19
Ampicillin	21	25	24	26	-	-	-	-
Fluconazole	-	-	-	-	24	26	23	25
DMF	-	-	-	-	-	-	-	-

Table 2. Anticonvulsant and neurotoxicity screening of compounds 4a-j.

Sr. No.	Treatment	Ar	MES screen[a]		Neurotoxicity screen[a]	
			0.5h	4h	0.5h	4h
1	4a	4-Cl	30	300	300	_
2	4b	2-Cl	30	300	_	300
3	4c	$3\text{-}NO_2$	30	300	_	_
4	4d	$4\text{-}OCH_3$	100	300	300	300
5	4e	$4\text{-}N(CH_3)2$	100	300	_	300
6	4f	phenyl	100	300	300	300
7	4g	2-Furyl	100	300	_	_
8	4h	4-Br	30	300	300	300
9	4i	4-OH	100	300	_	300
10	4j	$2,4\text{-}OCH_3$	30	300	_	_
11	Phenytoin	_	30	30	100	100
12	Carbamazepine	_	30	100	300	300

"a" Doses of 30, 100 and 300 mg/kg were administered. The figures in the Table indicate the minimum dose whereby bioactivity was demonstrated in half or more of mice. The animals were examined 0.5 and 4 h after injections were given. The dash "-" indicates an absence of activity at maximum dose administered (300 mg/kg).

Neurotoxicity screening (NT)

The minimal motor impairment was measured in mice by the rotorod test.[26] The Albino mice (20-25 g) were trained to stay on an accelerating rotorod that rotated at 10 rotations/min and its diameter was 3.2 cm. Only those mice were taken for the test which could stay on the revolving rod for at least one minute. Trained animals were injected intraperitoneally with the test compounds at doses of 300 mg/kg. Neurotoxicity was indicated by the inability of the animal to maintain equilibration on the rod for at least for one minute.

Anticancer activity

Anticancer activity of newly synthesized heterocycles were evaluated. Primarily compounds submitted at National Cancer Institute (NCI) Maryland, USA andselected compounds were screened for anticancer activity against 60 cell lines of different human tumor, representing leukemia, melanoma and cancers of the lung, colon, brain, ovary, breast, prostate, and kidney for one dose against the 60 cell lines at a single dose of 10^{-5}M. The mean growth %, range of growth % and growth % relative to most sensitive cell line is depicted in Table 3.

Results and discussion

The synthesis of 6-(substituted aryl)-4-(3,5-diphenyl-1*H*-1,2,4-triazol-1-yl)-1,6-dihydropyrimidine-2-thiol derivatives (4a-j)depicted in Figure 1. The compound1-(3,5-diphenyl-1*H*-1,2,4-triazol-1-yl)ethanone (2) on condensation with various aromatic aldehydes in NaOH solution yielded the corresponding chalcones (3a-j). These chalcones were further reacted with thiourea in the presence of KOH in ethanol, which led to the formation of dihydropyrimidine derivatives (4a-j) (Figure 2). The structural assessments of compounds 4a-j were carried out by IR, ^{1}H-NMR, Mass spectra and elemental analysis.Structures of compounds 4a-j were confirmed IR, ^{1}H-NMR, mass spectra and elemental analysis. Infrared spectrum of compounds 4a-j showed a sharp absorption band frequencies for-NO_2, -Cl, OCH_3, -N-$(CH_3)_2$, -OH and -Br groups. Compounds 4a-j showed appropriate ^{1}H-NMR signals for aromatic protons and multiplets were observed in the range of δ 7.06-8.59. The ^{1}H NMR spectra showed a downfield singlet at around 13.4 ppm attributed to SH group. Mass spectraof the compounds 4a-j showed molecular ion peaks with high abundance at m/z in agreement with their molecular formula. Compounds 4a-j evaluated for their *in vitro* antimicrobial, anticonvulsant and anticancer activity.

Table 3. Anticancer screening data of selected compounds.

Compound No.	60 Cell lines in assay in 1-dose 10^{-5} M concentration			
(NSC code)	Mean growth (%)	Range growth (%)	Most sensitive cell line	Growth of most sensitive cell line (%)
4a (764753/1)	106.85	-27.71-55.23	Non-Small Cell Lung Cancer (HOP 92)	- 27.71
4d (764754/1)	103.26	-19.05-50.25	Non-Small Cell Lung Cancer (HOP 92)	-19.05

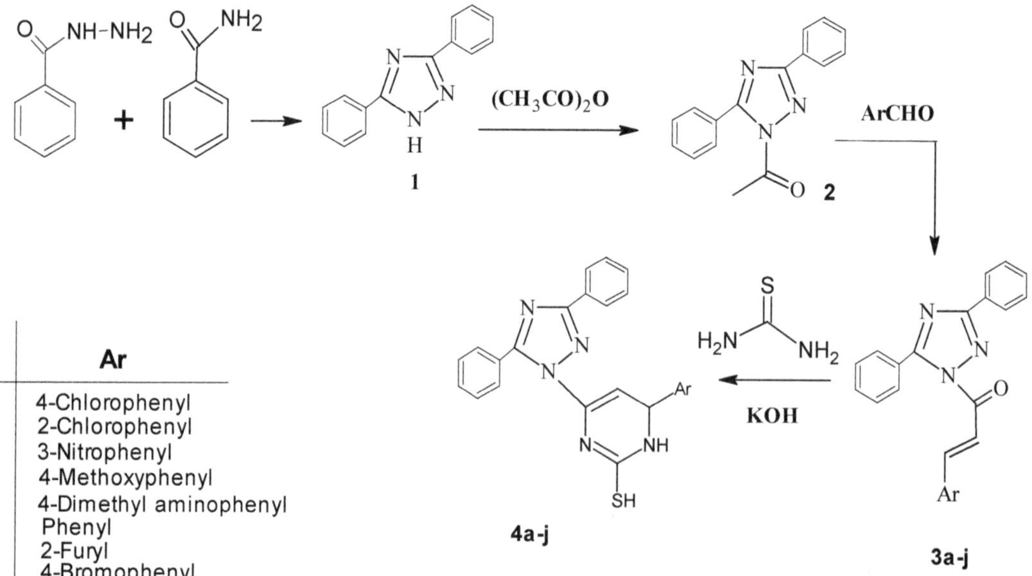

	Ar
3a and4a	4-Chlorophenyl
3b and4b	2-Chlorophenyl
3c and4c	3-Nitrophenyl
3d and4d	4-Methoxyphenyl
3e and4e	4-Dimethyl aminophenyl
3f and 4f	Phenyl
3g and4g	2-Furyl
3h and4h	4-Bromophenyl
3i and4i	4-Hydroxyphenyl
3j and4j	2, 4 -Dimethoxyphenyl

Figure 1. Synthesis of compounds 4a-j.

The *in vitro* antimicrobial activity of tested compounds was determined by agar well method. The results are summarized in Table 1. These antimicrobial data clearly indicated that the presence of methoxy, chloro, nitro and hydroxysubstitution on phenyl ring of the pyrimidine nucleus produced remarkable improvement in antimicrobial activity. Phenyl substitution is weakly active among the synthesized compounds. Compound 4c showed significant antibacterial activity against *S. aureus* and *E. coli*. Compound 4b showed fungicidal potential against *C. albicans* and *A. niger*. The *in vitro* antimicrobial study clearly reveals that pyrimidine derivatives (4a-j) were found to be significant antimicrobial agents probably due to pharmacologically active pyrimidine nucleus attached with 1,2,4-triazole.

The target compounds (4a-j) were tested for anticonvulsant activity by maximal electroshock induced seizure (MES) test. The anticonvulsant and neurotoxicity data of the compounds and standard drugs are presented in Table 2. The compounds that exhibited the most potent anti-MES activity included 4a, 4b, 4c, 4h and 4j which have activity comparable with Phenytoin and Carbamazepine. Minimal motor impairment was measured by the rotorod test. Compounds 4c, 4g, and 4j successfully passed the rotorod test without any sign of neurological deficit, whereas compounds 4d, 4f and 4h exhibited neurological deficit at the dose of 300 mg/kg *i.p.* Compounds with the electron withdrawing chloro substituent at the *ortho* and *para* position and bromo at *para* position on the phenyl ring of pyrimidine nucleus led to considerable increase in the activity but were relatively toxic. The presence of a bulkier electron donating methoxy group at *para* and *ortho* position on the phenyl ring of pyrimidine nucleus results increase in anticonvulsant activity. This may be due to the increase in lipophilicity of the compound. The nitro substituent at the *meta* position of the phenyl ring found to be equally active with chloro substitution but without sign of neurotoxity. The effect of the hydroxy, phenyl and furyl substitution were found to be less active compounds as compared to other tested compounds.

The compounds 4a and 4d were evaluated at single concentration of 10^{-5} M towards the panel of approximately 60 cancer cell lines derived from nine different cancer types. The mean growth %, range of growth % and growth % relative to most sensitive cell line is depicted in Table 3. The tested compounds showed a broad spectrum of growth inhibitory activity against human tumor cells, as well as some distinctive pattern of selectivity (Figure 3 and Figure 4). Compound 4a was found to be a highly active growth inhibitor of the Non-Small Cell Lung Cancer (HOP-92) and CNS Cancer cell line (SNB-75) with a growth % of most sensitive cell line to be - 27.71, whilst least active over other cell lines. The mean growth % for compound 4a was observed 106.85% and fall in a range - 27.71-55.23. Compound 4d showed selective antitumor sensitivity on Non-Small Cell Lung Cancer (HOP-92) and renal Cancer cell line (A498) with a growth % of most sensitive cell line to be -19.05, whilst least active over other cell lines. The mean growth % for compound 4d was observed 103.26% and fall in a range -19.05-50.25.

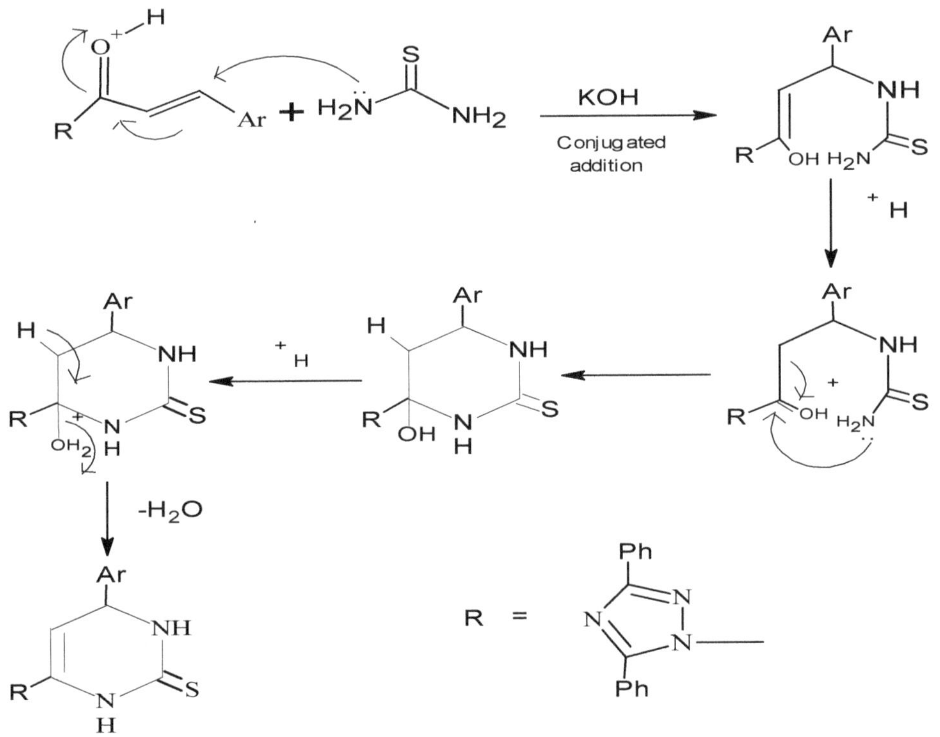

Figure 2. The possible mechanism involved in the formation of dihydropyrimidine derivatives (4a-j)from the respective chalcones is shown above.

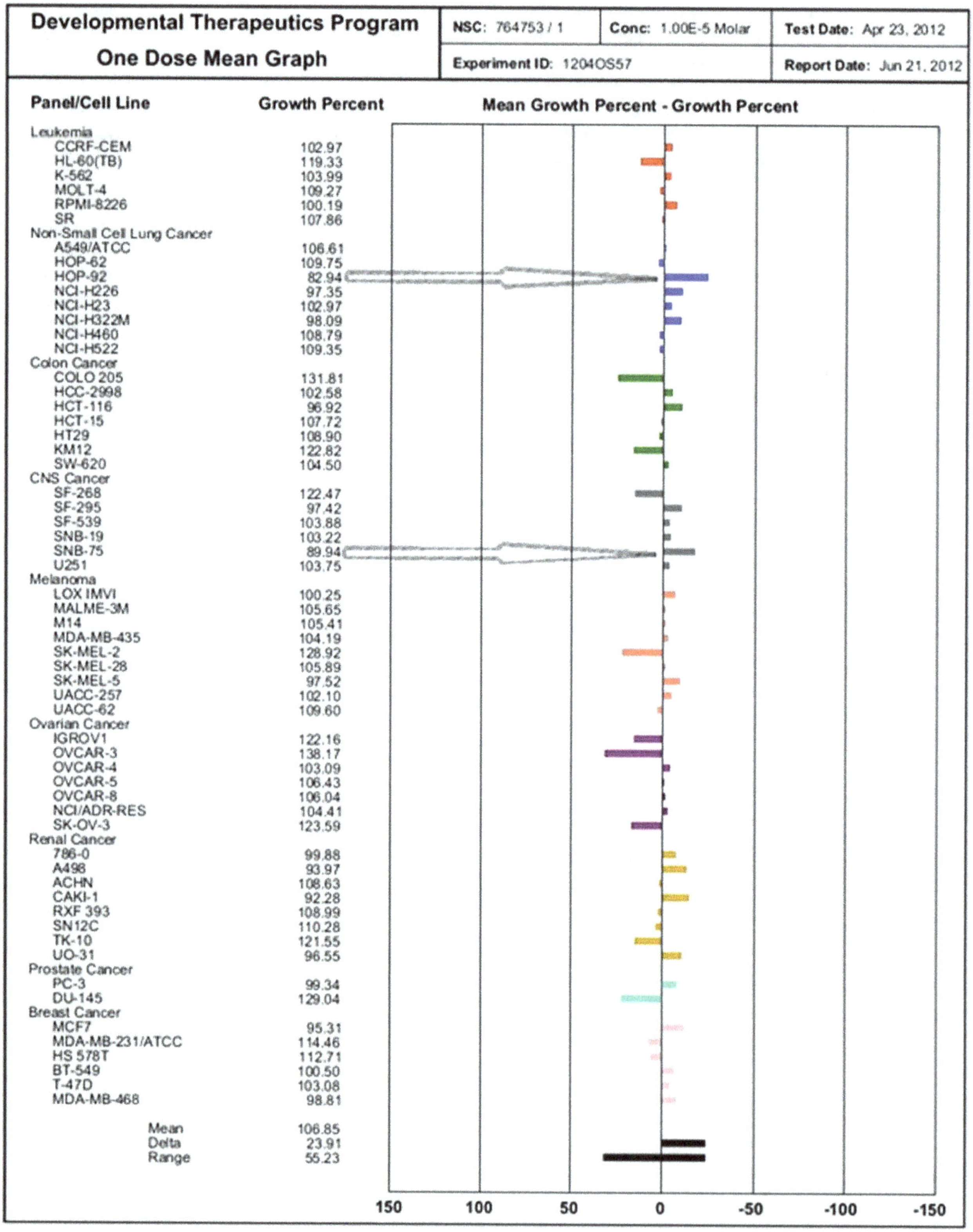

Figure 3. Selected NCI sixty cell screening data highlighting the potency of compound (4a: NSC: 764753/1) againstnon-Small Cell Lung Cancer (HOP-92) and CNS Cancer cell line (SNB-75). Bars to the right of the mean line represent cell lines more sensitive to test compound compared to mean, whereas bars to the left represent less sensitive cell lines.

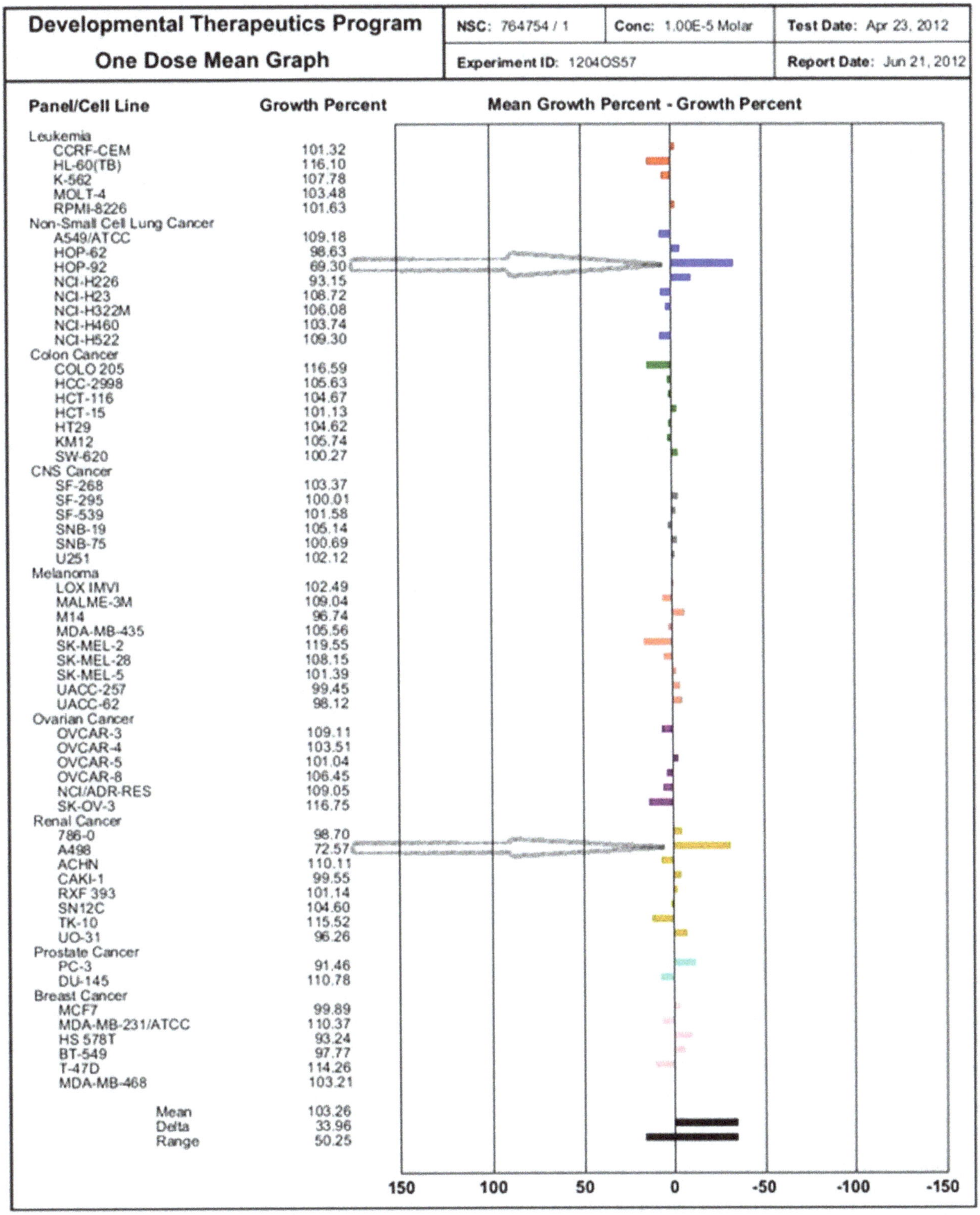

Figure 4. Selected NCI sixty cell screening data highlighting the potency of compound (4d: NSC: 764754/1) againstnon-Small Cell Lung Cancer (HOP-92) and renal Cancer cell line (A498). Bars to the right of the mean line represent cell lines more sensitive to test compound compared to mean, whereas bars to the left represent less sensitive cell lines.

Conclusion

In conclusion, new class of pyrimidine derivatives containing 1,2,4-triazole was synthesized and evaluated as antimicrobial, anticonvulsant and anticancer properties. The newly synthesized heterocycles exhibited promising antimicrobial activity against tested microorganisms. Compounds 4b, 4c, 4d, 4i and 4j were found to be the most active antimicrobial agents from synthesized series. From the anticonvulsant screening data it was found that of 6-(substituted aryl)-4-(3,5-diphenyl-1H-1,2,4-triazol-1-yl)-1,6-dihydropyrimidine-2-thiol derivatives (4a-j) have encouraging anticonvulsant activity in the MES screen. Compound 4a, 4b, 4c, 4h and 4j found to be effective anticonvulsant agent from tested compounds. In the present study two compounds (4a and 4d) were tested for anticancer activity and most of them displayed antitumor activity on cell lines of Non-Small Cell Lung Cancer, CNS Cancer and renal Cancer.These results suggest that novel triazolechalcones and pyrimidine derivatives are interesting lead molecules for further synthetic and biological evaluation.

Acknowledgments

We are highly thankful to IICT Hyderabad for providing spectral data, NCL Pune for providing micro organisms for this study, National Cancer Institute (NCI) Bethesda, USA for *in vitro* screening of our compounds in human cancer cell lines. We are also grateful of Principal M.E.S. College Pharmacy, Sonai and Prashant Patil Gadakh, Secreatary, Mula Education Society for providing excellent research facilities for this work.

Conflict of interest

The authors report no conflicts of interest.

References

1. Al-Soud YA, Al-Masoudi NA, Ferwanah AE. Synthesis and properties of new substituted 1,2,4-triazoles: Potential antitumor agents. Bioorg Med Chem 2003;11:1701-8.
2. Khanage SG, Mohite PB, Raju SA. Synthesis, Anticancer and Antibacterial Activity of Some Novel 1,2,4-Triazole Derivatives Containing Pyrazole and Tetrazole Rings. Asian J Res Chem 2011;4:567-73.
3. Lingappa B, Girisha KS, Kalluraya BN, Rai S, Kumari NS. Regioselective reaction: Novel Mannich bases derived from 3-(4,6-disubstituted-2-thiomethyl)3-amino-5-mercapto-1,2,4-triazoles and their antimicrobial properties. Ind J Chem 2008;47B:1858-64.
4. Rao G, Rajasekran S, Attimarad M. Synthesis and Antimicrobial activity of Some 5-phenyl-4-substituted amino-3-mercapto (4H) 1,2,4-triazoles. Ind J Pharm Sci 2000;6:475-7.
5. Jalilian AR, Sattari S, Bineshmarvasti M, Shafiee A, Daneshtalab M. Synthesis and in vitro antifungal and cytotoxicity evaluation of thiazolo-4H-1,2,4-triazoles and 1,2,3-thiadiazolo-4H-1,2,4-triazoles. Arch Pharm (Weinheim) 2000; 333:347-54.
6. Lazarevic M, Dimova V, Molnar GD, Kakurinov V, Colanceska RK. Synthesis of some N1-aryl/heteroarylaminomethyl/ethyl-1,2,4-triazoles and their antibacterial and antifungal activities. Hetero Comm 2001;7:577-82.
7. Chimirri A, Bevacqua F, Gitto R, Quartarone S, Zappala MD, Sarro A, et al. Synthesis and anticonvulsant activity of new 1-H-triazolo[4,5-c][2,3]benzodiaze-pines. Med Chem Res 1999;9:203-12.
8. Hunashal RD, Ronad PM, Maddi VS, Satyanarayana D, Kamadod MA. Synthesis, anti-inflammatory and analgesic activity of 2-[4-(substituted benzylideneamino)-5-(substitutedphenoxymethyl)-4H-1,2,4-triazol-3-yl-thio] acetic acid derivatives. Arab J Chem 2011;1-9.
9. Khanage SG, Mohite PB, Pandhare RB, Raju SA. Study of analgesic activity of novel 1,2,4-triazole derivatives bearing pyrazole and tetrazole moiety. J Pharm Res 2011;4:3609-11.
10. Kane MJ, Dudley MW, Sorensen MS, Miller FP. Synthesis of 1,2,4-Dihydro-3H-1,2,4-triazole-3-thiones as potential antidepressant agents. J Med Chem 1988;31:1253-8.
11. Husain MI, Amir M, Singh E. Synthesis and antitubercular activities of [5-(2furyl)-1,2,4-triazoles-3yl thio] acehydrazide derivatives. Ind J Chem 1987;26B:2512-54.
12. Khanage SG, Mohite PB, Pandhare RB, Raju SA. Investigation of pyrazole and tetrazole derivatives containing 3,5 disubstituted-4h 1,2,4-triazole as a potential antitubercular and antifungal agent. Bioint Res App Chem 2012;2:277-83.
13. Xiao Z, Waters NC, Woodard CL, Li PK. Design and synthesis of pfmrk inhibitors as potential antimalarial agents. Bioorg Med Chem Lett 2001;11:2875-8.
14. Deliwala CV, Mhasalkar MY, Shah MH, Pilankar PD, Nikam ST, Anantanarayan KG. Synthesis and hypoglycaemic activity of 3-aryl(or pyridyl)-5-alkyl amino-1,3,4, thiadiazole and some sulfonyl ureas derivatives of 4h-1,2,4 triazoles. J Med Chem 1971;14:1000-3.
15. Cieplik J, Stolarczyk M, Pluta J, Gubrynowicz O, Bryndal I, Lis T, et al. Synthesis and antibacterial properties of pyrimidine derivatives. Ac Polo Pharm Drug Res 2011;68:57-65.
16. Mohamed MS, Awad SM, Ahmed NM. Synthesis and Antimicrobial Activities of New Indolyl-Pyrimidine Derivatives. J App Pharm Sci 2011;1:76-80.
17. Richa M, Mishra B, Moorthy N. Synthesis and Antimicrobial Evaluation of Some 3,4-Dihydro Pyrimidine-2-one Derivatives. Tre App Sci Res 2008;3:203-8.
18. Morgan JR, Haritakul R, Keller PA. Antimalarial Activity of 2,4-Diaminopyrimidines. Lett Drug Des Discov 2008;5:277-80.
19. Naik TA, Chikhalia KH. Studies on Synthesis of Pyrimidine Derivatives and their Pharmacological Evaluation. E J Chem 2007;4:60-6.
20. Ramesh B, Kulakarni SV. Design, Synthesis and Anticancer Activity Of Some New Pyrimidine Derivatives. J Glo Pharma Tech 2010;2:110-2.

21. Sondhi SM, Dinodia M, Rani R, Shukla R, Raghubir R. Synthesis, antiinflammatory and analgesic activity evaluation of some pyrimidine derivatives. Ind J Chem 2009;49B:273-81.
22. Pore Y, Kuchekar B. Synthesis of novel N_1, 6-disubstituted 5-cyano-2-thiouracil Derivatives as antinociceptive agents. Dig J Nano Biostr 2008; 3:293-8.
23. Chitre TS, Kathiravan MK, Chothe AS, Rakholiya VK, Asgaonkar KD, Shital M, et al. Synthesis and Antitubercular activity of some substituted pyrimidine derivatives. J Pharm Res 2011;4:1882-3.
24. Khanage SG, Mohite PB, Pandhare RB, Raju SA. Synthesis and pharmacological evaluation of isoxazole derivatives containing 1,2,4-triazole Moiety. Mar Pharm J 2012;16:134-40.
25. Krall RI, Penry JK, White BG, Kupferberg HG, Swingard EA. Antiepileptic drug development II. Anticonvulsant drug screening. Epilepsia 1978; 19:409-28.
26. Kucukguzel I, Kucukguzel SG, Rollas S, Ozdemir O, Bayrak I, Stables JP. Synthesis of some 3-(aryl/alkylthio)-4-alkyl/aryl-5-(4-aminophenyl)-4h-1,2,4-triazole derivatives and their anticonvulsant activity. Farmaco 2004;59:893-901.

Preparation and Evaluation of Tretinoin Microemulsion Based on Pseudo-Ternary Phase Diagram

Eskandar Moghimipour [1,2], Anayatollah Salimi [1,2*], Fatemeh Leis [2]

[1] *Nanotechnology Research Center, Jundishapur University of Medical Sciences, Ahvaz, Iran.*

[2] *Department of Pharmaceutics, Faculty of Pharmacy, Jundishapur University of Medical Sciences, Ahvaz, Iran.*

ARTICLE INFO

Keywords:
Tretinoin
Phase diagram
Microemulsion
Differential scanning calorimetry

ABSTRACT

Purpose: The aim of the present research was to formulate a transparent microemolsion as a topical delivery system for tretinoin for the treatment of acne. ***Methods:*** Microemulsion formulations prepared by mixing appropriate amount of surfactant including Tween 80 and Labrasol, co-surfactant such as propylene glycol (PG) and oil phase including isopropyl myristate – transcutol P (10:1 ratio). The prepared microemolsions were evaluated regarding their particle size, zeta potential, conductivity, stability, viscosity, differential scanning calorimetry (DSC), scanning electron microscopy (SEM), refractory index (RI) and pH. ***Results:*** The results showed that maximum oil was incorporated in microemolsion system that was contained surfactant to co-surfactant ratio (Km) of 4:1. The mean droplets size range of microemulsion formulation were in the range of 14.1 to 36.5 nm and its refractory index (RI) and pH were 1.46 and 6.1, respectively. Viscosity range was 200-350 cps. Drug release profile showed 49% of the drug released in the first 8 hours of experiment belong to ME-7. Also, Hexagonal and cubic structures were seen in the SEM photograph of the microemulsions. ***Conclusion:*** physicochemical properties and in vitro release were dependent upon the contents of S/C, water and, oil percentage in formulations.Also, ME-7 may be preferable for topical tretinoin formulation.

Introduction

The word microemulsion was originally proposed by Hoar and Schulman in the earliest of the 1940s. They were generated a clear single-phase solution by titrating a milky emulsion with hexanol.[1] Microemulsions are thermodynamically stable, isotropic clear colloidal dispersion of oil, water and surfactant, frequently in combination with a co-surfactant which have high stability, ultra low interfacial tension, large interface area , low viscosity and ease of preparation.[2,3] Conventional microemulsions can be classified oil- in -water, (o/w), water- -in- oil (w/o) and bicontinuous phase microemulsions. Some advantages offered by microemulsions include improvement in poorly drug solubility, enhancement of bioavailability, protection of the unstable drugs against environmental conditions and a long shelf life.

Tretinoin is trans-retinoic acid and related to retinol (vitamin A). The drug in use decreases proliferation of acute promyelocytic leukemia APL cells in culture and in vivo. The drug is used for treatment of various skin disorders including acne, photo aged skin and severe condition like psoriasis, squamous cell carcinoma.[4,5] The main aim of our investigation was to develop and evaluate a microemulsion based tretinoin (0.05%, w/w) for topical delivery. The proposed tretinoin concentration is chosen on the basis of the marketed tretinoin formulations. The ability of microemulsion to improve photostability of tretinoin was also investigated in the present study.

Materials and Methods

Tretinoin was purchased from Sepidaj Company (Iran). Isopropyl myristate, Tween 80 and PG were obtained from Merck (Germany), Caprylocaproyl macrogoglycerides (Labrasol) and Diethylene glycol monoethyle ether (Transcutol P) were gift from Gattefosse Company (France). All chemicals and solvents were of analytical grade. Freshly distilled water was used in the experiments. Minitab15 software was used for experimental design and the evaluation of the effect of variables on responses. Sigma plot software was applied for providing tertiary phase diagrams.

Tretinoin assay

The quantitative determination of tretinoin was performed by UV spectrophotometry (BioWaveII,WPA) at $\lambda max = 362$ nm.

***Corresponding author:** Anayatollah Salimi (PhD), Nanotechnology Research Center, Jundishapur University of Medical Sciences, Ahvaz, Iran. E-mail: anayatsalimi2003@yahoo.com

Solubility of tretinoin

Solubility of tretinoin was determined in different oil (oleic acid, isopropyl myristate, transcutol P), surfactants (Span 80, Labrasol, Tween 80) and co-surfactant (Propylen glycol) by dissolving an excess amount of tretinoin in 3ml of oil, and other components using a stirrer at 37 ^{0}C ± 0.5 for 72 h.[6] The equilibrated samples were then centrifuged at 10000rpm for 30 min to remove the undissolved drug. The solubility of tretinoin was determined by analyzing the filtrate spectrophotometrically using nanospecterophotometry (Biochrom WPA Bioware) after dilution with methanol at 362 nm.

Pseudo-ternary phase diagram construction

To investigate concentration range of components for the existing boundary of MEs, pseudo-ternary phase diagrams were constructed using the water titration method. Three phase diagrams were prepared with the 2:1, 3:1, and 4:1 weight ratios of (Labrasol /Tween 80) Propylen glycol respectively. Oil phase (Oleic acid-Transcutol P) and the surfactant mixture were then mixed at the weight ratios of 1:9, 2:8, 3:7, 4:6, 5:5, 6:4, 7:3, 8:2, and 9:1.[7] These mixtures were diluted dropwise with double distilled water, under moderate agitation. The samples were classified as microemulsions when they appeared as clear liquids.[8] Several parameters influence on final properties of microemulsions. Full factorial design was used concerning with 3 variables at 2 levels for formulations Major variables take part in determination of microemulsion's properties includes surfactant/cosurfactant ratio (S/C), percentage of oil (% oil) and water percentage (%w). Eight different formulations with low and high values of oil (5% and 30%), water (5%, 15%), and S/Co mixing ratio (3:1, 4:1) were prepared for preparing of microemulsion formulation.

Preparation of tretinoin microemulsions

Various MEs were selected from the pseudoternary phase diagram with 3:1, and 4:1 weight ratio of Labrasol /Tween 80/Propylen glycol. Tretinoin(0.05%) was added to oil phase , then adding S/ CoS mixture and an appropriate amount of double distilled water was added to the mixture drop by drop and the MEs containing tretinoin were obtained by stirring the mixtures at ambient temperature.[9,10]

Differential scanning calorimetry (DSC)

DSC measurements were carried out by means of a Metller Toldo DSC1 star^R system equipped with refrigerated cooling system (Hubert Tc45). Approximately 10-15mg of microemulsion samples were weighted into hermetic aluminium pans and quickly sealed to prevent water evaporation from microemulsion samples. Simultaneously an empty hermetically sealed pan was used as a reference. Microemulsion samples were exposed in a temperature ranging from +30 ^{0}C to - 50 ^{0}C (scan rate: 100C/min).

In order to ensure accuracy and repeatability of data, DSC instrument was calibrated and checked under the conditions of use by indium standard. Changes of Enthalpy quantities (ΔH) were calculated from endothermic and exothermic transitions of thermograms by Eq1:[10-12]

$$\Delta H = \text{peak area/sample weight}$$

Scanning electron microscopy (SEM)

Scanning electron microscopy (SEM) was used to characterize microstructure of emulsions. SEM of samples were measured by LED 1455VP, Germany.

Zeta potential determination

Zeta potential of samples were measured by Zetasizer (Malvern instrument ltd ZEN3600, UK). Samples were placed in clear disposable zeta cells and results were recorded. Before putting the fresh sample, cuvettes were washed with methanol and rinsed using the sample to be measured before each experiment.

Particle size measurements

The average droplet size of samples was measured at 25 °C by SCATTER SCOPE 1 QUIDIX (South Korea) and their refractory indices were also calculated.

Determination of viscosity

The viscosity microemulsions were measured at 25 °C with a Brookfield viscometer (DV-II+Pro Brookfield., USA) using spindle no. 34. With shear rate 100 rpm.[13]

Conductivity measurements

The electric conductivity of ME was measured with a conductivity meter (Metrohm Model 712). This was done by using conductivity cell (with a cell constant of 1.0) consisting of two platinum plates separated by desired distance and having liquid between the platinum plate acting as a conductor.

Determination of pH

The pH values for microemolsion was determined at 25°C by pH meter (Mettler Toledo seven easy, Switzerland). All measurements were carried out in triplicate.

Surface tension measurement

The surface tension of microemulsion was measured at 25°C with a Torsion balance (WHITE ELEC Model NO. 83944E).

Stability study

The stability of microemulsions was studied regarding the temperature stability and centrifugation. Microemulsions were kept in various temperature ranges (4 °C, 25 °C and 37 °C) and observed for phase separation, flocculation or precipitation. Also, Microemulsions were centrifuged by high speed brushless centrifuge (MPV-350R, Poland at 10000 rpm for 30 minute at 25 °C and inspected for any change in their homogeneity.

Release study

Franz diffusion cells (area 3.4618 cm^2) with a cellulose membrane were utilized to determine the Release rate of tretinoin from different microemulsion formulations. The cellulose (molecular weight G12 000) membrane was first hydrated in the distilled water solution at 25 ^{0}C for 24 hours. The membrane was then clamped between the donor and receptor compartments of the cells Diffusion cell was filled with 25 ml of phosphate buffer (pH = 7.4) and methanol (1:2). The receptor fluid was constantly stirred by externally driven magnetic bars at 600 rpm throughout the experiment. Tretinoin microemulsion (5 g) was accurately weighted and placed in donor compartment. At 0.5, 1, 2, 3, 4, 5, 6, 7, 8 and 24 h time intervals, 2 ml sample was removed from receptor for spectrophotometric determination and replaced immediately with an equal volume of fresh receptor solution. Samples were analyzed by UV visible spectrophotometer (BioWaveII,WPA) at 362 nm. The results were plotted as cumulative released drug percent versus time.

Statistical methods

All the experiments were repeated three times and data were expressed as the mean value ± SD. Statistical data were analyzed by one-way analysis of variance (ANOVA) and $P < 0.05$ was considered to be significant with 95% confidence intervals.

Results and discussion

The maximum solubility of tretinoin was found in Isopropyl mirystate: Transcotol P (10:1) (4.85 ± 0.09) as compared to other oils (Table 1). In addition, the highest drug solubility of tretinoin in surfactants were found in Labrasol (3.232 ± 0.23), and Tween 80 (4.27 ± 0.12). Based on the solubility studies of tretinoin in oil, surfactant and co-surfactant and the preformulation studies we found IPM-Transcutol P, labrasol, Tween 80 and propylene glycol could be the most appropriate combination for preparation of microemulsion.

Pseudo-ternary phase diagrams of the investigated quaternary system water/ isopropyl mirystate, Transcotol P (10:1)/ Labrasole -Tween 80/ PG is showed in figure 1. Microemulsions were formed at ambient temperature. The phase diagrams clearly indicated that microemulsion existence region increased with increase in the weight ratio of surfactant/cosurfactant (km=2 - 4).

The ME formulations had the mean particle size in the range of 14-60 nm (Table 2). Particle size of selected ME and drug loaded ME were determined and there was no significant difference observed in average particle size after loading the drug. The ME 6 formulation had the lowest average particle size 14.1 ± 0.6 nm with polydispersity index (PI) of 0.362 ± 0.010 (Table 2). PI is a measure of particle homogeneity and it varies from 0.0 to 1.0. The closer to zero the PI value the more homogenous are the particles.

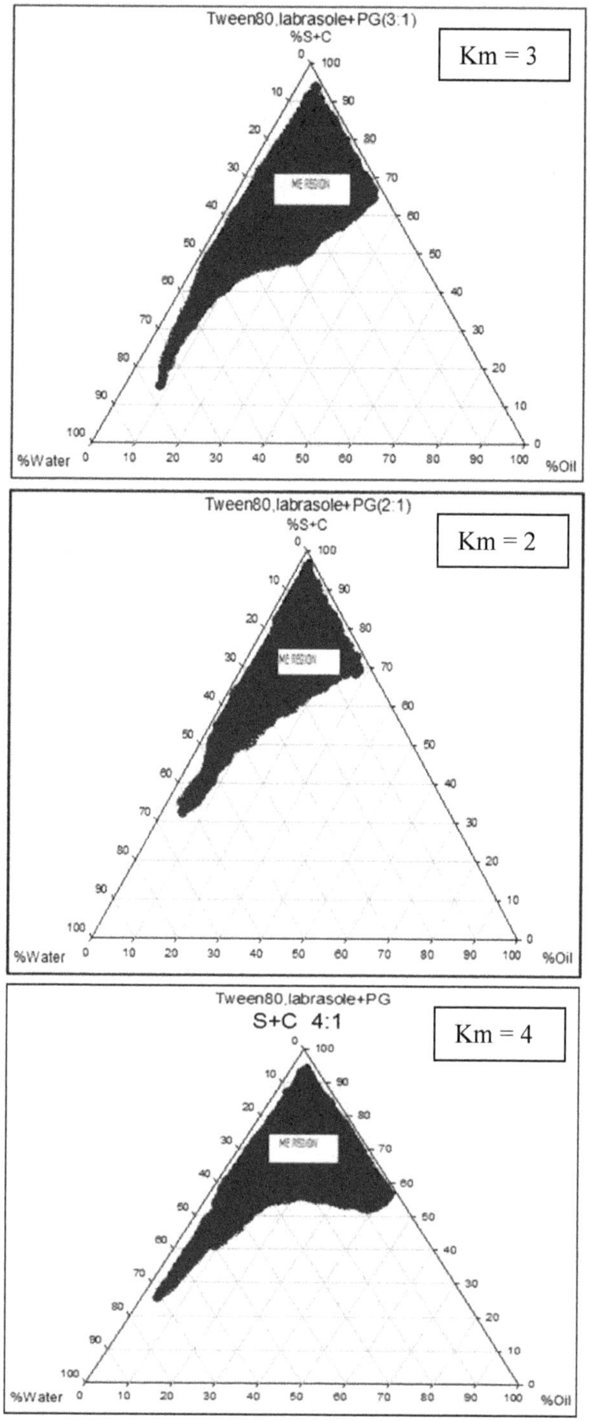

Figure 1. The pseudo-ternary phase diagrams of the oil-surfactant/cosurfactant mixture–water system at the 2:1, 3:1, and 4:1 weight ratio of labrasol /Tween 80/ Propylene glycol at ambient temperature, dark area show microemulsions zone.

The PI indicated that ME formulation had narrow size distribution. Analysis of variance is shown that correlation between mean particle size, PI and independent variables are not significant ($p > 0.05$).

The refractive index (RI) of the ME formulation was found 1.45 that is near to oil phase which indicates MEs formulations have water -in-oil structures. Analysis of variance is shown that correlation between RI and independent variables (%w) are significant ($p < 0.05$). Linear equation which indicates all the main effects for RI is: RI=1.45 + 0.0012s/c-0.000124 (%oil)-0.000625 (%water).

The ME formulations had the average conductivity in the range of 0.0447-0.0900 ms/cm.

The ME formulation had appropriate observed pH value (6.84 ± 0.11) that is best for topical application. Incorporation of tretinoin did not significantly affect the observed pH value of the ME formulations (Table 3).

Table 1. Solubility of Tretinoin in different oils, surfactant and co-surfactant (mean ± SD, n = 3)

Phase type	Excipient	Solubility (mg/ml)
oil	Oleic acid	3.61± 0.3
	Isopropyl Myristat	1.32 ± 0.091
	Oleic acid + Transcutol P	3.69 ± 0.046
	IsopropyMyristat +Transcutol P	4.85 ±0.09
surfactant	Tween 80	4.27 ± 0.12
	Span 80	2.494 ± 0.03
	labrasol	3.232 ± 0.23
co-surfactant	Propylene glycol	7.93 ± 0.06

Table 2. Compositions of Selected Microemulsions (% w/w) and Particle Size (mean ± SD, n=3)

Formulation	Factorial	S/C	Oil	S+C	water	Particle size(nm)	Polydispersity
ME-1	+ + +	4:1	30	55	15	15.3±0.5	0.362±0.032
ME-2	+ + -	4:1	30	65	5	53.9±1.3	0.411±0.015
ME-3	+ - +	4:1	5	80	15	20.8±0.8	0.372±0.024
ME-4	+ - -	4:1	5	90	5	31.7±1.05	0.352±0.016
ME-5	- - -	3:1	5	90	5	17.3±0.4	0.361±0.027
ME-6	- - +	3:1	5	80	15	14.1±0.6	0.362±0.010
ME-7	- + -	3:1	30	65	5	59.3±1.7	0.393±0.031
ME-8	- + +	3:1	30	55	15	36.5±1.2	0.381±0.022

+: high level; - : low level

Table 3. pH, Refractive index,Conductivity and Zeta potential of selected Tretinoin microemulsions (mean ± SD, n = 3)

Formulation	pH	Refractive index	Zeta potential(mv)	conductivity (ms/cm)
ME-1	6.1±0.15	1.4412±0.002	-2.30	0.0662±0.0011
ME-2	6.83±0.08	1.4450±0.008	-1.88	0.0593±0.0002
ME-3	6.72±0.1	1.4413±0.012	-2.19	0.0900±0.0012
ME-4	6.76±0.14	1.4505±0.003	-2.27	0.0634±0.0003
ME-5	6.87±0.18	1.4491±0.012	-3.45	0.0535±0.0008
ME-6	6.73±0.16	1.4409±0.009	-6.41	0.0447±0.0017
ME-7	6.84±0.11	1.4435±0.016	-3.24	0.0495±0.0009
ME-8	6.87±0.13	1.4397±0.019	-0.0674	0.00902±0.0015

The ME formulation had the average viscosity range (215.5 ± 5.2cps - 343.5 ± 8.3cps) (Table 4). The highest viscosity belongs to ME-8 formulation with bicontinueous structure. Multivariate regression was applied for the analysis of correlation between independent variables and MEs viscosity. The percent of water and s/c had more positive effect and negative effect on viscosity, respectively.

Table 4. Surface tension and viscosity of selected microemulsions (mean ± SD, n=3)

Formulation	Surface tension (dyne/cm)	Viscosity(cps)
ME-1	37.83±1.25	215.5±5.2
ME-2	38.16±1.04	228.4±6.3
ME-3	38.83±1.25	290.1±7.1
ME-4	37.83±1.25	226.2±7.8
ME-5	40±2.17	253.4±3.7
ME-6	39.66±0.76	271.3±5.8
ME-7	39.66±1.52	229.4±4.8
ME-8	38.16±1.04	343.5±8.3

Linear equation which shows all the main effects for viscosity is: Viscosity = 336-34.3s/c-0.24 (%oil) + 4.57(%water). There was no significant difference found between the viscosities of free drug and drug loaded MEs ($p > 0.05$).

The ME formulation had the zeta potential average (-0.0674-6.41mv) (Table 3). The highest zeta potential belongs to ME-6 formulation with micellar and bicontiuous structure the lowest belong to ME-8 with bicontinuous structure. Multivariate regression was used for the analysis of correlation between independent variables and MEs zeta potential. The S/C had more positive effect on zeta potential. There was no significant difference found between the zeta potential and independent variables ($p > 0.05$).

The MEs formulation had the surface tension average (37.83 ± 1.25 to 40 ± 2.17 dyne/cm) (Table 4).The surface tension data implies water –in-oil microemulsions because surface tension amounts of MEs is nearby to oil phase surface tension.

Figure 2 shows the release profiles of microemulsions of tretinoin MEs formulations. The cumulative amount of tretinoin that had permeated through the cellulose membrane (%) was plotted as a function of time (hours). In this study, ME-7 and ME-8 have the highest and lowest accumulative release percent, respectively. It was observed that there is a strong correlation between the water percent, S/C ratio and release percentage value of tretinoin ($p < 0.05$). Multivariate regression was used for the analysis of correlation between independent variables and MEs release. The percent of water and S/C ratio had more negative accumulative release percent, respectively. Linear equation which shows all the main effects for accumulative release percent is: %Release = 39.9-2.75S/C + 0.0206 (%oil) - 0.349(%water).

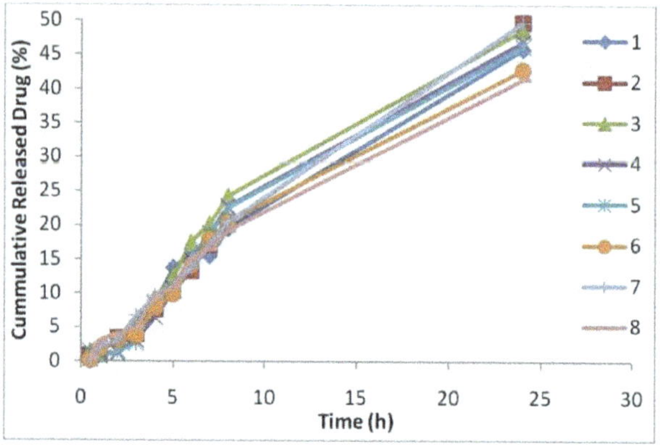

Figure 2. In vitro release profile of MEs formulation of tretinoin.

Figure 3 shows the SEM images of ME-7 and ME-8. DSC result implies important information about water state in microemulsions.[15] When water is mixed in to a microemulsion system it can be either bound (interfacial) or free (bulk) water depending of its state in the system. In cooling curves of the samples (ME_1-ME_2), DSC thermogram showed one exothermic peak at around -10 to -14 ^{0}C that indicate the freezing of internal or bound water in these formulations. The other exothermic peak at around – 19 to – 25 ^{0}C belong to oil phase freezing.[14,15] In cooling curves of ME-3 and ME-4 , DSC thermograms showed one exothermic peak at -33^{0}C (ME-3) and two exothermic peak at -1 and -34.4^{0}C for ME -4 which indicates bulk water(-1^0 C) and bound water (-33, -34.4 ^{0}C). DSC thermograms of ME-5 and ME-6 showed two exothermic peak at -2^{0}C (bulk water) and 39.8-40.9 ^{0}C (bound water. science the freezing temperature is very low, the water must be strongly bound or interacts with surfactants.[16] In cooling curves of ME-7 and ME-8, DSC thermogrms showed two exothermic peaks of around -9 to -15 ^{0}C and -22 to -24 ^{0}C, which indicates bound water and oil phase freezing, respectively. Figure 4 shows DSC cooling thermogram of ME-8 and ME-7 formulations. Pure oil peaks could be observed at -14 and -28 ^{0}C, and became smaller when the water concentration in creased. The peaks disappeared at 15% wt/wt water, suggesting that oil phase changed from external to internal phase.

The visual inspection test was performed for 3 months by drawing ME sample at weekly interval for the first month and monthly interval for the subsequent months. The visual observation showed no evidence of phase separation or any flocculation or precipitation.

These samples also revealed no sign of phase separation under stress when subjected to centrifugation at 10000 rpm for 30 min. The centrifugtion tests revealed that microemulsions were remained homogenous without any phase separation throughout the test indicates good physical stability of both preparations.

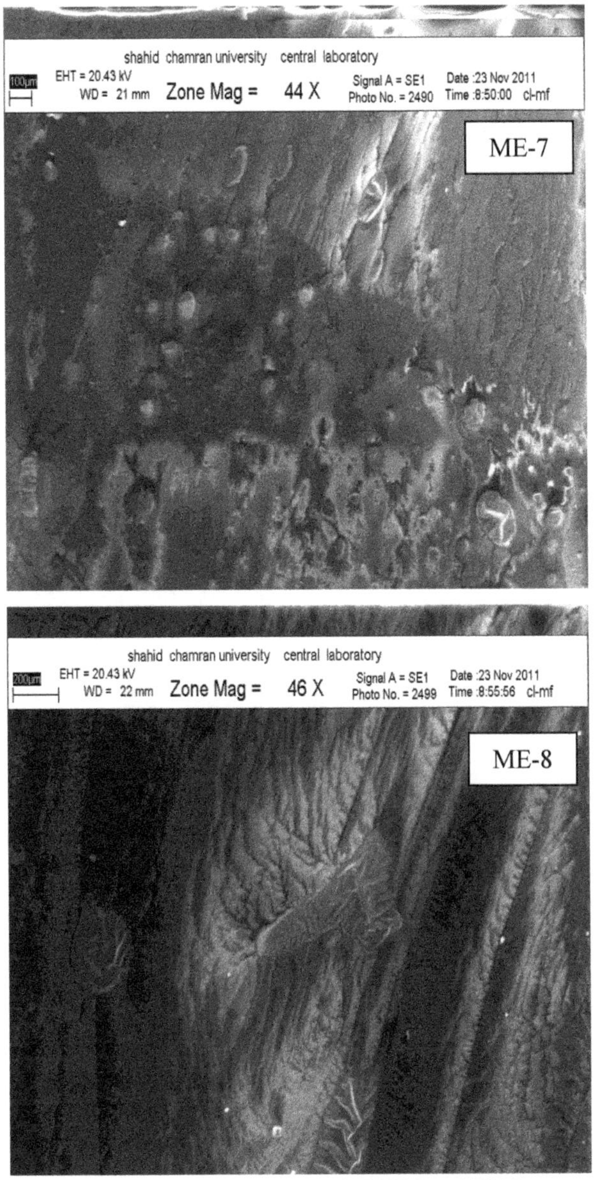

Figure 3. SEM photographs of of ME-7 and ME-8.

Conclusion

This study demonstrated that physicochemical properties and in vitro release were dependent upon the contents of S/C, water and, oil percentage in formulations. Phase diagrams indicated more width microemulsion region with a rise in S/C ratio. It seems that the effect of PG as co-surfactant in MEs release profile may be as retardant, since with decrease in S/C ratio and water and increase in oil phase ratio could be obtained high in vitro percentage release. ME-7 may be preferable for topical tretinoin formulation, however, significant work still needs to be carried out to elucidate the mechanisms of drug delivery into the skin.

Acknowledgment

This paper is extracted from pharm.D.thesis (Leis, F) and financial support was provided by Ahvaz Jundishapur University of Medical Sciences. The authors are very thankful to Faratin company Executive manager (Taheri, M, Iran) for providing gratis samples of Labrasol and Transcutol P from GATTEFOSSE (France) and also GATTEFOSSE company (France).

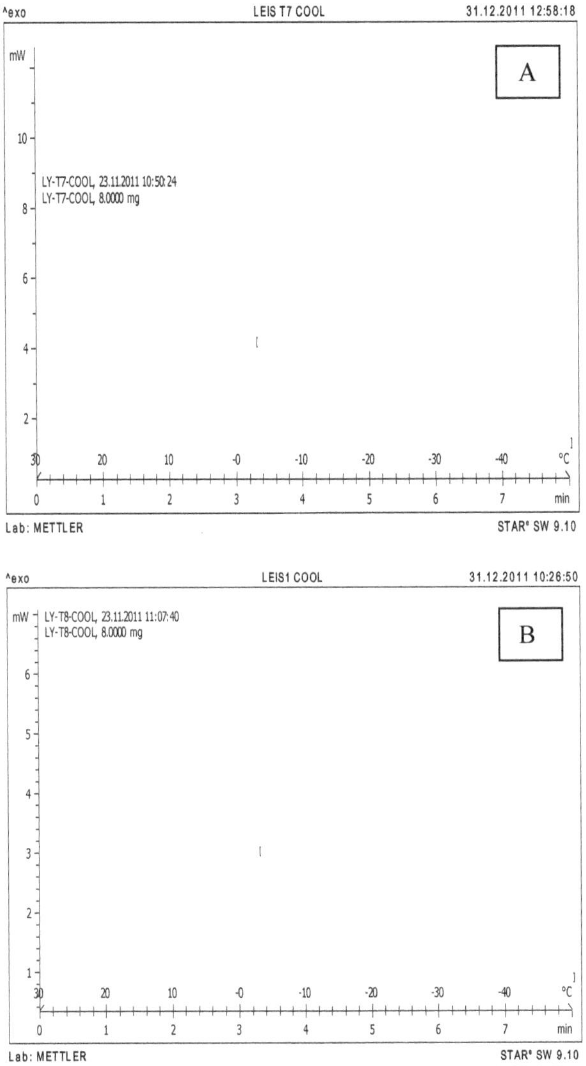

Figure 4. DSC cooling thermograms of ME-7(A) and ME-8(B) formulations.

Conflict of Interest

There is no conflict of interest in this study.

References

1. Fialho SL, Silva-Cvnha AD. New vehide based on a microemulsion for topical ocular administration of dexamethasone. Clin Exp Ophthalmol 2004;6:626-32.
2. Kreilgaard M. Dermal pharmacokinetics of microemulsions determined by in vivo microdialysis. Pharm Res 2001;18:367-73.
3. Keilgaard M. Influence of microemulsions on cutaneous drug delivery. Adv Drug Dliv Rev 2002;54:77-98.
4. Cohen BA, Prose N, Schachner LA. Acne. In: Schachner LA, Hansen RC, editors. Pediatric

Dermatology. New York: Churchill Livingstone; 1988. pp. 663-94.
5. Suthar M, Modi D, Patel P, Baria H. Microemulsion-Based gel formulation and evaluation of tretinoin for topical delivery. Int J Pharm Res 2009;1(4):28-34.
6. Sanjula B, Faiyaz S, Alka A, Javed A, Sheikh S. Design, development and evaluation of novel nanoemulsion formulation for transdermal potential of celecoxib. Acta Pharm 2007;57:315-32.
7. Wilk KA, Zielinska K, Hamerska-dudra A, Jeziershi A. Biocompatible microemulsions of dicephalic aldonamide–type surfactants: Formulation, structure and temperature influence. J Colloid Interf Sci 2009;334:87-95.
8. Sharif Makhmal zadeh B, Moghimi H. Formulation of microemulsion system for improvement of nitrofurazone permeation through silicon membrane as burn wound imitating coverage. Int J Pharmacol 2010;6(3):264-70.
9. Shafiq S, Faiyaz S, Sushma T, Farhan J, Khar R, Ali M. Development and bioavailability assessment of ramipril nanoemulsion formulation: In vitro and in vivo assessment. J Biomed Nanotechnol 2007;2:28-44.
10. Sharif Makhmal zadeh B, Torabi SH. Optimization of ibuprofen delivery through rat skin from traditional and novel nanoemulsion formulations. Iran J Pharm Res 2012;11(1):47-58.
11. Sharif Makhmal zadeh BS, Hasani MH. The effect of chemical and physical enhancers on trolamine salicylate permeation through rat skin. Trop J pharm Res 2010;9(6):541-8.
12. Gabbot P. Principles and applications of thermal analysis. Australia: Blackwell Publishing, 2008;2-49.
13. Lapasin R, Grassi M, Coceani N. Effects of polymer addition on the rheology of o/w microemulsions. Rheol Acta 2001;40:185-92.
14. Garti N, Aserin A, Tiunova I, Fanum M. A DSC study of water behavior in w/o microemulsions stabilized by sucrose esters and butanol. Colloid Surface 2000;120:1-18.
15. Podlogar F, Gasperlin M, Tomsic M, Jamnik A, Rogac MB. Structural characterisation of water-Tween 40/Imwitor 308-isopropyl myristate microemulsions using different experimental methods. Int J Pharm 2004;276:115-28.
16. Zhang J, Michniak-Kohn B. Investigation of microemulsion microstructures and their relationship to transdermal permeation of model drugs: ketoprofen, lidocaine and caffeine. Int J Pharm 2011;421:34-44.

Degenerative Effect of Cisplatin on Testicular Germinal Epithelium

Daryosh Mohammadnejad[1], Ali Abedelahi[2]*, Jafar Soleimani-rad [2], Ameneh Mohammadi-roshandeh[3], Morteza Rashtbar[2], Ayda Azami[1]

[1] *Drug Applied Research Center, Tabriz University of Medical Sciences, Tabriz, Iran.*

[2] *Department of Anatomical Sciences, Tabriz University of Medical Sciences, Tabriz, Iran.*

[3] *Department of Anatomical Sciences, Hamedan University of Medical Sciences, Hamedan, Iran.*

ARTICLE INFO

Keywords:
Cisplatin
Electron microscope
Apoptosis
Germinal epithelium

ABSTRACT

Purpose: The present study was designed to explore the effect of intraperitoneal administration of cisplatin in germinal epithelium of mice. There are few reports on the side effect of cisplatin on spermatogenesis when are used as anticancer drug. Therefore, in the present study the effect of cisplatin on spermatogenesis was evaluated by electron microscopy. ***Methods:*** Twenty balb/c mice aging 6-8 weeks was used in this study. The mice were divided into two groups, control and cysplatin treated. cysplatin was injected for five days as 2.5 mg /kg. The mice were sacrificed after 5 weeks and testicular specimens were removed, fixed in boueins, formaldeyd fixative and 2.5% Glutaraldehide then prepared for light and electron microscopic study. ***Results:*** Observation with optic microscope in treated group thickness of germinal epithelium was reduced a lot and increased the number of apoptotic cells. In some seminiferous tubules only sertoli cells were observed and nucleus of spermatogony cells was hetrochromatin. The electron microscopic observations showed some irregularity waviness and thickening in basal layer. Also myoid cells of this group were thick and contracted. In this group many apoptotic cells and damaged organelles were seen. ***Conclusion:*** It was indicated that cisplatin affected testicular germinal epithelium by both cytotoxic effect and induction of apoptosis.

Introduction

Infertility is one of the major problems following chemotherapy in cancer treatment.[1]In young male patients, chemotherapy regimes affect fertility by influence on testicular function. Although the cancer controlled by chemotherapy, the ability to have a normal child as a factor of life quality becomes a major issue. Testicular dysfunction is the most common long-term side effects of chemotherapy in men.

Spermatogenesis is influenced by radiotherapy and cancer cytotoxic drugs.[2-5] Recently, the Cisplatin is used for treatment of various malignancies including cancer of testis, ovary, lung, bladder and Hodgkin and non-Hodgkin lymphoma[6-10] The previous studies on the side effects of chemotherapeutic drugs such as procarbazine, cyclophosphamide and chlorambucil showed long-term (up to years) azoospermia after treatment.[3,11] There are a few reports on the side effect of Cisplatin on the spermatogenesis when they are used as anticancer drugs, in the literature.[12] Tumors are characterized by division, which is no longer controlled as it is in normal tissue. Cancer cells no longer have the normal checks and balances in place that control and limit cell division. The process of cell division, normal or cancerous cell, is through the cell cycle. The cell cycle goes from the resting phase, through active growing phases and then to mitosis (division). The ability of chemotherapy to kill cancer cells depends on its ability to halt cell division. So chemotherapy is most effective at killing cells that are rapidly dividing. Unfortunately, chemotherapeutic agents can not differentiate between the cancerous and the normal cells. It has been shown that one of the mechanisms in cell destruction following chemotherapy is apoptosis.[12-16] Some agents including genes factors, Testicular ischemia, heat stress, exposure to irradiation and toxic substances, could increase the rate of germ cell apoptosis in testis.[5,12-17]Cisplatin is not a classical DNA directed alkylation agent but it involve in transcription, translation and repairing of DNA (like alkylation agents) and currently used in high dose therapy approaches to the treatment of various malignancies including, testis, ovary, lung, bladder cancers and Hodgkin and non-Hodgkin lymphoma.[6-10] These studies have not provided enough information about ultra-structural changes in germinal epithelium of testis and spermatogenesis. On the other hand, the results of electron microscope in evaluating morphological pattern of nucleus, organelles, membrane and cell

***Corresponding author:** Ali Abedelahi (PhD), Department of Anatomical Sciences, Tabriz University of Medical Sciences, Tabriz, Iran.
Email: abedanatomy@yahoo.com

adhesion is more valuable in comparison to light microscope. In the meantime, the knowledge about the ultra structural changes of germinal stem cells and spermatogenic cells following the administration of Cisplatin can help to understand the mechanisms of action of Cisplatin.

Materials and Methods

Animals: Twenty balb/c mice aging 6-8 weeks was used in this study. The mice were divided into two groups, control and Cisplatin treated. Cisplatin was injected intraperitoneally for five days as 2.5 mg /kg. Since spermatogenic cycle in mice is 35 days, mice in both groups were sacrificed 35 days after last injection. The testes were removed from the abdominal cavity and separated from the epididymis with care by using a surgical blade and then half of testicular specimen from right testis was fixed in boueins fixative for 48 h for quantitative studies. For quantitative study, we used Motic Image plus 20 software. That is, in 20 microscopic fields in the cross sectioned seminiferous tubule the number of spermatogonia and sertoli cells, thickness of germinal epithelium and spermatogenesis index (SI) were determined. The obtained data were analysed with T-test and using spss.13 softwere. Another half of the testis fixed in formaldehyde for histochemical study by using apoptosis Kit for detection of apoptotic cells. Then both groups processed for light microscopy.

The specimens from the left testis were fixed in 2.5% Glutaraldehyde (Pro. Sci. Tech. Au) for 12 h and washed with 0.2 M phosphate buffer and post fixed with 2% osmium tetroxide (TAAB, UK) for 2 h. After Dehydration, Clearing and Infiltration they embedded in resin (Pro. Sci. Tech. Au) and sectioned using ultramicrotome (Richert-Jung, Au). Semithin stained with toluidine blue and studied with light microscope. The thin sections (80 nm thickness) were stained with uranyl acetate and lead citrate and were studied with Leo 906 transmission electron microscope (Leo, Germany).

Results

Light microscopy

The result from light microscopy revealed that in control group the germinal epithelium of seminiferous tubules composed of multilayer cells and showed features of active spermatogenesis. So the 12 stages of spermatogenesis could easily be realized according to morphological characteristics of germinal epithelium in the seminiferous tubules (Figure 1.A).

In experimental group, the thickness of germinal epithelium was reduced and / in many cases it was completely depleted and only sertoli cells were left. Therefore, the stages of spermatogenesis were not detectable (Figure 1.B,C).

Morphometric evaluation

Morphometric study showed that the mean number of spermatogonia/tubule in control group was 43.22±1.55 and in treated group was 21.42 ± 2.44. Statistical analysis showed that the mean number of spermatogonia in treated group in comparison to control group is significantly ($P<0.05$) reduced (table 1). Spematogenic Index (SI) in control group was 24.43±9.22, in treated group was 1.52±1.39. Statistical analysis showed that the SI values in control and treated group is significantly ($p=0.000$) different (Table 1). The mean number of sertoli/tubule cells in control group was 5.50±0.52, in treated group was 8.61±0.80. Statistical analysis showed that the difference between controle and treated group is significant ($P<0.05$) (Table 1). Thickness of germinal epithelium in control group was 57.33±4.1 µm but it reduced to 20.90±3.84 µm in treated group. Statistical analysis showed that the difference between control and treated group is significant ($P<0.05$) (Table 1).

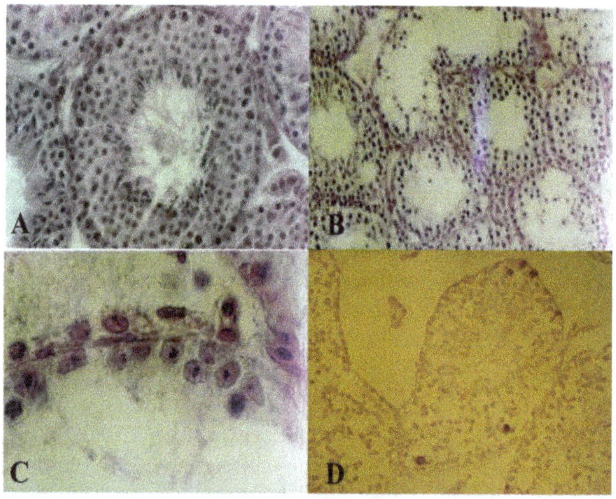

Figure 1. Photomicrography of seminiferous tubules of mice: A) in control group, Note different spermatogenenic cells in tubules. PAS staining .660 X. B) treated with cisplatin. Note the destroyed germinal epithelium and hyper chromic nuclei, PAS staining. 330 X. C) treated with cisplatin, sertoli cells are only observed inside tubules, PAS staining, 1650 X. D) which shows apoptotic cells in cisplatin receiving group Tunnel staining.660X.

Table 1. Comparison of different parameters in testis from control and cisplatin receiving group.

Groups	No. of Spermatogoniacells	No. of Sertoli cells	Thickness of germinal Epi (µm)	No. of Apoptotic cells	SI value
Control	43.22±1.55	5.50±0.52	57.33±4.1	1.27±0.20	24.43±9.22
Cisplatin	21.42±2.44*	8.61±0.80*	20.90±3.84*	7.21±0.90*	1.52±1.39*

*: Significantly different from control group

Histochemistery evaluation

The 3 micron samples was provided from fixed samples in formaldehyde and after deparafination, incubated in sodium citrate 0.1M buffer for 5 min, and then DNA fragmentation evaluated by Tunnel Kit based on instruction of company in order to show apoptotic cells. Histochemical study showed that the mean number of apoptotic cells/tubule in control group was 1.27±0.20 and in treated group was 7.21±0.90 which is significantly ($P<0.05$) different (table 1) and (Figure 1.D).

Electron microscopy

Ultrastructural studies revealed that in control group, the spermatogonia were regularly arranged and rested on basal lamina. The cells had a spherical or oval nucleus, with higher magnification they contained few mitochondria and poorly developed endoplasmic reticulum (Figure 2.A,B). Sertoli cells were also rested on basal lamina and had large nuclei with prominent nucleolus (Figure 2.A). The Junction between two adjacent sertoli cells was obvious (Figure 3.A). This structure has important role in normal spermatogenesis by forming Blood Testes Barrier (BTB) and is composed of three elements (Figure 3.A).

- Merged plasmalemma of adjacent sertoli cells in the center.
- Dilated endoplasmic reticulum in both sides.
- Bundles of filaments that are sandwiched between plasmalemma and endoplasmic reticulum.

Study of testis in the treated group showed that spermatogonia and sertoli cells were separated from basal lamina and neighboring cells by large spaces (Figure 2.C). Basement membrane was morphologically irregular and wavey. Myoid cells in the boundary tissue were thickened and condensed (Figure 2.D). BTB in this group was ruptured and appeared thinner than in the control group (Figure 3.B).

In this group also a lot of apoptotic cells in germinal epithelium were observed that they were recognized based on DNA fragmentation (Figure 4.A). In this group also interacellular granules in interstitial cells were dramatically increased (Figure 4.B).

Spermatogenic cells had also several damaged organelles such as vacuolated mitochondria (Figure 4.C). Due to destructive effect of Cisplatin different spermatogenic cells and stage of spermatogenesis was rarely observed.

Discussion

The aim of this study was to evaluate the adverse effect of cysplatin, as an anticancer drug, on germinal epithelium. The study revealed that in treated group which was received cysplatin the thickness of germinal epithelium, number of spermatogonial cells and SI were decreased. In addition, the nuclei of spermatogonial cells were dense in comparison to control group. This finding is similar to those obtained with other chemotherapeutic agents.[2,18]

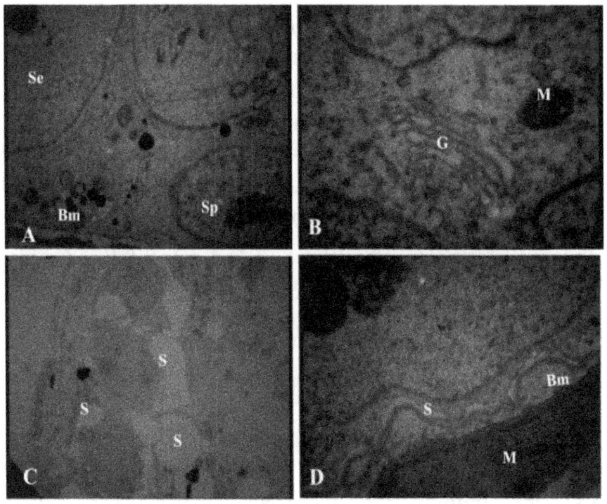

Figure 2. Electronmicrograph of seminiferous tubule in mice: control group (A, B) and experimental group (D, C). A) Spermatogonia (Sp) and sertoli cells (Se) on basement membrane (Bm), 3097 X. B) mitochondria (M) and Golgi (G), 12930 X. C) Note separation of cells from each other (s). D) Sertoli cell is separated from basement membrane (S). The basement membrane is wavey (Bm). A contracted myoid cell is shown in the figure (M). 3097 X.

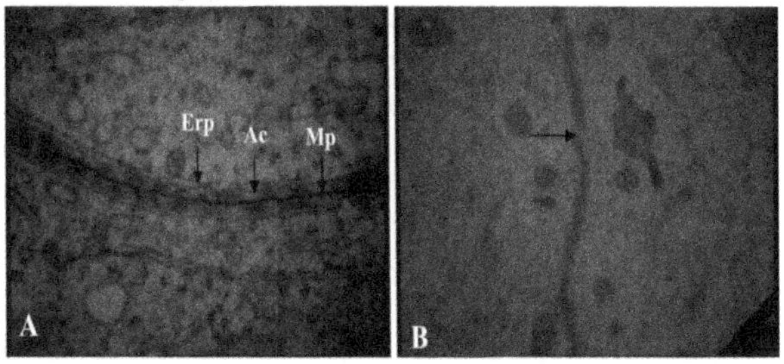

Figure 3. Electronmicrograph of Blood-Testes-Barrier: A) Control group, Mp: merged plasma membrane, Ac: actin filaments, Er: endoplasmic reticulum, 46460 X. B) experimental group, Note the rupture areas in BTB (arrow), 21560 X.

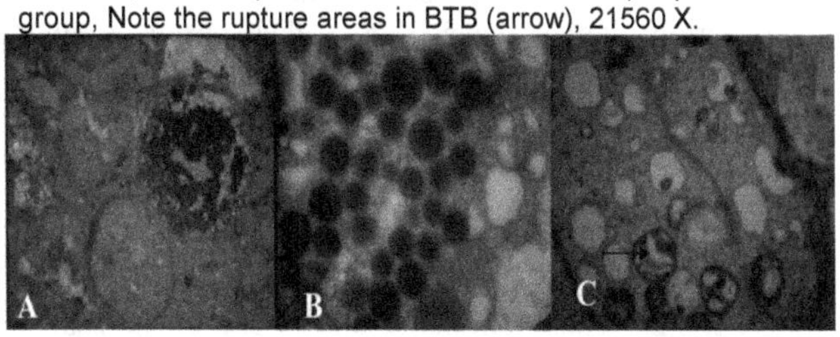

Figure 4. Electronmicrograph of: A) An apoptotic cell with fragmentation of DNA 10000 X, B) Interstitial cell of mice from experimental group. Note numerous secretary granules. 6000 X, D) Part of spermatogonial cell in the seminiferous tubule in of mice in experimental group. Note ruptured mitochondria (arrow). 3097 X.

Other findings of the present study were that cellular proliferation in the seminiferous tubules was reduced and nuclear hetrochromatin was increased. Both of which is indicating that decreased thickness of germinal epithelium in our study, is partly due to decreased cell division. In support of our finding other researcher has also been reported a reduction in mitosis and DNA changes following treatment with chemotherapeutic drugs.[19,20] On the other hands, it shown that the agents that are used in chemotherapy tend to act on activety dividing cells such as spermatogonia and cease their division.[3,21] Our results also showed that apoptotic cells were increased in cysplatin receiving group. In support of this finding there are some reports showing that anticancer drugs could induced apoptosis in germinal epithelium.[12-16] On the other hand, apoptosis has a critical role on the removal of damaged spermatogonial cells to prevent the formation of abnormal sperms.[22] It is also shown that spermatocytes that fail to complete their mitotic division are removed by apoptosis.[23] It appears that cysplatin as a chemotherapic agent induces apoptosis on spermatogenic cells. Other changes, such as separation of spermatogonial cells from each other and basal lamina could also be considered as preapoptotic sign. Other finding such as nuclear condensation, chromatin margination and mitochondrial vacuolization are additional evidence for appearance of apoptotic cells. There were also several separations between cells of germinal epithelium and between them and basal lamina. In this regard, it has been shown that cell adhesion enhances the survival of germ cells and cadherins mediated adhesion between sertoli and germ cells in vitro.[24]Cadherins as an important molecular system controls interaction between sertoli and germ cells and promotes the survival of germ cells. It has thought that cadherin based adhesion generates intracellular signaling cascades that control cell survival, migration and maturation.[25] In our TEM study both BM and myoid cells were altered structurally in experimental group. BM in the treated group was irregular and had some swirls. Similar findings were observed in irradiated rats[26] and after efferent ligation.[27] The swirls may be due to contraction of myoid cells or reduction of tubular diameter. In this study the BM was continuous even in the absence of germ cells. It means that germ cells are probably not involved in BM production. It has been shown that during tubular injury, for survival and regeneration of stem cells, the BM is produced.[26] Testicular BM is synthesized by both sertoli and myoid cells.[28] In our TEM study it appeared that the thickness of BM is increased in cysplatin treated group. Increasing of BM thickness similarly occurs in: aging,[29] efferent ligation[27] and after irradiation.[26] This alteration either is due to increasing of production by sertoli or myoid cells or reduction of proteolysis rate in ECM. In efferent ligation the gene expression of laminin is changed in sertoli cells and their protein synthesis is enhanced. According to our results intracellular granules in interstitial cells were increased in treated group. In this regard is appears that, interstitial cells are the only cells that have LH receptor and in response to LH secrets estrogen and testosterone. On the other hand it is shown that following chemotherapy, level of FSH, LH and testosterone increases.[3,21,30] Therefore it can be concluded that the increased granules in interstitial cells are a response to increased LH which results from cysplatin treatment. The nucleus of myoid cells in cysplatin treated groups was appeared shorter and had a contractile form in comparison to control group. Myoid cells contain abundant actin filaments which are distributed in the cells in a species specific manner. Myoid cells also have myosin, desmin and actinin.[31] In other words they are kind of smooth muscle cells.[32] Testosterone and several substances such as prostoglandins, oxytocin, TGF-β have been suggested to affect the contraction of these cells.[31] These finding suggest that probably after treatment with cysplatin, secretion of testosterone increased or damaging of epithelium stimulates secretion of some factors such as oxytocin or prostaglandins and cause myoid cells contraction.

Acknowledgment
The authors are thankful to Drug Applied Research Center, Tabriz University of Medical Sciences, for their financial support of the project.

Conflict of Interest
There is no conflict of interest in this study.

References

1. Nejad MD, Rad SJ, Roshankar L, Karimpor M, Ghanbari AA, Azami A, Valilou MR. Effect of Thiotepa on mice Spermatogenesis using light and electronic microscope. Pak J Biol Sci 2008;11:1929-34.
2. Codrington AM, Hales BF, Robaire B. Exposure of male rats to cyclophosphamide alters the chromatin structure and basic proteome in spermatozoa. Hum Reprod 2007;22:1431-42.
3. Howell SJ, Shalet SM. Spermatogenesis after cancer treatment: damage and recovery. J Natl Cancer Inst Monogr 2005;34:12-7.
4. Boekelheide K. Mechanisms of Toxic Damage to Spermatogenesis. J Natl Cancer Inst Monogr 2005;34:6-8.
5. Liu GP, Gong P, Bernstein LR, Bi Y, Gong S, Cai L. Apoptotic cell death induced by low-dose radiation in male germ cells: Hormesis and adaptation. Crit Rev Toxicol 2007;37:587-605.
6. Duale N, Lindeman B, Komada M, Olsen A, Andreassen A, Soderlund EJ, et al. Molecular portrait of cisplatin induced response in human testis cancer cell lines based on gene expression profiles. Mol Cancer 2007;6:1-27.
7. Helm CW, States JC. Enhancing the efficacy of cisplatin in ovarian cancer treatment – could Arsenic have a role. J Ovarian Res 2009;2:2.
8. Noda K, Nishiwaki Y, Kawahara M, Negoro S, Sugiura T, Yokoyama A, etal. Irinotecan plus cisplatin compared with etoposide plus cisplatin for extensive small-cell lung cancer. N Engl J Med 2002;346:85-91.
9. Shipley WU, Prout GR Jr, Einstein AB, Coombs LJ, Wajsman Z, Soloway MS, et al. Treatment of invasive bladder cancer by cisplatin and radiation in patients unsuited for surgery. JAMA 1987;258:931-5.
10. Velasquez WS, Cabanillas F, Salvador P, Mclaughlin P, Fridrik M, Tucker S, et al. Effective

salvage therapy for lymphoma with cisplatin in combination with high-dose Ara-C and dexamethasone (DHAP). Blood 1988;71:117-22.
11. Sieniawski M, Reineke T, Nogova L, Josting A, Pfistner B, Diehl V, Engert A. Fertility in male patients with advanced Hodgkin lymphoma treated with BEACOPP: A report of the German Hodgkin Study Group (GHSG). Blood 2008;111:71-6.
12. Sawhney P, Giammona CJ, Meistrich ML, Richburg JH. Cisplatin-induced long-term failure of spermatogenesis in adult C57/Bl/6J mice. J Androl 2005;26:136-45.
13. Andriana BB, Tay TW, Maki A, Awal MA, Kanai Y, Kurohmaru M, Hayashi Y. An ultrastructural study on cytotoxic effects of mono (2-ethylhexyl) phthalate (MEHP) on testes in Shiba goat in vitro. J Vet Sci 2004;5:235-40.
14. Bakalska M, Atanassova N, Koeva Y, Nikolov B, Davidoff M. Induction of male germ cell apoptosis by testosterone withdrawal after ethane dimethanesulfonate treatment in adult rats. Endocr Regul 2004;38:103-10.
15. Habermehl D, Kammerer B, Handrick R, Eldh T, Gruber C, Cordes N, et al. Proapoptotic activity of ukrain is based on Chelidonium majus L. alkaloids and mediated via a mitochondrial death pathway. BMC Cancer 2006;6:14.
16. Hou M, Chrysis D, Nurmio M, Parvinen M, Eksborg S, Soder O, et al. Doxorubicin induces apoptosis in germ line stem cells in the immature rat testis and amifostine cannot protect against this cytotoxicity. Cancer Res 2005;65:9999-10005.
17. Sakallioglu AE, Ozdemir BH, Basaran O, Nacar A, Suren D, Haberal MA. Ultrastructural study of severe testicular damage following acute scrotal thermal injury. Burns 2007;33:328-33.
18. Kasper DL, Braunwald E, Fauci AS, Hauser SL, Longo DL, Jameson JL. Harrisons Principles of Internal Medicine. 16th ed. New York:McGraw Hill Medical Publishing Division; 2005.
19. Khilkevich LV, Kurilo LF. The gametatoxic effect of antenatal exposure to thiotepa in mice. Ontogenez 1992;23:401-6.
20. Evenson Dp, Baer RK, Jost LK, Gesch RW. Toxicity of thiotepa on mouse spermatogenesis as determined by dual-parameter flow cytometry. Toxicol Appl Pharmacol 1986;82:151-63.
21. Howell SJ, Shatel SM. Testicular function following Chemotherapy. Hum Reprod Update 2001;7:363-9.
22. Cai L, Hales BF, Robaire B. Induction of apoptosis in the germ cells of adult male rats after exposure to cyclophosphamide. Biol Reprod 1997;56:1490-7.
23. Print CG, Loveland KL. Germ cell suicide: New insights into apoptosis during spermatogenesis. Bioessays 2000;22:423-30.
24. Newton SC, Blaschuk OW, Millette CF. N-cadherin mediates Sertoli cell-spermatogenic cell adhesion. Dev Dyn 1993;197:1-13.
25. Honecker F, Kersemaekers AM, Molier M, Van Weeren PC, Stoop H, De Krijger RR, et al. Involvement of E-cadherin and beta-catenin in germ cell tumours and in normal male fetal germ cell development. J Pathol 2004;204:167-74.
26. Sawada H, Esaki M. Electron microscopic observation of 137Cs-irradiated rat testis: production of basal laminae for germ cells, despite their absence. J Electron Microsc (Tokyo) 2003; 52: 391-7.
27. Richardson LL, Kleinman HK, Dym M. Altered basement membrane synthesis in the testis after tissue injury. J Androl 1998;19:145-55.
28. Skinner MK, Tung PS, Fritz IB. Cooperativity between Sertoli cells and testicular peritubular cells in the production and deposition of extracellular matrix components. J Cell Biol 1985;100:1941-7.
29. Siu MK, Cheng CY. Extracellular matrix: Recent advances on its role in junction dynamics in the seminiferous epithelium during spermatogenesis. Biol Reprod 2004;71:375-91.
30. Shetty G, Wilson G, Huhtaniemi I, Shuttlesworth GA, Reissmann T, Meistrich ML. Gonadotropin-releasing hormone analogs stimulate and testosterone inhibits the recovery of spermatogenesis in irradiated rats. Endocrinology 2000;141:1735-45.
31. Maekawa M, Kamimura K, Nagano T. Peritubular myoid cells in the testis: Their structure and function. Arch Histol Cytol 1996;59:1-13.
32. Virtanen I, Kallajoki M, Narvanen O, Paranko J, Thornell LE, Miettinen M, et al. Peritubular myoid cells of human and rat testis are smooth muscle cells that contain desmin-type intermediate filaments. Anat Rec 1986;215:10-20.

Protective Effect of Ginger on Gentamicin-Induced Apoptosis in Testis of Rats

Afshin Zahedi [1], Fatemeh Fathiazad [2*], Arash Khaki [3], Behnam Ahmadnejad [4]

[1] *Faculty of Veterinary Medicine, Islamic Azad University, Rasht Branch, Rasht, Iran.*

[2] *Department of Pharmacognosy, faculty of Pharmacy, Tabriz University of Medical Sciences, Tabriz, Iran.*

[3] *Women's Reproductive Health Research Center, Tabriz University of Medical Sciences, Tabriz, Iran.*

[4] *Faculty of Veterinary Medicine, Islamic Azad University, sciences & Research campus Branch, Tehran, Iran.*

ARTICLE INFO

Keywords:
Gentamicin
Ginger
Apoptosis
Antioxidant
Zingiber officinale
Testis

ABSTRACT

Purpose: Ginger, the rhizome of *Zingiber officinale*, is one of the most widely used spices for various foods and as an herbal medicine in Asian countries. It has been shown that ginger has antioxidant power. Gentamicin is an aminoglycoside antibiotic with a very broad spectrum against microbial pathogens, especially the gram-negative. Many studies revealed that gentamicin induces an oxidative stress-status in the testis by increasing free radical formation and lipid peroxidation. The present study was designed to investigate on the effects of Ginger as a natural anioxidant on testis apoptosis after treatment with gentamicin in rats. ***Methods:*** In order to study the recovery effects of ginger on testis apoptosis after treatment with gentamicin 40 adult Wistar male rats were selected and randomly divided into four groups. Normal salin control (group I) (n=10), gentamicin control (group II), ginger control (group III) and gentamicin + ginger (group IV) each 10 rats. There was observation of negative effect of Gentamicin on testis histology in rats. ***Results:*** The results revealed that there was a significant increase in apoptosis in group III when compared with other groups ($P<0.05$).However, ginger could decrease apoptosis in group IV that received 100mg/kg/rat of Ginger. ***Conclusion:*** Regarding the results, it is recommended that administration of ginger with gentamicin might be beneficial in men who receive gentamicin to treat infections.

Introduction

Ginger root (actually the rhizome, family: zingiberaceae), is a common kitchen spice widely used worldwide as powder or as the whole fresh root. The surface of the rhizome is grayish-white with pale brown rings. Ginger has a long history of medicinal use in Chinese traditional medicine and Ayurvedic medicine for conditions such as headaches,toothache, nausea, rheumatism, colds and to improve circulation to the limbs. The main constituents of ginger are the essential oil (1-3%) and pungent compounds, including zingibere, sesquiphellandrene and beta-bisabololene, gingerols and shogaols.

Early animal studies demonstrated the antiinflamatory activity of ginger. Ginger and its extract inhibit cyclooxygenase and lipooxygenase enzymes in biosynthesis of prostaglandin and leukotriene. It helps in lowering blood cholesterol, blood clotting and pressure.The effectiveness of ginger as an antiemetic agent was also proved in several studies for motion sickness, postoperative nausea and vomiting during pregnancy. It was found ginger is an effective treatment for rheumatic disorders.[1] Research suggests the antioxidant activity of ginger, ginger extract and its pungent components.[2] Since, lipooxygenase inhibitors are strong antioxidant, such activity might be expected. Androgenic activity of ginger was also reported in animal models.[3]

The spermatozoa are susceptible to oxidative stress induced damage because of the large polyunsaturated fat content in their membranes.[4] In recent years, many studies revealed that gentamicin induces an oxidative stress-status in the testis by increasing free radical formation and lipid peroxidation.These biochemical changes manifest as structural and cytotoxic changes in the testis. Further, gemtamicin and Ofloxacin affects the spermatozoa by affecting their number, motility and morphology.[5,6] The sperm count and sperm motility were decreased and abnormality was increased. Gentamicin induced structural changes such as sloughing of somniferous epithelium, vacuoles and

***Corresponding author:** Fatemeh Fathiazad (PhD), Department of Pharmacognosy, faculty of Pharmacy, Tabriz University of Medical Sciences, Tabriz, Iran. E-mail: fathiazad@tbzmed.ac.ir

gaps in the epithelium, nuclear pyknosis and atrophic changes in a few tubules.[5,7] Antibiotics such as gentamicin, neomycin, streptomycin and ofloxacin are routinely used by urologists, andrologist and to treat infections prior to in vitro fertilization treatment or when high concentration of leukocytes is present in the semen of these patients.[8-10] Therefore, the present study was designed to investigate the protective effects ginger rhizome on toxicity of gentamicin on testis of rats.

Materials and Methods

Plant material

Ginger rhizome was purchased from local market in Tabriz and grounded before commencing experiments.

Animals

Forty adult male wistar rats weighting 200±10 g were used in this study. They were fed with standard diet pellets and allowed food and water for an acclimation period of two weeks. The animals were maintained in a strictly controlled temperature (18± 1°c). Humidity was kept at 50% and the lighting cycle was 7.00-19.00 h light and 19.00-7.00 h dark with adequate ventilation. Animals were handled with human care in accordance with the national institutes of health guidelines. The rats were randomly divided into 4 groups each consisting of ten animals. Group I received normal salin, group II received 50 mg/kg (i.p.) gentamycin, group III received 100mg/kgBW/day of ginger rhizome via gavages for 30 days at an interval of 24 hr between subsequent treatments and group IV received gentamicin (50 mg/kg, i.p.) and ginger (100mg/kgBW/day). Animals were sacrificed on day 30, testes were removed and then tissue preparation was performed to investigate apoptosis by TUNEL.

TUNEL analysis of apoptosis

The in-situ DNA fragmentation was visualized by TUNEL method.[11] Briefly, dewaxed tissue sections were predigested with 20 mg/ml proteinase K for 20 min and incubated in phosphate buffered saline solution (PBS) containing 3 % H_2O_2 for 10 min to block the endogenous peroxidase activity. The sections were incubated with the TUNEL reaction mixture, fluorescein-dUTP (in situ Cell Death Detection, POD kit, Roche, Germany), for 60 min at 37°C. The slides were then rinsed three times with PBS and incubated with secondary antifluorescein- POD-conjugate for 30 min. After washing three times in PBS, diaminobenzidine-H_2O_2 (DAB, Roche, Germany) chromogenic reaction was added on sections and counterstained with hematoxylin. As a control for method specificity, the step using the TUNEL reaction mixture was omitted in negative control serial sections, and nucleotide mixture in reaction buffer was used instead. Apoptotic cells were quantified by counting the number of TUNEL stained nuclei per testis tissues cross sections. Cross sections of 100 testis tissues per specimen were assessed and the mean number of TUNEL positive apoptotic cells per cross- section was calculated.

Statistical analysis

Statistical analysis was done using the ANOVA and test for comparison of data in the control group with the experimental groups. The results were expressed as mean ± S.E.M (standard error of means). P-value less than 0.05 were considered significant.

Results

Compared to the control group, apoptotic cells percent decreased following administration of 100mg/kgBW/day of ginger rhizome. Administration of 50 mg/kg/day gentamicin caused a significant increase in the apoptotic cells percent. When gentamicin at dose of 50 mg/kg (i.p.) was administrated with 100 mg/kg/rat/day of ginger rhizome, apoptotic cells percent was significantly ($P<0.05$) decreased from 22.11± 1.11 to 15.05± 1.11 indicating the protective effect of ginger rhizome against gentamicin- induced apoptosis (Table 1).

Table 1. Apoptotic cells percent of male rats exposed to ginger rhizome.

groups	Gentamicin + Ginger	Ginger	Gentamicin	Control
Apoptotic cell (%)	15.05±1.11	0.15±0.14	22.11±1.11	6±2.11

Discussion

Infertility is one of the major problems in match's life. About 25 and 35 percent of infertility is regarded to man and woman respectivity.[12] The importance of many of these factors is not yet clearly understood. A better understanding of underlying mechanisms in fertility and better study results clarifying the effectiveness of nutritional and biochemical factors importance to improve diagnosis and treatment. Smart choices for better foods might prevent body from many diseases.[13,14] As all spermatogenesis stages occur in seminiferous tubule of testis, it is possible to evaluate the extent of spermatogenesis by determination of number of spermatozoa produced per one gram of testicular parenchyma.[15] The sperm count is considered as an important parameter to assess the effects of chemicals on spermatogenesis.[16] It has also been reported that there is a direct correlation between the epididymal sperm count and motility with fertility in animals.[17-19] The oxidative damage, elevated lipid peroxidation and the alteration of memberane properties. This subsequently can lead to germ cell death at different stages of development and the sperm count decrease.[20] Accordingly, it is expected that antioxidant therapy acts as a protective defense against oxidative stress and improve fertility parameters. The ability of antioxidants such as ascorbic acid in semen to protect spermatozoa from oxidative damage has been shown by researchers Oxidants and antioxidants have attracted widespread interest in nutrition research, biology and medicine. It has become clear that constant generation of pro-oxidants, including oxygen free radical, is an essential attribute of aerobic life.[15] A disturbance in the pro-oxidant/antioxidant system has been defined oxidative stress. Reactive oxygen species (ROS) are very reactive molecules ranked as free radicals owing to the presence of one unpaired electron such as a superoxide ion, nitrogen oxide and hydroxyl radical.[18]

The most reported effects of ginger are immunomodulatory, anti-tumorigenic, anti-inflammatory, anti-apoptotic, anti-hyperglycemic, anti-lipidemic and anti-emetic activity. Ginger is a powerful antioxidant and may either mitigate or prevent generation of free radicals. It is considered as a safe herbal medicine with only few and insignificant adverse side effects.[17] Gentamicin is able to generate destructive reactive oxygen species including superoxide, hydrogen peroxide and hydroxyl radical and frequently used to produce oxidative and necrotic damages.[6] Gentamicin can reduce the sperm count.[8] The role of gentamicin in the induction of apoptosis and oxidative damage has been reported. Recently, researchers also reported that ciprofloxacin, gentamicin, neomycin, streptomycin and ofloxacin induce apoptosis in testis.[21] Accordingly, the administration of carrot seed extract with gentamicin showing the effectiveness of this extract in the prevention of cell necrosis and apoptosis.[22] This could be indicative of free radical scavengering properties of carrot seeds which has been reported previously.[19] The results of other study showed the ability of ginger in the enhancement of caudaepididymal sperm reserves of rats resulting from increased testicular resulting from decreasing of apoptosis in testis. In fact, administration of ginger with gentamicin was able to counterbalance the negative effect of gentamicin on sperm count.[5] This study demonstrated that the administration of ginger can overcome toxicity of gentamicin on testis tissue and can protect testicular tissue from the detrimental effects of gentamicin.

Acknowledgment

We would like to thank of Islamic Azad University, Rasht branch, Rasht, Iran, for their financial support.

Conflict of interest

The authors report no conflicts of interest in this work.

References

1. Mills S, Bone K. Principle and practice of phytotherapy. London-UK: Churchill Livingstone; 2000.
2. Nassiri M, Khaki A, Gharachurlu S, Ashteani A, Rastegar H, Rezazadeh S. Effects of ginger on spermatogenesis in streptozotocin-induced diabetic rat. Iranian J Med Plants 2009;8(31):118-24.
3. Kirtikar KR, Basu BD. Indian Medicinal Plants. 2nd edition. New Delhi-India: Periodical Export; 1991.
4. Kumar R, Gautam G, Gupta NP. Drug therapy for idiopathic male infertility: rationale versus evidence. J Urol 2006;176:1307-12.
5. Khaki A, Fathiazad F, Nouri M, Khaki AA, Ozanci CC, et al. The effects of ginger on spermatogenesis and sperm parameters of rat. Iran J Reprod Med 2009;7(1):7-12.
6. Khaki A, Ghaffari Novin M, Khaki AA, Fathiazad F, Khabiri M, Hossinchi J. Ultra structural study of gentamicin and ofloxacin effect on testis tissue in rats: light and transmission electron microscopy. Afr J Pharm Pharmacol 2009;3(4):105-9.
7. Kilarkaje N. An aminoglycoside antibiotic gentamycin induces oxidative stress, reduces antioxidant reserve and impairs spermatogenesis in rats. J Toxicol Sci 2008;33(1):85-96.
8. Khaki A, Khaki AA, Iraj S, Bazi P, Imani SAM, Kachabi H. Comparative study of aminoglycosides (gentamicin and streptomycin) and (fluoroquinolone ofloxacin) antibiotics on testis tissue in rats: light and transmission electron microscopic study. Pak J Med Sci 2009;25(4):624-9.
9. Khaki A, Heidari M, Ghaffari Novin M, Khaki AA. Adverse effects of ciprofloxacin on testis apoptosis and sperm parameters in rats. Iran J Reprod Med 2008;6(2):14-20.
10. Mosher WD, Pratt WF. Fecundity and infertility in the United States: incidence and trends. J Fertil Steril 1991;56(2):192-3.
11. Huang HFS, Linsenmeyer TA, Li MT, Giglio W, Anesetti R, Von Hagen J, et al. Acute effects of spinal cord injury on the pituitary-testicular hormone axis and Sertoli cell functions: a time course study. J Androl 1995;16:148-157.
12. Carlsen E, Giwercman A, Keiding N, Skakkebaek NE. Evidence for decreasing quality of semen during past 50 years. BMJ 1992;12(305):609-13.
13. Reddy PS, Pushpalatha T, Reddy PS. Reduction of spermatogenesis and steroidogenesis in mice after fentin and fenbutatin administration. Toxicol Lett 2006;166:53-59.
14. Suryavathi V, Sharma S, Saxena P, Pandey S, Grover R, Kumar S, et al. Acute toxicity of textile dye wastewaters (untreated and treated) of Sanganer on male reproductive systems of albino rats and mice. Reprod Toxicol 2005;19:547-56.
15. Achary UR, Mishra M, Patro J, Panda MK. Effect of vitamins C and E on spermatogenesis in mice exposed to cadmium. Reprod Toxicol 2008;25:84-8.
16. Yousef MI. Protective role of ascorbic acid to enhance reproductive performance of male rabbits treated with stannous chloride. Toxicology 2005;207:81-9.
17. Dawson EB, Harris WA, Teter MC, Powell LC. Effect of ascorbic acid supplementation on the sperm quality of smokers. Fertil Steril 1992;58:1034-9.

18. Timmermans LM. Modifications in permatogenesis following antibiotic therapy. Acta Urol Belg 1989;57:35-46.
19. Yu LL, Zhou KK, Parry J. Antioxidant properties of cold-pressed black caraway, carrot, cranberry, and hemp seed oils. Food Chem 2005; 91:723-9.
20. Bestas A, Bayar MK, Akpolat N, Okuducu MN. Effect of sevoflurane anesthesia on the severity of renal histopathologic changes in rabbits pretreated with gentamicin: A controlled, investigator-blinded, experimental study. Curr Therap Res 2006;67:386-95.
21. Hong SH, Park SK, Cho YS, Lee HS, Kim KR, Kim MG, et al. Gentamicin induced nitric oxide-related oxidative damages on vestibular afferents in the guinea pig. Hear Res 2006,211:46-53.
22. Nouri M, Khaki A, Fathiazad F, Rashidi MR. The protective effects of carrot seeds extract on spermatogenesis and cauda epididymal sperm reserves in gentamicin treated rats. Yakhteh Med J 2009;11:327-33.

22

Modified Synthesis of Erlotinib Hydrochloride

Leila Barghi[1,2], **Ayuob Aghanejad**[3,4], **Hadi Valizadeh**[1,5], **Jaleh Barar**[1,3], **Davoud Asgari**[1,3*]

[1] *Faculty of Pharmacy, Tabriz University of Medical Sciences, Tabriz, Iran.*

[2] *Student Research Committee, Tabriz University of Medical Sciences, Tabriz, Iran.*

[3] *Research Center for Pharmaceutical Nanotechnology, Tabriz University of Medical Sciences, Tabriz, Iran.*

[4] *Faculty of Pharmacy, Tehran University of Medical Sciences, Tehran, Iran.*

[5] *Drug Applied Research Center, Tabriz University of Medical Sciences, Tabriz, Iran.*

ARTICLE INFO

Keywords:
Tyrosine kinase
Erlotinib
Palladium/Charcoal (Pd/C)

ABSTRACT

Purpose: An improved and economical method has been described for the synthesis of erlotinib hydrochloride, as a useful drug in treatment of non-small-cell lung cancer. ***Methods:*** Erlotinib hydrochloride was synthesized in seven steps starting from 3, 4-dihydroxy benzoic acid. In this study, we were able to modify one of the key steps which involved the reduction of the 6-nitrobenzoic acid derivative to 6-aminobenzoic acid derivative. An inexpensive reagent such as ammonium formate was used as an *in situ* hydrogen donor in the presence of palladium/charcoal (Pd/C) instead of hydrogen gas at high pressure. ***Results:*** This proposed method proceeded with 92% yield at room temperature. Synthesis of erlotinib was completed in 7 steps with overall yield of 44%. ***Conclusion:*** From the results obtained it can be concluded that the modified method eliminated the potential danger associated with the use of hydrogen gas in the presence of flammable catalysts. It should be mentioned that the catalyst was recovered after the reaction and could be used again.

Introduction

Although there are wide range of cytotoxic drugs with different mechanismsof action, most of them could not distinguish between cancerous and normal cell types. Growth factor signaling pathways have major role in regulating key cellular functions including cellproliferation,differentiation, metastasis and survival. An important mediator of growth factor signaling pathways is the human epidermal receptors (HERs).[1] Tyrosine kinase receptors, which belong to (HER) family, are over expressed in various types of solid tumors, including non-small-cell lung cancer (NSCLC).These receptors are cell membrane bound proteins that consist of three regions: an extracellular ligand binding site; an intracellular domain with tyrosine kinase activity and regulatory functions; and a region that binds the receptor to the cell membrane.[2-4] Phosphorylation of tyrosine residues on HERs is an important stage in signal transduction, leading to cell proliferation for major human carcinomas. Therefore, interruption of this growth signal is a potential target for anticancer treatment.[5] Erlotinib, a 4-anilinoquinazoline, is a potent inhibitor of tyrosine kinase. It reversibly and selectively binds to the adenosine triphosphate (ATP) binding site of the tyrosine kinase domain associated with HERs. Consequently phosphorylation of the tyrosine kinase is inhibited and thereby it can interfere with cell communication, signal transduction and ultimately cellular growth. [6] The common method for preparation of 4-anilinoquinazolines such as erlotinib involves the construction of suitable 4-chloroquinazoline intermediate and then reacting of this intermediate with suitable substituted aniline in acidic media. The 4-chloroquinazolines are key intermediates and their preparation involve a series of reaction and the use of highly flammable gas such as hydrogen at high pressure, and costly reagents such platinum oxide.[7] Erlotinib hydrochloride was synthesized in seven steps starting from 3, 4-dihydroxy benzoic acid. In this study, we were able to modify one of the key steps which involved the reduction of the 6-nitrobenzoic acid derivative to 6-aminobenzoic acid derivative. An inexpensive reagent such as ammonium formate was used as an *in situ* hydrogen donor in the presence of palladium/charcoal (Pd/C) instead of hydrogen gas at high pressure. This modified method eliminated the potential danger associated with the use of hydrogen gas in the presence of flammable catalysts. Furthermore catalyst could be recovered and used again.

Materials and methods

Etynyl aniline was purchased from Sigma-Aldrich. Other chemicals were purchased from Merck Chemical

***Corresponding author:** Davoud Asgari (PhD), Research Center for Pharmaceutical Nanotechnology, and Faculty of Pharmacy, Tabriz University of Medical Sciences, Tabriz, Iran. E-mail: dasgari@tbzmed.ac.ir

Company (Darmstadt, Germany). Melting points were determined by a Gallenkamp capillary apparatus. H NMR spectra were obtained with a Bruken-Spectrospin 400 MHz spectrometer (Varian, Switzerland).

3,4-bis(2-methoxyethoxy)-benzoic acid (3)

A suspension of 3,4-dihydroxy benzoic acid (23 g), potassium carbonate (82.5 g) and tetrabutyl ammonium iodide (5.51 g) in DMF (120 ml) was stirred for 1 h at 100 °C. The reaction mixture was cooled to 50 °C, and then 1-chloro-2-methoxyethane (54.18 ml) was added and the reaction mixture was heated to 85 °C and stirred for 20 h at this temperature. The reaction mixture was filtered and the solid material was washed with ethyl acetate (300 ml). The combined filtrates were evaporated under reduced pressure to afford a yellow residue (2). Without any further isolation and purification, the ester residue was dissolved in a solution of ethanol (200 ml), water (70 ml) and potassium hydroxide (33.5g) and stirred for 4 h at room temperature. Ethanol was removed under reduced pressure, and the pH of the solution was adjusted to ~3 by adding a solution HCl (2 N) at 0 °C. A solid was precipitated which was filtered, washed with cold water, and dried (Na_2SO_4) to afford carboxylic acid (3: 40 g, 99.27%) as a white solid; R_f (20% n-hexane/ethyl acetate) 0.25; Mp: 101-103 °C, ^{1}H-NMR ($CDCl_3$): 0.95-0.99 (t, 3H, CH_3CH_2, ^3J= 7.10 Hz), 3.43 (d, 6H, 2x OCH_3), 3.78-3.81 (m, 4H, 2x CH_2O), 4.18-4.27 (q, 2H, CH_2, 3J=7.10 Hz), 6.90-6.92 (d, 1H, HAr, ^3J=8.41 Hz), 7.60 (d, 1H, HAr), 7.62-7.71 (dd, 1H, HAr,^3J=8.41 Hz, ^4J=1.96 Hz).

Ethyl 3,4-bis(2-methoxyethoxy)-benzoate (4)

To 3,4-bis(2-methoxyethoxy)-benzoic acid (40 g) in ethanol (300 ml) was added sulfuric acid (3 ml). The mixture was stirred under N_2 at reflux for 24 hours. The solvent was removed in vacuo and the residue was extracted with ethyl acetate. Then the organic phase was washed with sodium bicarbonate solution and brine, dried over sodium sulfate, filtered and concentrated in vacuo to afford ethyl 3,4-bis(2-methoxyethoxy)-benzoate (31.65 g, 71.63%); Mp: 56.5-57.5°C, ^{1}H-NMR ($CDCl_3$): 1.30-1.33 (t, 3H, CH_3CH_2, ^3J= 7.10 Hz), 3.44 (s, 6H, 2x OCH_3), 3.76-3.73 (m, 4H, 2x CH_2O), 4.16-4.21 (m, 4H, 2 x CH_2O), 4.31-4.36 (q, 2H, CH_2, 3J=7.10 Hz), 6.89-6.92 (d, 1H, HAr, ^3J=8.41 Hz), 7.50-7.52 (d, 1H, HAr,^4J=1.96 Hz), 7.60-7.62 (dd, 1H, HAr,^3J=8.41 Hz, ^4J=1.96 Hz).

Ethyl 4,5-bis(2-methoxyethoxy)-2-nitro-benzoate (5)

The product of previous step (30g) in acetic acid (90 ml)was treated drop wise with conc. HNO_3 (25ml) at 5 °C, and the solution was stirred 24 hours before pouring in to the ice. The solvent was removed in vacuo and the residue was extracted with ethyl acetate. Then the organic phase was washed with sodium bicarbonate solution and brine and concentrated in vacuo to afford Ethyl 4,5-bis(2-methoxyethoxy)-2-nitro-benzoate (32 g, 92.75%); ^{1}H-NMR ($CDCl_3$): 1.32-1.36 (t,3H, CH_3CH_2, ^3J= 7.20 Hz), 3.44 (s, 6H, 2x OCH_3), 3.71-3.81(m, 4H, 2x CH_2O), 4.23-4.27 (m, 4H, 2x CH_2O), 4.34-4.36 (q, 2H, CH_2, ^3J=7.20 Hz),7.13 (s, 1H, HAr,), 7.50 (s, 1H, HAr).

2-amino-4,5-bis (2-methoxyethoxy)-benzoate (6)

2-Propanol (350 ml) was added to a flask containing Pd/C (9.32 g). Ammonium formate (55.14 g) in water (35 mL) was transferred to the same flask. The reaction mixture was stirred for 1 min to activate Pd/C. Next, Ethyl 4,5-bis(2-methoxyethoxy)-2-nitro-benzoate (30 g) were added, and the reaction mixture was stirred at room temperature (20 min). The reaction mixture was filtered and the solid material was washed with ethyl acetate and 2-propanol. The filtrate was evaporated under reduced pressure and the residue was extracted with ethyl acetate, dried over sodium sulfate, filtered and concentrated in vacuo to afford 2-amino-4,5-bis (2-methoxyethoxy)-benzoate (25.270 g, 92.33%); ^{1}H-NMR ($CDCl_3$):1.34-1.37 (t, 3H, CH_3CH_2, ^3J= 7.10 Hz), 3.43 (s, 6H, 2x OCH_3), 3.71-3.77 (m, 4H, 2x CH_2O), 4.06-4.10 (m, 4H, 2x CH_2O), 4.26-4.31 (q, 2H, CH_2, ^3J=7.10 Hz), 5.65 (br, 2H, NH_2), 6.14 (s, 1H, HAr,),7.41 (s, 1H, HAr).

6,7- bis (2-methoxy-ethoxy) quinazolone (7)

2-amino-4,5-bis (2-methoxyethoxy)-benzoate(25g) and ammonium formate(5g) were dissolved in formamide(38ml) and the stirred mixture was heated to 160-165 °C under an atmosphere of N_2 for 2 hours. Cold H_2O was added and precipitated product was recovered by filtration, washed with cold H_2O and dried in oven. The filtrate was extracted with $CHCl_3$ and the organic extracts were washed with brine, dried over sodium sulfate and concentrated in vacuo. The residue and quinazolone precipitate were combined, treated with ether and filtered to afford 6,7- bis (2-methoxy-ethoxy) quinazolone (20.45, 87.1%); Mp: 190-191°C, ^{1}HNMR ($CDCl_3$): 3.48 (s, 6H, OCH_3), 3.81-3.87 (m, 4H, 2x OCH_2), 4.27-4.29(m, 4H, 2x OCH_2), 7.15(s, 1H, HAr), 7.59 (s, 1H, HAr), 8.04 (s, 1H, HAr).

4-chloro-6,7-bis- (2-methoxy-ethoxy)- quinazoline (8)

To 6,7- bis (2-methoxy-ethoxy) quinazolone (18.5g) in $CHCl_3$ (470 ml) containing 2.5 ml DMF was added oxalylchloride (19 ml) in four portions over 20 minutes. Once foaming ceased the solution was refluxed 2 hours. The solvent was evaporated under reduced pressure and the residue was dissolved in dichloromethane and washed with brine, sodium bicarbonate and water. The organic phase was dried over sodium sulfate and concentrated in vacuo to give 4-chloro-6,7-bis- (2-methoxy-ethoxy)- quinazoline (19.5g, 99.1%); Mp: 107-108 °C, ^{1}H-NMR ($CDCl_3$): 3.49 (s, 3H, OCH_3), 3.50 (s, 3H, OCH_3), 3.88-3.90 (m, 4H, 2x OCH_2), 4.32-4.39 (m, 4H, 2x OCH_2), 7.36 (s, 1H, HAr),7.44 (s, 1H, HAr), 8.88 (s, 1H, HAr).

Erlotinib hydrochloride (9)

4-chloro-6,7-bis- (2-methoxy-ethoxy)- quinazoline (19.5 g) was suspended in 300 ml water and 3-ethynylaniline (8.4 g)and 37% hydrochloric acid (5.2 ml) was added at 25-30 °C. The reaction mixture was heated at 40 °C and stirred for 1.5 hours. After cooling, obtained solid material was filtered and washed with water and ethylacetate:n-hexane (50:50) and was dried in oven at 40 °C to afford erlotinib hydrochloride(22.26g, 83%); Mp: 225-227 °C, ^{1}H NMR (DMSO-d6) δ 11.13 (s, 1H, NH), 8.70 (s, 1H, H-Ar), 8.14 (s,1H, H-Ar), 7.70-7.81 (m, 2H, H-Ar), 7.28-7.51 (m, 3H, HAr),4.31-4.32 (m, 4H, 2 CH2O), 3.74-3.77 (m, 4H, 2 CH2O), 3.67 (s, 1H, ethynyl), 3.33-3.34 (d, 6H, 2 OCH3).

Results and Discussions

The synthesis of erlotinib (Figure 1) was started from 3,4-dihydroxy benzoic acid. O-alkylation of 3,4-dihydroxy benzoic acid with 4.0 equivalent of 1-chloro-2-methoxyethane in hot DMF afforded intermediate methoxyethoxy-3,4-bis(2-methoxyethoxy)-benzoate in quantitative yield. DMF was then removed and basic hydrolysis of the ester was performed in the same batch to afford the 3,4-bis(2-methoxyethoxy)-benzoic acid in 99.27% overall yield. No further purification was performed in this step. Esterification of carboxylic acid in acidic ethanol gave ethyl 3,4-bis (2-methoxy-ethoxy)benzoate. Nitration of ethyl 3,4-bis(2-methoxyethoxy)-benzoate in nitric acid and glacial acetic acid at 0 °C afforded the single nitro product in 92.75% yield. No purification was performed in this step.[8] There have been reports on the reduction of nitro compounds to their corresponding derivatives using ammonium formate as in situ hydrogen donor.[9]So, the reduction of the nitro group of ethyl 3,4-bis(2-methoxyethoxy)-2-nitro-benzoate, by using ammonium formate and Pd/C catalyst in aqueous alcoholic solvent at room temperature gave 2-amino-4,5-bis (2-methoxyethoxy)-benzoate. The cyclization of this product and construction of 6,7- bis (2-methoxy-ethoxy) quinazoloneby using formamide and ammonium formate was the next step. Then chlorination of quinazolone carried out by using oxalylchloride. The reaction mixture was refluxed 1.5 hours and 4-chloro-6,7-bis- (2-methoxy-ethoxy)-quinazoline was formed. Finally erlotinib hydrochloride was prepared in aqueous medium by using 3-ethynylaniline under acidic condition. The proposed method for reduction of 6-nitrobenzoic acid derivative proceeded with 92.33% yield at room temperature. Synthesis of erlotinib was completed in 7 steps with overall yield of 44%.

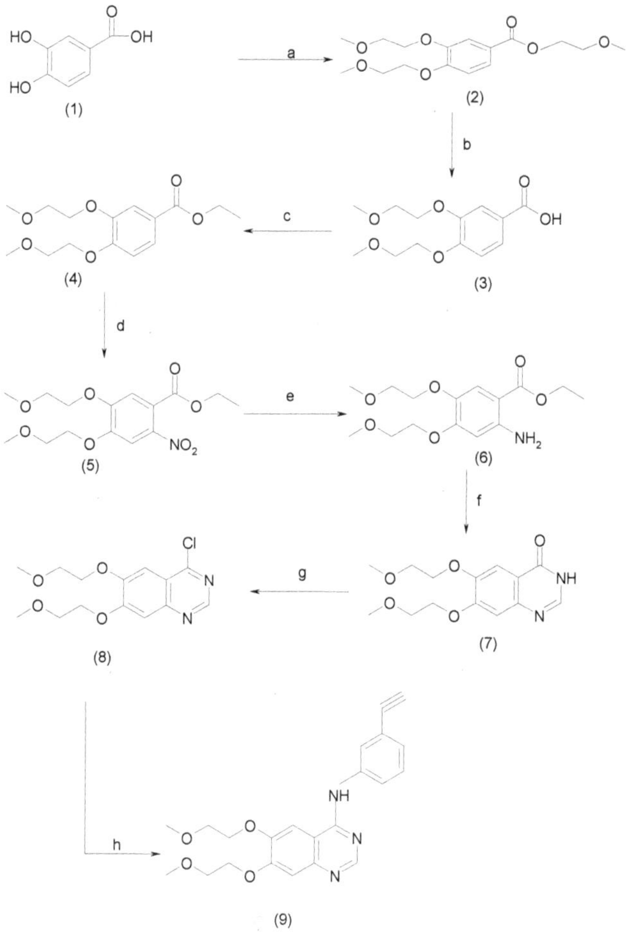

Figure 1. a) K_2CO_3, $ClCH_2CH_2OCH_3$, TBAI, DMF, 85 °C, 20h; b) KOH, CH_3CH_2OH, H_2O, 4h; C) CH_3CH_2OH,H_2so_4,90°C; d) HNO_3, glacial acetic acid, 0 °C, 2h; e)ammonium formate, Pd/C,2-propanol,25°C,20 min; f)ammonium formate, formamide, 160°C, 2h; g)$CHCl_3$, DMF, oxalylchloride,80°C, 1.5h; h)H_2O,3-ethynylaniline, HCl, 25°C, 1.5h.

Conclusion

An improved and economical method has been described for the synthesis of erlotinib hydrochloride, which is used as a second- and third-line treatment of advanced or metastatic NSCLC. One of the key steps of erlotinib formation which involved the reduction of the 6-nitrobenzoic acid derivative to 6-aminobenzoic acid derivative was modified. An inexpensive reagent such as ammonium formate was used as an in situ hydrogen donor in the presence of Pd/C instead of hydrogen gas at high pressure. This modified method eliminated the potential danger associated with the use of hydrogen gas in the presence of flammable catalysts. Furthermore catalyst could be recovered and used again.

Acknowledgement

The authors would like to thank research center for pharmaceutical nanotechnology. This article was a part of a thesis submitted for PhD degree (No.51) in Faculty of Pharmacy, Tabriz University of Medical Sciences, Tabriz, Iran.

Conflict of interest
The authors report no conflicts of interest.

References

1. Chandregowda V, Kush AK, Chandrasekara Reddy G. Synthesis and in vitro antitumor activities of novel 4-anilinoquinazoline derivatives. *European Journal of Medicinal Chemistry* 2009;44(7):3046-3055.
2. Danielle M G. Molecular targets in cancer therapy. *Seminars in Oncology Nursing* 2003;19(3):193-205.
3. Janine S. Erlotinib: Small-molecule targeted therapy in the treatment of non-small-cell lung cancer. *Clinical Therapeutics* 2005;27(10):1513-1534.
4. Ullrich A, Schlessinger J. Signal transduction by receptors with tyrosine kinase activity. *Cell* 1990;61(2):203-212.
5. Lepper ER, Swain SM, Tan AR, Figg WD, Sparreboom A. Liquid-chromatographic determination of erlotinib (OSI-774), an epidermal growth factor receptor tyrosine kinase inhibitor. *Journal of Chromatography* 2003;796(1):181-188.
6. Clay D, Lipman YM, Bonk ME. Erlotinib (Tarceva): A brief overview.*P and T* 2005;30(10):561-562, 571-572, 602.
7. Rodney CaughrenSchunr, Arnold LD. Inventors; Pfizer Inc. New york,N.Y, assignee. Alkynyl and Azido substituted 4-Anilinoquinazolines. US patent 5747498, 1998.
8. Asgari D, Aghanejad A, Mojarrad JS. An Improved Convergent Approach for Synthesis of Erlotinib, a Tyrosine Kinase Inhibitor, via a Ring Closure Reaction of Phenyl Benzamidine Intermediate. Bull Korean Chem Soc. 2011;32(3):909
9. Byun E, Hong B, De Castro KA, Lim M, Rhee H. One-pot reductive mono-N-alkylation of aniline and nitroarene derivatives using aldehydes. *J Org Chem* 2007;72(25):9815-9817.

23

Iontophoretic Permeation of Lisinopril at Different Current Densities and Drug Concentrations

Ashish Jain [1]*, Satish Nayak [1], Vandana Soni [2]

[1] *Bansal College of Pharmacy, Kokta, Anand Nagar, Bhopal-462021, India.*

[2] *Department of Pharmaceutical Sciences, Dr H.S.Gour Vishwavidyalaya, Sagar 470003, M.P. India.*

ARTICLE INFO

Keywords:
Lisinopril
Iontophoresis
Current densities
Pigskin
Transdermal drug delivery

ABSTRACT

Purpose: The purpose of the present work was to assess iontophoretic permeation of Lisinopril at different current densities and concentrations for development of patient-controlled active transdermal system. ***Methods:*** *In vitro* iontophoretic transdermal delivery of Lisinopril across the pigskin was investigated at three different drug concentrations and three different current densities (0.25- 0.75 mA/cm^2) in the donor cell of the diffusion apparatus, using cathodal iontophoresis along with the passive controls. ***Results:*** For passive permeation, the steady state flux significantly increased with the increasing of donor drug concentration. At all concentration levels, iontophoresis considerably increased the permeation rate compared to passive controls. Iontophoretic transport of Lisinopril was to be found increase with current densities. Flux enhancement was highest at the lowest drug load and lowest at the highest drug load. ***Conclusion:*** The obtained results indicate that permeation rate of Lisinopril across the pigskin can be considerably enhanced, controlled or optimized by the use of Iontophoresis technique.

Introduction

Transdermal delivery of drugs through the skin to the systemic circulation provide a convenient route of administration to the delivery of drugs for prolonged therapy in diseases like hypertension and diabetes.[1] Cardiovascular diseases account for a large proportion of all deaths and disability worldwide. Global Burden of Disease study reported that in 1990 there were 5.2 million deaths from cardiovascular diseases in economically developed countries and 9.1 million deaths from the same causes in developing countries.[2,3] Worldwide frequency estimates for hypertension may be as much as 1 billion individuals, and approximately 7.1 million deaths per year may be attributable to hypertension.[4]

There are many oral drugs used in the treatment of hypertension. However problem may arise with oral delivery due to uneven bio-distribution throughout the body, a lack of drug targeting specificity, the necessity of a large dose to achieve high blood concentration and adverse side effects due to such high doses. It is also noted that difficulties in the treatment of hypertension does not necessarily lie in the inadequacies pharmacological therapeutics but it may be due to poor patient compliances during lifelong administration. Approximate 50 % of hypertensive patients do not fulfill with their prescribed treatment.[5] Reason suggested for this complication includes intolerable side effects, complex treatment and lake of reminders.[5]

Lisinopril is an angiotensin-converting enzyme inhibitor used for the treatment of hypertension. It is available only in the form of oral tablets in the market with slow and incomplete absorption after oral administration with a bioavailability of 25–30%.[6-7] Lisinopril is an ideal candidate for transdermal study because of low oral dose (2.5–20 mg), low molecular mass (405.5 g/mol), and low oral bioavailability (25%). This study investigated the iontophoretic permeability of lisinopril through excised pig skin to assess its potential for the development of a patient-controlled active transdermal system.

The first commercial patch was approved for scopolamine in 1979. Some other available transdermal patches in world drug market are: nitroglycerin, nicotin, clonidine, fentanyl, estradiol, testosterone, lidocain, and oxbutinin. Skin has been recognized as a route of drug administration for decades but limited permeability of human skin is still a basic problem, restraining its widespread therapeutic use also limiting suitability of number of drug candidates for this route. So it is the very big challenge of creating effective transdermal system because it involves adequate drug permeability through the stratum corneum.[8] Introduction of the physical enhancement techniques like iontophoresis combined with the prospect of the programmed delivery has contributed significantly in the expansion of transdermal research. Iontophoresis

***Corresponding author:** Ashish Jain, Bansal College of Pharmacy, Kokta, Anand Nagar, Bhopal, India.
Email: aashish.pharmatech@gmail.com

may be defined as facilitated movement of compounds, in particular charged moiety, into or across a membrane by the application of an externally applied electrical potential difference across the membrane.[9] Iontophoresis has provided a non-invasive delivery system for local or systemic delivery of drugs. Beside the common benefit of transdermal delivery iontophoresis presents a unique opportunity to provide programmed drug delivery.[10] The enhancement of permeation by the iontophoresis results from a possible mechanism including electro-osmosis, electro repulsion or current induced.[11,12] Iontophoretic products have already been launched in the US market and gained growing acceptance for the topical delivery of drugs[13,14] hence attempts have been undertaken to develop transdermal iontophoretic system for lisinopril.

Materials and Methods

Lisinopril was a gift sample from Lupin laboratories Bhopal. Silver plates (purity 99.99%, 5 mm diameters) were obtained from a goldsmith shop Bhopal, India. Sodium Chloride AR, octanol, isopropyl alcohol, silver chloride were obtained from SD Fine-Chem (Mumbai, India). Franz-diffusion cell was designed by Peekay scientific glass wares, Bhopal, All the reagents/chemicals used were of analytical grade. Experiments were conducted with ultra pure water (resistivity, 18.2 MW cm) obtained from Milli-Q Academic System.

Equipment

Iontophoretic DC source (digital display, current 0-10 mA, voltage 0-25 V) was purchased from C-tech Psu-2510/lab (Mumbai, India) and iontophoretic diffusion cell was fabricated by Navin Scientific Glass Product (Bangalore, India) as per given specifications. Silver/silver chloride electrode was prepared as per the standard procedure.[14] Silver wire (99.99% pure, 1.0 mm thickness) was used as connecting wire. U-V Visible Spectrophotometer- Shimadzu UV-1700 PC Shimadzu Corporation, Japan was used for analysis.

Experimental Design

Iontophoretic transdermal permeation study of Lisinopril was carried out at different concentrations and current densities. Different systems having different concentration (current density 0.5 mA/cm^2) had been designed as System A, System B, System C having concentration 25 mg/ml, 50 mg/ml and 75 mg/ml respectively. Moreover system with different current densities (concentration 25 mg/ml) designed as System A1, System A2, SystemA3 having current densities 0.25, 0.5 and 0.75 mA/cm^2 respectively.

Preparation of skin membrane

From a local abattoir, ear was obtained from freshly slaughtered pigs. The skin was removed carefully from the outer regions of the ear and separated from the underlying cartilage with a scalpel. After separating the full thickness skin, the fat adhering to the dermis side was removed using a scalpel and isopropyl alcohol. Finally the skin was washed with tap water and stored at refrigerator in aluminum foil packing and was used within two days.[15]

In vitro passive permeation studies

The *in vitro* passive permeation studies were performed using vertical type Franz diffusion cell having a receptor compartment capacity of 10 ml. The excised skin was mounted between the half-cells with the dermis in contact with receptor fluid (Phosphate buffer pH 7.4) and equilibrated for 1 h. The area available for diffusion was about 1.21cm^2. The donor cell was covered with an aluminum foil to prevent the evaporation of vehicle. The fluid in the receptor compartment was maintained at 37±0.5 °C. Under these conditions, the temperature at the skin surface was approximately 32 °C. Different solution of lisinopril in phosphate buffer pH 7.4 (each one ml) was placed in the donor compartment. The entire assembly was kept on a magnetic stirrer and the solution in the receiver compartment was stirred continuously using a magnetic bead. The sample solution was withdrawn from the receptor compartment at regular intervals and assayed for drug content.[16]

Procedure of iontophoretic diffusion

For the iontophoretic study, diffusion cell was modified according to Glikfield et al.[17] The apparatus essentially consisted of a glass molded large receiving chamber provided with two parallel ports on the topside and a sampling port on the side. Two upper chambers are made from open-ended cylindrical glass tubes, the outer diameters of which were equivalent to the inner diameter of the parallel ports. The lower 10 mm of these tubes were slightly constricted to allow a clearance of 1 to 1.5 mm on the side. This ensured easy fitting. After the skin was tied at this constricted end, the effective diameter increased and became exactly equal to inner diameter of the extended ports. Once slipped into parallel ports, they stay attached by glass joints forming two separate chambers with skin at the base. Both the skin touched the receptor solution at the same depth and each chamber housed one electrode. Once the battery was switched on, current flowed through the skin placed in anodal compartment into receiving solution below and reached the cathodal electrode through the skin tied to cathodal end. Donor solution was filled in one of the top chambers depending on the polarity of the drug and the other serve as return electrode chamber. For our study, silver/silver chloride electrode was inserted into the donor compartment whereas silver plate was inserted into anodal chamber as return electrode. Direct current (0.25-0.75 mA cm^{-2}) was used throughout experiment. The receptor fluid (5 ml) was withdrawn at regular intervals and replaced with fresh buffer to maintain sink condition. Samples were assayed by the U-V spectrophotometrically.

Solubility determination

Excess amounts of drug were taken into glass vials and dissolved in measured amount of different solvent to get saturated solutions. The solutions were kept at rest for 24 h to assist the attainment of equilibrium with the undissolved drug particles. From these solutions, the supernatant was filtered to separate the undissolved drug particles and diluted suitably and the concentrations were measured.[18]

Partition coefficient

The octanol / phosphate buffer partition coefficient of the lisinopril was determined by shaking equal volume of octanol and phosphate buffer in a separating funnel for 10 min and allowing to stand for 24 h. Aqueous phase was assayed before and after partitioning to get the partition coefficients.[18,19] Skin/vehicle partition coefficient was determined by dipping the skin in known concentrations of drug in phosphate buffer for 24 h, assaying aqueous phase remaining drug for estimation of concentration after partitioning.

Data analysis

The cumulative amount permeated was plotted against time, and the slope of the linear portion of the plot was estimated as the steady state flux. Permeability coefficient and diffusion coefficient were calculated using following formulas[20]:

$$KP = JSS / Cd \qquad (1)$$

$$D = KP\, h / K \qquad (2)$$

where Kp represents permeability coefficient, Jss is the steady-state flux, Cd is the concentration of drug in donor compartment, D is the diffusion coefficient, K is the skin/vehicle partition coefficient and h the thickness of the skin. Flux enhancement was calculated by dividing iontophoretic steady state flux by the corresponding passive steady state flux.

Statistical analysis

Statistical analysis was carried out using 2- way ANOVA. The effect of concentration on steady state flux was separately evaluated by one-way ANOVA followed by Bonferroni's test.[21] At 95% confidence intervals, p values less than 0.05 were considered to be significant.

Results and Discussion

Permeability of drug through skin is strongly influenced by its physicochemical parameters. Molecular weight for ideal candidate of transdermal drug delivery suggested around 200-500 Da by Doh and co-workers.[22] Lisinopril having molecular weight 405.5 fits into this category. Physicochemical parameters of lisinopril were investigated and the results were listed in Table 1. The drug showed good solubility in water (90.47 mg/ml). Phosphate buffer (pH 7.4) was used as receiver fluid in our study, by this basis saturation solubility was also determined in this media. Solubility of Lisinopril in phosphate buffer (pH 7.4) was found 90.68 mg/ml which is very close to solubility of Lisinopril in water. The octanol–water partition coefficient is a measure of the relative lipophilicity of a compound. The experimentally determined partition coefficient (octanol/phosphate buffer pH 7.4) was found to be 0.675 ± 0.0124, which indicated that the drug had less affinity towards the lipids compared to phosphate buffer. However, the lipophilicity of a drug moiety is an intrinsic character and cannot be changed.

At pH 7.4 mammalian skins are negatively charged and ionic forms have low affinity toward skin. Lisinopril, being an acidic drug with the pKa value of 3.85, was largely ionized which reduced its affinity toward the skin.[23] In iontophoresis, the ionized moieties actively propelled through natural pore pathways of skin while the unionized fraction could pass the unbroken horny layers by passive permeation resulting in enhanced permeation.[24] To simulate the physiological condition, the diffusion cell was modified where both the electrodes were place on the same side of skin. The receiving chamber with phosphate buffer reflected the body. The permeability and diffusion parameters are very important for comparison purpose.[25] It is evident that as the concentrations increases in donor the permeability coefficients decrease. Result for the permeability and diffusion coefficients of lisinopril in different systems in our study for passive diffusion and iontophoresis are provided in Table 2, which found to be obey above hypothesis.

Table 1. Physicochemical Parameters of Lisinopril

Trial No.	Solubility (mg/ml)		Partition Coefficient	Molecular Weight
	Phosphate buffer 7.4 pH	Water	Octanol/Phosphate Buffer 7.4 pH	(g/mol)
1	90.12	93.22	0.671	
2	92.14	90.87	0.689	405.5
3	89.78	87.34	0.665	
Mean±SD	90.68±1.2757	90.47±2.9596	0.675±0.0124	

Table 2. Comparison of Permeation & Diffusion coefficients of Lisinopril in different Systems by Passive and Iontophoresis

Donor System	Permeability Coefficient (cm/hr)		Diffusion coefficient (cm^2/s)	
	Passive	Iontophoretic	Passive	Iontophoretic
System- A	0.0252	0.0797	$0.1147 * 10^{-5}$	$0.3629 * 10^{-5}$
System-B	0.0250	0.0789	$0.1138 * 10^{-5}$	$0.359 * 10^{-5}$
System-C	0.0235	0.0543	$0.1070 * 10^{-5}$	$0.247 * 10^{-5}$

Among the various factors that affect passive permeability, the concentration of the actives in the donor system is most crucial. To evaluate this effect, the experiment was design at three different drug concentrations. Results show that overall iontophoretic permeability at all concentration level significantly higher that of passive values. The passive and iontophoretic permeation profiles of lisinopril at different donor concentrations are shown in Figures 1 and 2. The passive profiles are linear at all concentration levels indicating the permeation kinetics was more or less zero order. In the passive process, both the rate and extent of permeation increased with increasing donor drug concentrations. This was expected as increase in the donor drug concentration enhanced the concentration gradient, which was the driving force of mass transport.[26] In contrasts iontophoretic profiles were less linear indicating the involvement of multitude of factors. When the concentration of the drug was raised from low (System A) to medium (System B), the permeation rate increased but there no significant increase was found at the highest concentration (System C) over that of next lower concentration. This was in agreement with the hypothesis that in the drug concentration increases iontophoretic delivery upto a certain point, but at still higher concentrations, the flux may become independent of concentration.[27] In iontophoresis though ionic repulsion is the dominant force, convective flow of solutes toward the direction of current, influences the permeation rate. Permeability of skin also changes under influences of current.[28]

The total flux of a solute during iontophoresis is the sum of fluxes due to electro-repulsion, convective flow, and passive diffusion.[24] Lisinopril (pKa 3.85) at pH 7.4 acquires a negative charge and was delivered from cathodal chamber. Since the isoelectric point of the skin varies between 3 and 4, at physiological pH, the volume flow was directed toward the cathode. Hence at pH 7.4, only passive and electro-repulsive fluxes were likely to contribute to the overall permeation. Electro-osmotic flow may even oppose the permeation from the cathodal compartment.[29] The iontophoretic profile showed the initial permeation was high but the permeation rate declined in the later hours. This was unexpected as the voltage gradually dropped with time and hence the magnitude of electro-osmotic opposition was expected to be lesser in the later part of the study. The opposite result suggested the involvement of a factor that negatively influenced the permeation as time progressed. It is possible that during the passage of current, the cathodal electrode (Ag/AgCl) received a steady flow of electron, which resulted in the liberation of negatively charged chloride ions. As time progressed, the concentration of this newly released chloride ions were likely to increase in the cathodal compartment. Since the drug was negatively charged, chloride ions served as competitor. A chloride ion, being much smaller than the drug ion, was a powerful competitor, which reduced the transport efficiency of lisinopril.[30]

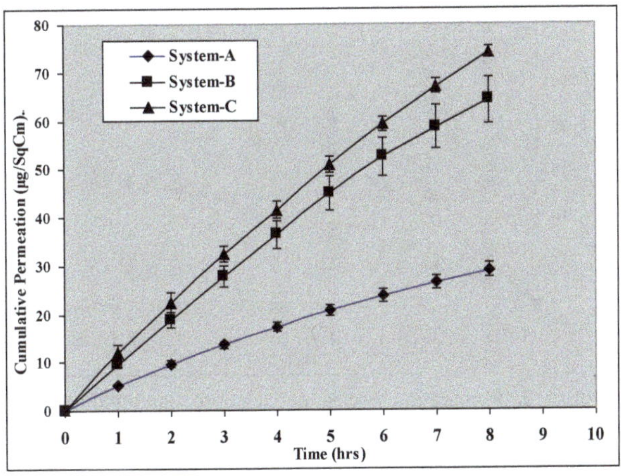

Figure 1. Permeation profile of Lisinopril (Iontophoresis) at different donor concentrations (n=3).

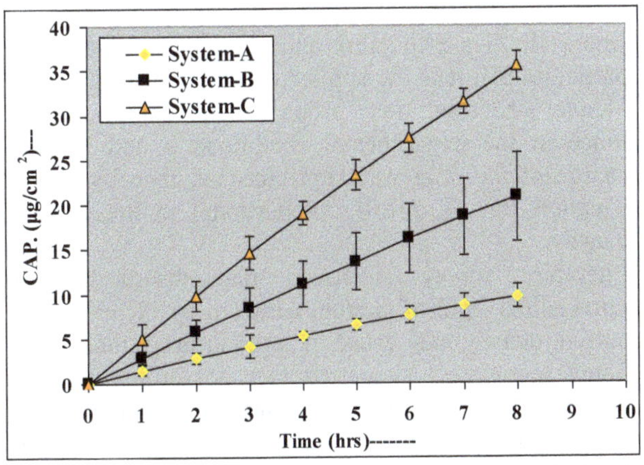

Figure 2. Permeation profile of Lisinopril (passive) at different donor concentrations (n=3).

Table 3 depicts the enhancement in iontophoretic flux compared to the passive flux of same donor concentration. Enhanced permeation was highest at the lowest drug load and lowest at the highest drug load. The iontophoretic contribution was found to be slightly more at higher donor concentrations.

Table 3. Enhancement Ratio and Benefit by iontophoresis

Donor Systems	Steady State flux (μg/ hr.cm2)		Benefit by Iontophoresis (μg/hr.cm2)	Enhancement Ratio (R)
	Passive	Iontophoretic		
System-A	1.429	4.517	3.088	3.160
System-B	2.841	8.636	5.795	3.0397
System-C	3.998	9.227	5.229	2.3079

The effect of current densities on the transport of lisinopril through pig ear skin, experiment was carried out at three different current densities and result was found that iontophoretic drug transport of lisinopril increased with the increasing current densities. (Figure 3).

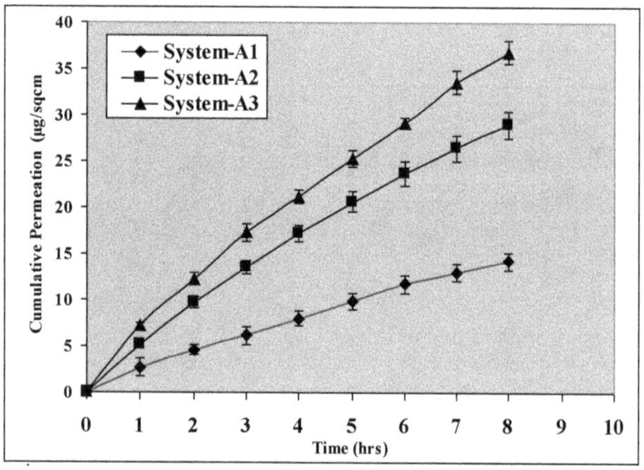

Figure 3. Permeation Profile of Lisinopril (Iontophoretic) at different Current Densities (n=3).

The relationship between current density and flux of lisinopril may be described by Faraday's law which is represent by following equation[31]

$$Ji = ti\ It / Zi\ F$$

where Ji, Zi are the flux and charge of lisinopril at particular pH, It is the applied current density, F is the Faraday's constant, ti is a proportionality constant.

Since in the experimental conditions ti and Zi i.e., charge of the drug was kept constant, then by above equation flux is directly proportional to the current density.

Literature survey suggested that disordering of intracellular lipid of stratum corneum by increasing of current density may cause increase in drug transport.[32]

Some researchers suggested that possibility may be also that the electro-osmotic volume flow increase with an increase an current densities[33] which leads to increase in the flux of the drug.

Experimental data indicate that by proper selection of donor solution current density and some other related factors, extent of lisinopril transport across skin can be manipulated.

Conclusion

The present work shows that the iontophoretic approach was feasible to enhance and control the rate of transdermal drug delivery of lisinopril. Study show that iontophoretic drug delivery increase with the current densities and concentration, but in case of concentration permeation increase up to certain points, afterwards flux may become independent of concentration. It can be said that lisinopril is a promising candidate for transdermal delivery and its delivery can be manipulates, controlled and optimized by iontophoresis.

Conflict of interest

The authors report no conflicts of interest.

References

1. Jain A, Ghosh B, Nayak B, Soni V. A Study of Transdermal Delivery of Glibenclamide Using Iontophoresis. Int J Health Res 2009; 2(1): 83-91.
2. Pravilo VS, Belov VV. Risk factors of cardiovascular diseases, cerebral hemodynamics and psychological features of personality: correlation in young males depending on prognosis of essential hypertension. Ter Arkh 2007;79(1):43-6.
3. Jorgensen T, Willaing I, Thomson TF. Cardiovascular diseases from epidemiology to prevention . Ugeskr laeger 2005;167(10) : 1170-3.
4. Alderman MH. Hypertension Control: Improved, but not enough. Am J Hypertens 2007;20(4): 347.
5. Foster SB, Kousch D. Adherence to therapy in hypertensive patients. Nurs Clin North Am 1981; 16(2): 331-41.
6. Marc H. Angiotensin converting enzyme inhibitors, angiotensin and calcium channel blockers. In: Williams AD, Thamas LL, editors. Foye's principles of medicinal chemistry. 5th ed. Baltimore, MD: Lippincott Williams and Wilkins; 2002. 533-61.

7. Barry BW. Mode of action of penetration enhancers in human skin. J Control Release 1987; 68:85-97.
8. Jain A, Mishra A, Nayak A, Soni V. Transdermal Delivery of Antihypertensive Agents: A tabular update. Int J Drug Deliv 2010;3: 1-13.
9. Nair VB, Panchagnula R. Effect of iontophoresis and fatty acids on permeation of arginine vasopressin through rat skin. Pharmacol Res 2003; 47(6): 563-9.
10. Kalia YN, Naik A, Garrison J, Guy RH. Iontophoretic drug delivery. Adv Drug Deliv Rev 2004; 56(5): 619-58.
11. Wang Y, Thakur R, Fan Q, Michniak B. Transdermal iontophoresis: combination strategies to improve transdermal iontophoretic drug delivery. Eur J Pharm Biopharm 2005; 60(2): 179-91.
12. Pillai O, Nair V, Panchagnula R. Transdermal iontophoresis of insulin: IV. Influence of chemical enhancers. Int J Pharm 2004; 269(1): 109-20.
13. Jamakandi VD, Ghosh B, Desai BG, Khanam J. Recent Trends in Transdermal Cardiovascular Therapy. Ind J Pharma Sci 2006; 68(5): 556-61.
14. Kanikkannan N, Singh J, Ramarao P. In vitrotransdermal iontophoretic transport of timolol maleate: effect of age and species. J Cont Rel 2001; 71: 99-105.
15. Suwanpidokkul N, Thongnopnua P, Umprayn K. Transdermal delivery of zidovudine: The effects of vehicles, enhancers, and polymer membranes on permeation across cadaver pig skin. AAPS Pharm Sci Tech 2004;5(3):48.
16. Mutalik S, Udapa N. Pharmacological evaluation of membrane-moderated transdermal system of glibenclamide. Clin Exp Pharmacol Physiol 2006;33:17-26.
17. Glikfield P, Cullander C, Hinz R, Guy R. A new system for in vitro studies of iontophoresis. Pharm Res 1988;5:443-6.
18. Ghosh B, Reddy LH. Effect of physicochemical parameters on skin permeability of antihypertensives. Ind J Exp Biol 2001;39(7):710-4
19. Silcocks CG. The Physical Chemistry. 3rd Ed. London: Macdonald and evans; 1980.
20. Sung KC, Fang JY, Hu OYP. Delivery of nalbuphine and its prodrugs across skin by passive diffusion and iontophoresis. J Cont Rel 2000; 67:1-8.
21. Bolton S. Pharmaceutical analysis practical and clinical application. 3rd ed. New York: Marcel Dekker; 1999.
22. Doh HJ, Cho WJ, Yong CS, Choi HG, Kim JS, Lee CH, et al. Synthesis and evaluation of ketorolac ester prodrugs for transdermal delivery. J Pharm Sci 2003; 92: 1008–17.
23. Modamio P, Lastra CF, Marino EL. A comparative in vitro study of percutaneous preparations of b-blockers in human skin. Int J Pharm 2000;194: 249-59.
24. Sieg A, Guy RH, Delgado-Charro MB. Electro-osmosis in transdermal iontophoresis: implications for non-invasive and calibra- tion-free glucose monitoring. Biophys J 2004;84: 3344-50.
25. Huang JF, Sung KC, Hu OYP, Wang JJ, Lin YH, Fang JY. The effects of electrically assisted methods on transdermal delivery of nalbuphine benzoate and sebacoyl dinalbuphine ester from solutions and hydrogels. Int J Pharm 2005;297: 162-271.
26. Panchagnula R, Bokalial R, Sharma P, Khandavilli S. Transdermal delivery of naloxone: skin pharmacokinetic, irritancy and stability studies, permeation. Int J Pharm 2005;293: 213-23.
27. Banga AK. Electrically assisted transdermal and topical delivery. London: Taylor and Francis ltd; 1998.
28. Pikal MJ. The role of electro osmotic flow in transdermal iontophoresis. Adv Drug Deliv Rev 2001;46: 281-305.
29. Alvarez-Figueroa MJ, Delgado-Charro MB, Blanco-Mendez J. Passive and iontophoretic transdermal penetration of methotrexate. Int J Pharm 2001;212(1):101-7.
30. Mudry B, Guy RH, Delgado-Charro MB. Transport number in transdermal iontophoresis. Biophys J 2006;90: 2822-30.
31. Phipps JB, Gyory JR. Transdermal ion migration. Adv Drug Del Rev 1992; 9: 137-76.
32. Bernard I. Percutaneous absorption. J Pharm Sci 1975; 64(6): 901-24.
33. Craane-Van Hinsberg IW, Verhoef JC, Spies F, Bouwstra JA, Gooris GS, Junginger HE, et al. Electroperturbation of the human skin barrier in vitro: II. Effects on stratum corneum lipid ordering and ultrastructure. Microsc Res Tech 1997;37(3): 200-13.

24

Lactose Engineering for Better Performance in Dry Powder Inhalers

Yahya Rahimpour [1], **Hamed Hamishehkar** [2*]

[1] *Biotechnology Research Center and Student Research Committee, Tabriz University of Medical Sciences, Tabriz, Iran.*

[2] *Pharmaceutical Technology Laboratory, Drug Applied Research Center, Tabriz University of Medical Sciences, Tabriz, Iran.*

ARTICLE INFO

Keywords:
Carrier
Dry powder inhaler
Pulmonary drug delivery
Lactose

ABSTRACT

Dry powder *inhaler* (DPI) is generally formulated as a powder mixture of coarse carrier particles and micronized drug with aerodynamic diameters of 1-5 µm. Carrier particles are used to improve drug particle flowability, thus improving dosing accuracy, minimizing the dose variability compared with drug alone and making them easier to handle during manufacturing operations. Lactose is the most common and frequently used carrier in DPIs formulations and nowadays various inhalation grades of lactose with different physico-chemical properties are available on the market. Therefore, the purpose of this manuscript is to review evolution of lactose as a carrier in inhalable formulations, their production and the impact of its physico-chemical properties on drug dispersion. This review offers a perspective on the current reported studies to modify lactose for better performance in DPIs.

Introduction

Pressurized metered-dose inhaler (MDI), nebulizer and dry powder inhaler (DPI) are main delivery systems in pulmonary delivery.[1] Among these, DPI appears to be the most promising for future use.[2] They are propellant-free, portable, easy to operate and low-cost devices with improved stability of the formulation as a result of the dry state.[3-5] Spinhaler®, the first dry powder inhaler, came into the market in 1970 and since then a new are started in the subject of pulmonary drug delivery. DPIs and dry powder inhalation technology became the second most frequently used inhalation devices for pulmonary drug administration after Montreal Protocol in 1987 in limitation of using CFC in products. DPIs have even become the first choice of inhalation devices in European countries.[6] They are a widely accepted inhaled delivery dosage form where they are currently used by an estimated 40% of patients to treat asthma and chronic obstructive pulmonary disease.[7] Using the DPI system, respiratory delivery of potent drugs such as insulin,[8] antibiotics,[9,10] drugs for neurological disorders like Parkinson's disease,[11] antihypertensive nifedipine,[12] anticoagulant heparin,[13] opioids and fentanyl for cancer pain[14-16] and delivery of atropine sulphate nanoparticle as an antidote for organophosphorus poisoning with better bioavailability[17] have been studied. DPIs have to overcome various physical difficulties for effective drug delivery either local or systemic purposes.[4] First, small size of inhalable particles subjected them to forces of agglomeration and cohesion, resulting in poor flow and non-uniform dispersion.[18] Drug deposition in the lung is mainly controlled by its aerodynamic diameter.[19] Particles larger than 5 µm are mostly trapped by oropharyngeal deposition and incapable of reaching the lungs while smaller than 1 µm are mostly exhaled without deposition.[20,21] Particles with aerodynamic diameters between 1 and 5 µm are expected to efficiently deposit in the lung periphery.[22] The effective inhalation performance of dry-powder products is dependent on the drug formulation and the inhaler device. Dry powder formulations are usually prepared by mixing the micronized drug particles with larger carrier particles. The aerosolization efficiency of a powder is highly dependent on the carrier characteristics, such as particle size distribution, shape and surface properties. The main objective in the inhalation field is to achieve reproducible, high pulmonary deposition. This could be achieved by successful carrier selection and careful process optimization.[23]

The role of carrier on DPI performance

DPI is generally formulated as a powder mixture of coarse carrier particles and micronized drug particles with aerodynamic particle diameters of 1–5 µm.[24] Carrier particles are used to improve drug particle flowability, thus improving dosing accuracy and minimizing the dose variability observed with drug formulations alone while making them easier to handle during manufacturing operations.[1,25] With the use of carrier particles, drug particles are emitted from capsules and devices more readily, hence, the inhalation efficiency increases.[26] Moreover, usually no more than a few milligrammes of a drug needs to be

***Corresponding author:** Hamed Hamishehkar (PhD), Email: hamishehkar.hamed@gmail.com delivered (e.g., between 20 μg and 500 μg of corticosteroids for asthma therapy), and thus carrier provides bulk, which improves the handling, dispensing, and metering of the drug.[23] The presence of the carrier material is the taste/sensation on inhaling, which can assure the patient that a dose has been taken.[4] Consequently, the carrier forms an important component of the formulation and any change in the physico-chemical properties of the carrier particles has the potential to alter the drug deposition profile.[27] Therefore, the design of the carrier particle is important for the development of DPIs.[28] Carrier particles should have several characteristics such as physico-chemical stability, biocompatibility and biodegradability, compatible with the drug substance and must be inert, available and economical. During insufflation, the drug particles are detached from the surface of the carrier particles by the energy of the inspired air flow that overcomes the adhesion forces between drug and carrier. The larger carrier particles impact in the upper airways, while the small drug particles go through the lower parts of lungs.[23] Unsatisfactory detachment of drug from the carrier due to strong inter-particulate forces may be one of the main reasons of inefficient drug delivery encountered with most DPIs.[29,30] Therefore, in the best case, the adjusted balance between adhesive and cohesive forces provides enough adhesion between drug and carrier to produce a stable formulation (homogeneous mixture with no powder segregation and proper content uniformity) yet allows for easy separation during inhalation. Consequently, it has been stated that the efficiency of a DPI formulation is extremely dependent on the carrier characteristics and the selection of carrier is a crucial determinant of the overall DPI performance.[23] Obviously, the effect of the carrier material on DPI formulation should be carefully evaluated. The range of materials which can be proposed to be as carriers in inhaled products are restricted for toxicological reasons. Lactose and other sugars have been studied and used, therefore modifications to these materials may allow further formulation optimization.[4]

Lactose as the most frequently used carrier in DPIs

Lactose, 4-(b-D-galactosido-)-D-glucose, can be obtained in either two basic isomeric forms, α and β-lactose, or as an amorphous form.[31] Historically, lactose monohydrate was an obvious choice for use as a carrier excipient. Lactose accompanying with glucose and mannitol is allowed as carriers in DPIs by the US Food and Drug Administration department.[32] Lactose is the most common and frequently used carrier in DPI formulations accordingly nowadays various inhalation grades of lactose with different physico-chemical properties are available on the market. The advantages of lactose are its well-investigated toxicity profile, physical and chemical stability, compatibility with the drug substance, its broad availability and relatively low price.[33,34] α-lactose monohydrate is the most common lactose grade used in the inhalation field. Almost all DPI formulations on the market are based on α-lactose monohydrate as a carrier. Therefore, wealth of literatures refers to the optimization of lactose carrier particles for better inhalation performance. More than 250 articles have been published in the past 40 years regarding the role of lactose in adhesive mixtures used in DPIs. However, in spite of these extensive investigations, the relationship between physico-chemical properties of the lactose in adhesive mixtures and the performance of the DPIs remains largely indistinct.[6]

Lactose engineering for application in DPIs

Surface modification

Iida et al. prepared lactose carrier particles for dry powder inhalations by its surface modification with aqueous ethanol solution and evaluated the inhalation efficiency of salbutamol sulfate from its mixture with modified lactose. The degree of adhesion between drug particles and carrier particles and the separation characteristics of drug particles from carrier particles in air flow were assessed by the ultracentrifuge separation and the air jet sieve methods, respectively. It was shown that the average adhesion force between the surface-treated lactose carrier and drug particles was considerably lower than that of powder mixed with the un-treated lactose carrier, indicating better drug separation from carrier and consequently an improvement of in vitro inhalation properties. The authors claimed that surface-smoothing of lactose by aqueous ethanol solution resulted a well balanced drug-carrier adhesion force so that the drug particles could be emitted together with the carrier particles and efficiently separated in airflow after emission.[35] Fine lactose particles were immobilized on the lactose surface by spray coating with liquid suspensions consisting of micronized lactose dispersed in isopropyl alcohol and/or water mixtures to modify surface of lactose. The produced lactose was used as a carrier in the formulation of inhalable salbutamol sulfate powder. It was found that the roughness of the lactose surface established by immobilization of fine lactose increased the FPF and dispersibility of the drug. The authors claimed that unlike crevices and valleys, these microscopic undulations did not accommodate the drug particles and instead enhanced the detachment of drug from the lactose surface and improved the drug inhalation efficiency.[36] Spray dried amorphous, spray dried crystallized and fluidized bed granulated lactose were prepared and used as carrier for inhalation of pranlukast hydrate. Fluidized bed granulated lactose emitted drug particles effectively from the inhalation device, whereas most part of drug captured in the upper stage of twin impinger, resulting in lower inhalation efficiency, due to strong adhesion of drug to the carrier lactose. The spray dried amorphous lactose, smoothed sphere particle, did not so improve the inhalation efficiency as expected, because of fairly strong adhesion between drug and lactose particles. But the spray dried crystallized lactose having lots of microscopical projection on its surface increased the respirable particle percent of the emitted particles. The conclusion was that the surface roughness should be optimized to gain improved inhalation efficiency of particles.[37] In the other study, a Wurster fluidized bed was used for surface-coating of lactose particles with lactose aqueous solution containing hydroxypropyl methyl cellulose. The authors could be able to increase the inhalation performance of salbutamol sulfate 2.5 times more than commercial lactose (Pharmatose®200M) and reported that surface coating of carrier particles may be an effective technique for improving the inhalation performance of DPI.[38] Lactose carrier particles were layered with vegetable magnesium stearate by physical mixing and their effect of on the dry powder inhalation properties of salbutamol sulfate was investigated. The in vitro inhalation performance of drug was enhanced compared with the powder mixed with unlayered lactose carrier. It was stated that using this surface layering system would thus be valuable for increasing the inhalation properties of dry powder inhalation.[39] For example, increasing the surface smoothness of lactose carrier particles was shown to improve the potentially respirable fraction of albuterol sulfate from the Rotahaler®.[40]

Shape modification

Lactose crystallization from Carbopol gel in different conditions (named Carbo lactose) produced a more regular shape lactose with smoother surface as compared with the control lactose. The Carbo lactose caused a higher and reproducible salbutamol sulphate emission and fine particle fraction after aerosolisation via a Rotahaler® tested in multi-stage impinge. It was concluded that engineered crystal growth under controlled conditions can enhance the potential inhalable fraction of drug from dry powder inhalers.[41] More recently, the use of more elongated crystals of lactose was also found to produce a higher inhalation efficiency of albuterol sulfate.[29] However, the improvement in drug dispersion that can be achieved by increasing the elongation ratio of the carrier particles is limited.[42]

Composite lactose

Lactose carrier particles were prepared by fusing sub units of lactose (either 2, 6 or 10 μm prepared by spray drying) in saturated lactose slurry, sieve fractioned to obtain a 63–90 μm carriers and used for inhalation of salbutamol sulfate. The surface morphology and physico-chemical properties of the composite carriers were considerably different from regular α-lactose monohydrate. In all cases, the composite carriers resulted in improved drug aerosol performance. It was suggested that composite based carriers are a potential route to control drug-carrier adhesion forces and variability thus allowing more precise control of formulation performance.[43]

Engineered lactose-mannitol mixture

Mannitol and lactose were co-crystallised to prepare crystals with more desirable characteristics than either lactose or mannitol alone appropriate for application as carriers in the formulations of salbutamol sulfate DPIs. In vitro deposition evaluation showed that crystallized carriers resulted more efficient delivery of salbutamol sulphate compared to formulations containing commercial grade carriers. It was concluded that simultaneous crystallization of lactose-mannitol can be a new approach to enhance inhalation performance of DPI formulations.[44]

Expert Opinion and Final Remarks

Interest in DPIs has increased in the last decade due to its numerous advantages over other pulmonary drug delivery dosage forms. Currently, the inhalation performance of DPIs are being improved by changing formulation strategy, drug and carrier particle engineering. Regarding formulation development, micronized drug particles are cohesive with poor flow properties. Addition of large carrier particles, mostly lactose, into powders to enhance their flow characteristics has been an appropriate approach. The main goal in the inhalation field is to obtain reproducible, high pulmonary deposition which can be highly effected by physico-chemical characteristics of lactose. Technologies for engineering lactose particle shape, density, and size will continue to develop to enhance the effectiveness of pulmonary drug formulations. This approach may enable more drugs to be delivered through this route for local treatment of lung diseases or systemic therapy.

References

1. Timsina MP, Martin GP, Marriott C, Ganderton D, Yianneskis M. Drug delivery to the respiratory tract using dry powder inhalers. Int J Pharm 1994;101(1-2):1-13.
2. Todo H, Okamoto H, Iida K, Danjo K. Effect of additives on insulin absorption from intratracheally administered dry powders in rats. Int J Pharm 2001;220:101-10.
3. Carpenter JF, Pikal MJ, Chang BS, Randolph TW. Rational design of stable lyophilized protein formulations: some practical advice. Pharm Res 1997;14:969-75.
4. Prime D, Atkins PJ, Slater A, Sumby B. Review of dry powder inhalers. Adv Drug Deliv Rev 1997;26(1):51-8.
5. Hamishehkar H, Emami J, Najafabadi AR, Gilani K, Minaiyan M, Mahdavi H, et al. Influence of carrier particle size, carrier ratio and addition of fine ternary particles on the dry powder inhalation performance of insulin-loaded PLGA microcapsules. Powder Technol 2010;201: 289-95.

6. Marriott C, Frijlink HW. Lactose as a carrier for inhalation products: breathing new life into an old carrier. Adv Drug Deliv Rev 2012;64(3):217-9.
7. Atkins PJ. Dry powder inhalers: an overview. Resp Care 2005;50(10):1304-12.
8. Hamishehkar H, Emami J, Najafabadi AR, Gilani K, Minaiyan M, Hassanzadeh K, et al. Pharmacokinetics and pharmacodynamics of controlled release insulin loaded PLGA microcapsules using dry powder inhaler in diabetic rats. Biopharm Drug Dispos 2010;31(2-3):189-201.
9. Geller DE, Konstan WK, Smith J, Noonberg SB, Conrad C. Novel tobramycin inhalation powder in cystic fibrosis subjects: pharmacokinetics and safety. Pediatr Pulm 2007;42:307-13.
10. Hickey AJ, Lu D, Ashley ED, Stout J. Inhaled azithromycin therapy. J Aerosol Med 2006;19:54-60.
11. Stoessl AJ. Potential therapeutic targets for Parkinson's disease. Expert Opin Ther Tar 2008;12:425-36.
12. Plumley C, Gorman EM, El-Gendy N, Bybee CR, Munson EJ, Berkland C. Nifedipine nanoparticle agglomeration as a dry powder aerosol formulation strategy. Int J Pharm 2009;369(1-2):136-43.
13. Rawat A, Majumder QH, Ahsan F. Inhalable large porous microspheres of low molecular weight heparin: in vitro and in vivo evaluation. J Control Release 2008;128(3):224-32.
14. Farr SJ, Otulana BA. Pulmonary delivery of opioids as pain therapeutics. Adv Drug Deliv Rev. 2006;58(9):1076-88.
15. Kleinstreuer C, Zhang Z, Donohue JF. Targeted drug-aerosol delivery in the human respiratory system. Annu Rev Biomed Eng 2008;10:195-220.
16. Fleischer W, Reimer K, Leyendecker P. Opioids for the treatment of the chronic obstructive pulmonary disease. Luxembourg: Euro-Celtique S.A; 2005.
17. Ali R, Jain GK, Iqbal Z, Talegaonkar S, Pandit P, Sule S, et al. Development and clinical trial of nano-atropine sulfate dry powder inhaler as a novel organophosphorous poisoning antidote. Nanomedicine 2009;5(1):55-63.
18. Crowder TM, Rosati JA, Schroeter JD, Hickey AJ, Martonen TB. Fundamental effects of particle morphology on lung delivery: Predictions of Stokes' law and the particular relevance to dry powder inhaler formulation and development. Pharm Res 2002;19(3):239-45.
19. Wolff RK, Dorato MA. Toxicologic testing of inhaled pharmaceutical aerosols. Crit Rev Toxicol 1993;23:343-69.
20. Sakagami M. In vivo, in vitro and ex vivo models to assess pulmonary absorption and disposition of inhaled therapeutics for systemic delivery. Adv Drug Deliv Rev 2006;58(9):1030-60.
21. Emami J, Hamishehkar H, Najafabadi AR, Gilani K, Minaiyan M, Mahdavi H, et al. Particle size design of PLGA microspheres for potential pulmonary drug delivery using response surface methodology. J Microencapsul 2009;26(1):1-8.
22. Heyder J, Gebhart J, Rudolf G, Schiller CF, Stahlhofen W. Deposition of particles in the human respiratory tract in the size range 0.005 - 5 µm. J Aerosol Sci 1986;17(5):811-25.
23. Pilcer G, Wauthoz N, Amighi K. Lactose characteristics and the generation of the aerosol. Adv Drug Deliv Rev 2012;64: 233-56.
24. Iida K, Hayakawa Y, Okamoto H, Danjo K, Luenberger H. Effect of surface covering of lactose carrier particles on dry powder inhalation properties of salbutamol sulfate. Chem Pharm Bull 2003;51(12):1455-7.
25. Schiavone H, Palakodaty S, Clark A, York P, Tzannis ST. Evaluation of SCF-engineered particle-based lactose blends in passive dry powder inhalers. Int J Pharm 2004;281(1):55-66.
26. Iida K, Hayakawa Y, Okamoto H, Danjo K, Leuenberger H. Evaluation of flow properties of dry powder inhalation of salbutamol sulfate with lactose carrier. Chem Pharm Bull 2001;49(10):1326-30.
27. Zeng XM, Pandhal KH, Martin GP. The influence of lactose carrier on the content homogeneity and dispersibility of beclomethasone dipropionate from dry powder aerosols. Int J Pharm 2000;197:41-52.
28. Hamishehkar H, Emami J, Najafabadi AR, Gilani K, Minaiyan M, Mahdavi H, et al. Effect of carrier morphology and surface characteristics on the development of respirable PLGA microcapsules for sustained-release pulmonary delivery of insulin. Int J Pharm 2010;389(1-2):74-85.
29. Zeng XM, Martin GP, Marriott C, Pritchard J. The influence of carrier morphology on drug delivery by dry powder inhalers. Int J Pharm 2000;200:93-106.
30. Zhou QT, Morton DAV. Drug-lactose binding aspects in adhesive mixtures: controlling performance in dry powder Inhaler formulations by altering lactose carrier surfaces. Adv Drug Deliv Rev 2012;64(3):275-84.
31. Zeng XM, Martin GP, Marriott C, Pritchrd J. The Influence of crystallization conditions on the morphology of lactose intended for use as a carrier for dry powder aerosols. J Pharm Pharmacol 2000;52:633-43.
32. Labiris NR, Dolovich MB. Pulmonary drug delivery. Part II: the role of inhalant delivery devices and drug formulations in therapeutic effectiveness of aerosolized medications. Br J Clin Pharmacol 2003;56(6):600-12.
33. Steckel H, Bolzen N. Alternative sugars as potential carriers for dry powder inhalations. Int J Pharm 2004;270(1):297-306.
34. Pilcer G, Amighi K. Formulation strategy and use of excipients in pulmonary drug delivery. Int J Pharm 2010;392:1-19.
35. Iida K, Hayakawa Y, Okamoto H, Danjo K, Leuenberger H. Preparation of dry powder

inhalation by surface treatment of lactose carrier particles. Chem Pharm Bull 2003;51(1):1-5.
36. Chan LW, Lim LT, Heng PWS. Immobilization of fine particles on lactose carrier by precision coating and its effect on the performance of dry powder formulations. J Pharm Sci 2003;92(5):975-84.
37. Kawashima Y, Serigano T, Hino T, Yamamoto H, Takeuchi H. Effect of surface morphology of carrier lactose on dry powder inhalation property of pranlukast hydrate. Int J Pharm 1998;172(1):179-88.
38. Iida K, Todo H, Okamoto H, Danjo K, Leuenberger H. Preparation of dry powder inhalation with lactose carrier particles surface-coated using a Wurster fluidized bed. Chem Pharm Bull 2005;53(4):431-4.
39. Iida K, Hayakawa Y, Okamoto H, Danjo K, Luenbergerb H. Effect of surface layering time of lactose carrier particles on dry powder inhalation properties of salbutamol sulfate. Chem Pharm Bull 2004;52 (3):350-3.
40. Littringer EM, Mescher A, Schroettner H, Achelis L, Walzel P, Urbanetz NA. Spray dried mannitol carrier particles with tailored surface properties – The influence of carrier surface roughness and shape. Eur J Pharm Biopharm 2012;82(1):194-204.
41. Zeng XM, Martin GP, Marriott C, Pritchard J. The use of lactose recrystallised from carbopol gels as a carrier for aerosolised salbutamol sulphate. Eur J Pharm Biopharm 2001;51(1):55-62.
42. Zeng XM, Martin GP, Marriott C, Pritchard J. Lactose as a carrier in dry powder formulations: the influence of surface characteristics on drug delivery. J Pharm Sci 2001;90(9):1424-34.
43. Young PM, Kwok P, Adi H, Chan H-K, Traini D. Lactose composite carriers for respiratory delivery. Pharm Res 2009;26(4):802-10.
44. Kaialy W, Larhrib H, Martin GP, Nokhodchi A. The effect of engineered mannitol-lactose mixture on dry powder inhaler performance. Pharm Res 2012; 29(3):2139-56.

Determination of the Mutagenicity Potential of Supermint Herbal Medicine by Single Cell Gel Electrophoresis in Rat Hepatocytes

Heibatullah Kalantari, Mohsen Rezaei, Masoud Mahdavinia, Mojtaba Kalantar, Zivar Amanpour, Golnaz Varnaseri *

Faculty of Pharmacy, Toxicology Research Center, Ahvaz Jundishapur University of Medical Sciences, Ahvaz, Iran.

ARTICLE INFO

Keywords:
Toxicity tests
Comet assay
Herbal medicine
Supermint

ABSTRACT

Purpose: The increasing use of herbal drugs and their easy availability have necessitated the use of mutagenicity test to analyze their toxicity and safety. The aim of this study was to evaluate the genotoxicity of Supermint herbal medicine in DNA breakage of rat hepatocytes in comparison with sodium dichromate by single cell gel electrophoresis technique or comet assay. ***Methods:*** Hepatocytes were prepared from male wistar rats and were counted and kept in a bioreactor for 30 minutes. Then cells were exposed to the Supermint herbal medicine at doses of 125, 250 and 500 µl/ml. Buffer 4 (incubation buffer) and sodium dichromate were used as negative and positive control for one hour respectively. Then cell suspension with low melting point agarose were put on precoated slides and covered with agarose gel. Then lysing, electrophoresis, neutralization and staining were carried out. Finally the slides were analyzed with fluorescence microscope. The parameter under this analysis was the type of migration which was determined according to Kobayashi pattern. ***Results:*** With increased dose of Supermint herbal medicine the DNA damage was slightly increased (P<0001). ***Conlusion:*** In overall compared to the positive control significant differences is observed which convinced that the crude extract of Supermint in vitro did not have mutagenic effect.

Introduction

Fossils date human use of plants as medicine to approximately 60000 years ago. Today, almost 65% of the world's population relies on plants as an integral part of their primary health care. Also there have been many validations of traditional remedies through scientific research and in addition, the use of ethnomedical information has contributed to health care worldwide through the isolation of bioactive compounds for direct use in medicine. The adverse effects of widely used plants are not well documented in the literature. Based on their long-term use by human one might expect plants used in traditional medicine to have low toxicity. However, recent investigations have revealed that many plants used as food or in traditional medicine have mutagenic effects in *in vitro* assay this raises concern about the potential mutagenic hazards resulting from the long-term use of medicinal plants.[1-9]
In Iranian folk medicine, Supermint is an example of plants that are widely used and today, Supermint oral drop contains Essential oil of *Mentha spicata* which is widley used as Carminative, Gastrointestinal analgesic, antispasmodic, Dyspepsia treatment and Stomachic.[10] Therefore, one of the objectives of our study was to evaluate the saftey activity of Supermint as herbal medicine to evaluate the safety by in vitro method on hepatocytes.
In the evaluation of in vitro methods for natural products the biological activity determination has changed in the past few years, one of the recent developments is comet assay, which gives a ratio between the viable cells in the cell culture to total cells in the culture. These techniques are considered rapid and economical for the evaluation of mutagenicity or genotoxicity of compounds.[11-12] In view of the potential therapeutic use of Supermint herbal medicine and the absence of any data on its genetic toxicity in eukaryotes, the study described in this paper was under-taken to evaluate the potential in vitro mutagenic effects in terms of DNA damage in rat hepatocytes by Single Cell Gel Electrophoresis technique.

Materials and Methods

Animal used in this experiment was wistar rat (250 – 300 g weight) obtained from the animal house of Razi Institute, Iran. Rat was housed in polyethylene cage in a climate controlled environment with a 12 hours (07.00 to 19.00) day length and ad libitum access to food and water. Hepatocyte extraction was prepared by IP injection of ketamin 90 mg/kg and xylazine 10

***Corresponding author:** Golnaz Varnaseri, School of Pharmacy, Department of Pharmacology and Toxicology, Ahvaz Jundishapur University of Medical Sciences, Ahvaz, Iran. Email: g_varnaseri@yahoo.com

mg/kg for anesthesia. Then rat was dissected and IV injection of heparin the canulation of liver was made. Liver was washed with washing buffer for 10 minutes and then with perfusion buffer (colagenase buffer) for 12 minutes. The isolated liver was transferred in to a petri dish containing washing buffer to separate hepatocytes, then the cell suspension filtered and the filtrate was centrifuged for 3 minutes at 1500 rpm. The upper layer was discarded and to the lower layer 10 ml of washing buffer was added, mixed well and then from this mixture 100 μl was mixed with 200 μl of incubation buffer and 300 μl of trypan blue for counting cells. From this cell suspension little amount poured on Neubar slide and start counting the cells. Mean of the viable cells and dead cells were calculated as follow; % of viable cells = (mean of viable cells/total cells) × 100. Then hepatocytes were counted until we got the ratio 10^6 cells.[13] From this cell suspension a desired amount were kept in bioreactor bath at 37 C° atmosphere of 10 % O_2, 85 % N_2 and 5 % CO_2 for 30 minutes and then to five bioreactor flasks containing hepatocytes. After this step the hepatocytes were exposed to Supermint herbal medicine (was purchased from barijessence . co. Iran) for one period of 60 minute at doses of 125, 250 and 500 μl/ml (test groups) respectively. Buffer 4 (which contains HEPES 0.75 g and Krebs 250 ml) was used as negative control and 1000 μM of sodium dichromate used as positive control. Then from each bioreactor flask 1 ml of the hepatocyte cell suspension was taken and diluted to 10 ml with low melting point agarose and then 100 μl of this suspension were poured on precoated slides and covered with cover slips. Slides were kept for 15 to 20 minutes in a horizontal placed iced tray till to become solidified. The next step, the cover slips were removed from the slides and kept them in a lysing solution for one hour and then they were removed from lysing solution and washed by D-ionized water, kept for 20 minutes in electrophoresis buffer and did electrophoresis at 25 V and 300 mA for 20 minutes and then washed with neutralized buffer for five minutes for three times. Slides were immersed in ethidium bromide solution for five minutes and according to the method described by Speit and Hartmann,[14] which is based on the original work of Singh *et al.*[15] slides were analyzed by fluorescence microscope. The extent and distribution of DNA damage indicated by comet assay was evaluated by examining cells. The cells were visually scored into comet classes according to tail size class[16-18] Class 0 = no tail, Class 1 = tail shorter than the diameter of the head (nucleous), Class 2 = tail length 1 to 2x the diameter of the head and Class 3 = tail longer than 2x the diameter of the head. Comet without head and those with nearly all the DNA in the tail or with a very wide tail were excluded from the evaluation because they probably represented dead cells[19-20] tail length and the mutagenic Index is calculated according the following formula MI = (0NMC+ 1SMC+ 2MMC+ 3LMC) /200, or we can express it such as NMC = No migration cells (score 0), SMC = Short migration cells (score) MMC = Medium migration cells (score 2), LMC = Long migration cells (score 3).

Results and Discussion

In Iran like other countries, the use of herbal medicine in the treatment of diseases is very common; therefore, their safety like the mutagenecity potential should be evaluate by techniques like single cell gel electrophoresis. This technique is a sensitive, reliable and an important tool for evaluating the in vitro and in vivo genotoxic potential of bioactive compounds.

Table 1 demonstrates the percentage of frequency of comet pattern of rat hepatocytes at different doses of Supermint herbal medicine in comparison with positive control (sodium dichromate) in 60 minutes after exposure. Similarly, as can be seen in Table 2 the percentage of mutagenic index (MI) and damaged cells treated with Supermint herbal medicine at different doses are significantly lower that of positive control (sodium dichromate) in 60 minutes after exposure (P<0.0001).

The microscopic photograph 1 to 4 present the comet in scoring pattern from 0 score to score 3 which indicate the comet length (Figure 1). Comets from the broken ends of a negatively charged DNA molecule became free and migrated towards the anode in the electric field. The assay provided direct determination of the extent of DNA damage in individual cells and the extent of DNA damage have been assessed from the length of DNA migration. As it was expected, the results obtained from positive control were statistically significant in comparison to the negative control.

Table 1. The percentage of rat hepatocytes comet pattern frequency at different doses of Supermint herbal medicine and its comparison with positive control (sodium dichromate) in 60 minutes after exposure (P<0.0001)

Substance	Score 0	Score 1	Score 2	Score 3
Sodium dichromate 1000 μM	8.5 ± 1.21	16 ± 1.3	28.5 ± 1.38	47 ± 1.67
Supermint 0 μl/ml	94 ± 1.62	5.5 ± 1.09	0.5 ± 0.57	0 ± 0
Supermint 125 μl/ml	87 ± 1.22	10 ± 0.81	3 ± 0.4	0 ± 0
Supermint 250 μl/ml	82 ± 0.81	12 ± 0.81	6 ± 0	0 ± 0
Supermint 500 μl/ml	81 ± 2.1	12 ± 1.7	7 ± 0.66	0 ± 0

Table 2. Mutagenic index (MI) and damaged cells treated by Supermint at different doses and its comparison with positive control (sodium dichromate) in 60 minutes after exposure (P<0.0001).

Substance	MI (%)	Damaged cells (%)
Sodium dichromate 1000 μM	53.5 ± 1.38	75.5 ± 1.67
Supermint 0 μl/ml	1.6 ± 0.51	0.5 ± 0.57
Supermint 125 μl/ml	4 ± 0.81	3 ± 0.4
Supermint 250 μl/ml	6 ± 0.81	6 ± 0
Supermint 500 μl/ml	6. 5 ± 1.66	7 ± 0

The data are expressed as the means ± SE

The results obtained in this study indicated that the mutagenicity index of positive control was 53.5 % and the mutagenicity index for the lower dose of Supermint herbal medicine after 60 minutes was 4 % and the mutagenicity index of higher dose of the Supermint herbal medicine after 60 minutes was 6.5 %. These findings indicated that with the increase of the dose of the Supermint herbal medicine mutagenicity index was increased. However it was not significant as compared with positive control P<0.0001. Based on genotixicity study by comet assay the present study provided additional confirmation to our previous study, that high doses of Supermint herbal medicine did not produce significant DNA damage.

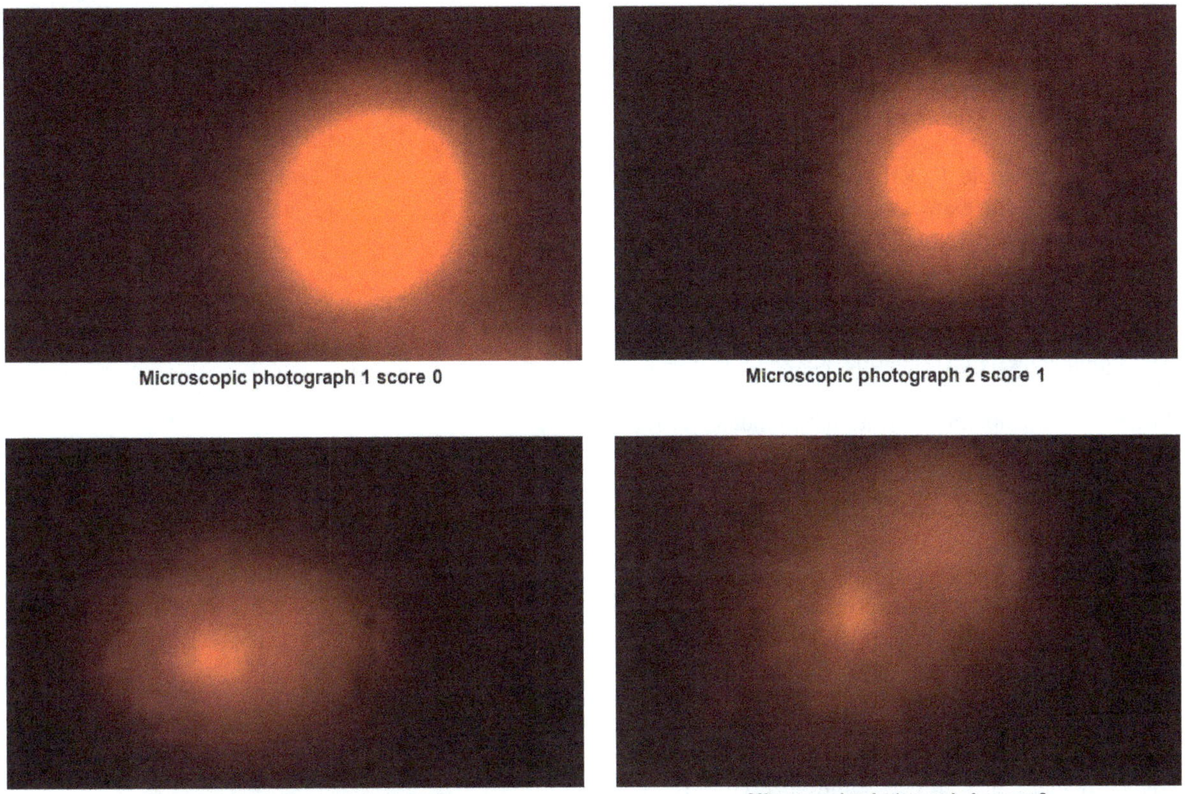

Microscopic photograph 1 score 0 | Microscopic photograph 2 score 1

Microscopic photograph 3 score 2 | Microscopic photograph 4 score 3

Figure 1. The extent and distribution of DNA damage indicated by comet assay.

As the herbal medicine contains antioxidant agents may protect the DNA damage by chemicals and prevent mutagenicity. In conclusion these results indicated that by increasing the dose of Supermint herbal medicine the DNA damage is lightly increases but in overall as compared to the positive control significant differences is observed which convinced that the Supermint herbal medicine in vitro did not have mutagenic effect.

Acknowledgement

This work was supported by a grant (NO. MPRC009) from Deputy of Research of Ahvaz Jundishapur University of Medical sciences Ahvaz Iran.

Conflict of interest

The authors declare there is no Conflict of interest in the content of this study.

References

1. Ahn HS, Jeon TI, Lee JY, Hwang SG, Lim Y, Park DK. Antioxidative activity of persimmon and grape seed extract: in vitro and in vivo. Nutr Res 2002;22(11):1265-73.
2. Fabricant DS, Farnsworth NR. The value of plants used in traditional medicine for drug discovery. Environ Health Persp 2001;109(Suppl 1):69-75.
3. Higashimoto M, Purintrapiban J, Kataoka K, Kinouchi T, Vinitketkumnuen U, Akimoto S, et al.

Mutagenicity and antimutagenicity of extracts of three spices and a medicinal plant in Thailand. Mutat Res 1993;303(3):135-42.
4. Kassie F, Parzefall W, Musk S, Johnson I, Lamprecht G, Sontag G, et al. Genotoxic effects of crude juices from Brassica vegetables and juices and extracts from phytopharmaceutical preparations and spices of cruciferous plants origin in bacterial and mammalian cells. Chem Biol Interact 1996;102(1):1-16.
5. Liu RH. Health benefits of fruit and vegetables are from additive and synergistic combinations of phytochemicals. Am J Clin Nutr 2003;78(3 Suppl):517S-20S.
6. McGaw LJ, Jager AK, van Staden J. Antibacterial, anthelmintic and anti-amoebic activity in South African medicinal plants. J Ethnopharmacol 2000;72(1-2):247-63.
7. Rabe T, Van Staden J. Screening of Plectranthus species for antibacterial activity. S Afr J Botany 1998;64(1):62-5.
8. Schimmer O, Hafele F, Kruger A. The mutagenic potencies of plant extracts containing quercetin in Salmonella typhimurium TA98 and TA100. Mutat Res 1988;206(2):201-8.
9. Schimmer O, Kruger A, Paulini H, Haefele F. An evaluation of 55 commercial plant extracts in the Ames mutagenicity test. Pharmazie 1994;49(6):448-51.
10. Barijessence. Supermint. [Internet].[Update 2012 May 3]. Available from http://www.barijessence.com.
11. Rubinstein LV, Shoemaker RH, Paull KD, Simon RM, Tosini S, Skehan P, et al. Comparison of in vitro anticancer-drug-screening data generated with a tetrazolium assay versus a protein assay against a diverse panel of human tumor cell lines. J Natl Cancer Inst 1990;82(13):1113-8.
12. Moneef MA, Sherwood BT, Bowman KJ, Kockelbergh RC, Symonds RP, Steward WP, et al. Measurements using the alkaline comet assay predict bladder cancer cell radiosensitivity. Br J Cancer 2003;89(12):2271-6.
13. Berry MN, Phillips JW. The isolated hepatocyte preparation: 30 years on. Biochem Soc Trans 2000;28(2):131-5.
14. Speit G, Hartmann A. The comet assay (single-cell gel test). A sensitive genotoxicity test for the detection of DNA damage and repair. Methods Mol Biol 1999;113:203-12.
15. Singh NP, McCoy MT, Tice RR, Schneider EL. A simple technique for quantitation of low levels of DNA damage in individual cells. Exp Cell Res 1988;175(1):184-91.
16. Jalali M, Hatami A, Kalantari H, Kalantar E. Mutagenicity Assessment of Two Herbal Medicines, Urtan and Carmint in Human Leukocytes by Single Cell Gel Electrophoresis. Saudi Pharm J 2006;14(2):129.
17. Junqueira APF, Perazzo FF, Souza GHB, Maistro EL. Clastogenicity of Piper cubeba (Piperaceae) seed extract in an in vivo ma mmalian cell system. Genet Mol Biol 2007;30:656-63.
18. Kalantari H, Jalali M, Moein E. In Vitro Evaluation of Mutagenic Effect of Vitagnus and Shirafza in Human Leukocytes by Single Cell Gel Electrophoresis. Jundushapur J Nat Pharm Prod 2007;1(1):26-31.
19. Hartmann A, Speit G. The contribution of cytotoxicity to DNAeffects in the single cell gel test (comet assay). Toxicol Lett 1997;90(2-3):183-8.
20. Kalantari H, Panahi M, Izadinajafabadi A, Mohammadi E. Genotoxicity Determinations of Coriander Drop and Extract of Coriander Sativum in Cultured Fibroblast of Rat Embryo by CometAssay. Saudi Pharm J 2008;16(1):85.

Fluoxetine Improves the Effect of Levodopa on 6-Hydroxy Dopamine-Induced Motor Impairments in Rats

Javad Mahmoudi [1], **Alireza Mohajjel Nayebi** [2,3*], **Siyamak Reyhani-Rad** [4], **Morteza Samini** [1]

[1] *Department of Pharmacology, Science and Research Branch, Islamic Azad University, Tehran, Iran.*

[2] *Department of Pharmacology and Toxicology, Faculty of Pharmacy, Tabriz University of Medical Science, Tabriz 51664, Iran.*

[3] *Drug Applied Research Center, Tabriz University of Medical Sciences, Tabriz 51664, Iran.*

[4] *Department of laboratory sciences, Marand Branch, Islamic Azad University, Marand, Iran.*

ARTICLE INFO

Keywords:
L-DOPA
Fluoxetine
$5\text{-}HT_{1A}$ receptor
Catalepsy
Motor imbalance
Rat

ABSTRACT

Purpose: Long term L-DOPA therapy in Parkinson's disease is associated with troublesome motor fluctuations such as L -DOPA Induced dyskinesia and wearing off effect. Our recent study showed that activation of $5\text{-}HT_{1A}$ receptors could improve the anti-cataleptic effect of L-DOPA in parkinsonian rats. In this study we investigated the effect of fluoxetine on anti-parkinsonian effect of L-DOPA in 6-hydroxydopamine (6-OHDA)-lesioned rats. ***Methods:*** Catalepsy and motor incoordination were induced by unilateral injection of 6-OHDA (8μg/2μl/rat) into the central region of the sabstantia nigra pars compacta (SNc). After 3 weeks as a recovery period, these rats injected intraperitoneally (i.p.) L-DOPA (15 mg/kg) twice daily for 20 consecutive days, and anti-parkinsonian effect of L-DOPA was investigated by bar-test and rotarod on days 5, 10, 15 and 20. ***Results:*** The results showed that L-DOPA is able to improve motor coordination in rotarod only until day 15 and these effects of L-DOPA were abolished on the day 20. On day 21, rats were co-injected with fluoxetine (0.1, 0.5 and 1mg/kg, i.p.) and L-DOPA (15 mg/kg, i.p.). Fluoxetine increased anti-cataleptic effect of L-DOPA at the dose of 1 mg/kg, while fluoxetine had not any impact on the effect of L-DOPA in rotarod test. The effect of fluoxetine (1 mg/kg, i.p.) on anti-cataleptic effect of L-DOPA (15 mg/kg, i.p.) was reversed by 1-(2-methoxyphenyl)-4-(4-phthalimidobutyl) piperazine hydrobromide (NAN-190; 0.5 mg/kg, i.p.), as a $5\text{-}HT_{1A}$ receptor antagonist. ***Conclusion:*** According to the results, it may be concluded that fluoxetine improves 6-OHDA-induced catalepsy and motor imbalance in L-DOPA- treated rats through activation of $5\text{-}HT_{1A}$. Further studies should be designed to clarify the precise mechanism of interaction between $5\text{-}HT_{1A}$ and dopaminergic neurons.

Introduction

Parkinson's disease (PD) is considered as a movement and neurodegenerative disorder.[1-2] Nearly 1% of populations over 60 years old are affected by this disease.[3] The main cause of this disease is the degeneration of nigrostriatal pathway, leading to reduction of dopamine levels in the striatum[4] that subsequently induces motor dysfunctions, such as muscle rigidity, akinesia, tremor at rest and bradykinesia.[5-6] Replacement therapy with L-3,4-dihydroxyphenylalanine (L-DOPA) commonly is used for treatment of PD motor symptoms.[7-8] This strategy is effective in the early stages of disease, but long-term use of L-DOPA causes motor fluctuations such as L-DOPA- induced dyskinesia (LID)[7,9] and wearing off phenomenon.[7] The mechanism(s) underlying of these motor disorders are weakly understood and there are not comprehensive data about these mechanisms. It has been shown that following destruction of dopaminergic neurons by 6-OHDA in rats, hyperinnervation of serotonergic (5-HT) fibers occurs within the affected area.[10] It seems these serotonergic neurons are able to compensate some effects of lost dopaminergic neurons.[11] In normal conditions, dopaminergic neurons are able to convert L-DOPA to dopamine. Accordingly this process is mediated by aromatic amino acid decarboxylase (AADC) and mono amine vesicular transporter 2 (VAMT 2) that are responsible for synthesis of dopamine from L-DOPA and loadingof dopamine from intra-neural space into vesicles within the dopaminergic neurons, respectively.[1,12] Serotonergic neurons possess both essential components, AADC and VAMT 2, for processing of L-

***Corresponding author:** Alireza Mohajjel Nayebi (PhD), Deapartment of Pharmacology and Toxicology, Faculty of Pharmacy, Tabriz University of Medical Science, Tabriz 51664, Iran. E-mail: nayebia@tbzmed.ac.ir

DOPA to dopamine.[13-14] Existence of these components enables 5-HT neurons to decarboxylate L-DOPA to dopamine as well as its loading into vesicles.[14] In serotonergic neurons dopamine is co-stored with serotonin in the same vesicles and is known as a false transmitter.[15]

Dopamine is released from dopaminergic neurons in a physiological level,[13] while it is released from serotonergic neurons in an activity dependent fashion.[13,16] This paradigm results in fluctuation of striatal dopamine levels.[14] It is therefore plausible that in PD dopamine receptors are faced to fluctuated levels of dopamine.[17] All components of basal ganglia receive serotonergic neurons from dorsal raphe nucleus.[18] Hence it seems that serotonergic system has an axial role in regulation of normal movement.[6] 5-HT_{1A} receptors are found throughout the basal ganglia.[6] It has been reported that activation of these receptors may exert anti-parkisonian effect.[2] Studies have shown that stimulation of these receptors results in improving of dyskinesia.[13] Anti-cataleptic effect of 5-HT_{1A} agonists in rodent model of PD has been shown.[6,19] We have shown that fluoxetine attenuates catalepsy in 6-OHDA-lesioned rats.[20] Furthermore, activation of 5-HT_{1A} receptors could improve anti-cataleptic effect of L-DOPA in hemiparkinsonian rats.[12] However there is not any report about effect of fluoxetine on anti-cataleptic and motor-balance improving effect of L-DOPA in 6-OHDA-lesioned rats. This study was designed to investigate effect of fluoxetine and L-DOPA co-treatment on 6-OHDA-induced motor impairments in rats.

Materials and Methods

Chemicals

All chemicals were purchased from Sigma Chemical Co. (USA). L-DOPA and Carbidopa were donated by Ramopharmin Co, Iran. Solutions were made freshly on the days of experimentation by dissolving drugs in physiological saline (0.9% NaCl). The drugs were injected intraperitoneally (i.p.) except for 6-hydroxydopamine (6-OHDA) which was injected into subestentia nigra pars compacta (SNc). Movement disorders were assessed by bar test and rotarod 5, 60, 120 and 180 min after drug administration.

Animals

The experiments were carried out on male Wistar rats weighing between 200-220 g. Animals were housed in standard polypropylene cages, four per cage, under a 12:12 light/dark program and at a temperature of 25 ± 2°C, with free access to food and water. Animals were acclimated to the testing conditions 2 days before the behavioral investigations were done. All of the procedures were carried out under the ethical guidelines of Tabriz University of Medical Sciences for the care and use of laboratory animals.

Surgical procedures

The animals were anesthetized by intraperitonel injection of ketamine (50 mg/kg) and xylazine (5 mg/kg). After they were deeply anaesthetized, rats were fixed in a stereotaxic frame in the flat skin positions. Scalp hairs of the rats were completely shaved with a standard electric shaving machine, swabbed with 70% ethanol and a central incision made to reveal skull. A 0.7 millimeter bar hole was drilled and 23 gauge sterile stainless steel cannula, as a guide cannula inserted for subsequent injection of 6-OHDA in to SNc. The coordinates for this position were determined according to the rat brain in stereotaxic coordinates:[21] anteroposterior from bregma (AP) = -5 mm, mediolateral from the midline (ML) = -2.2 mm and dorsoventral from the skull (DV) = -8.8 mm. Desipramine (25 mg/kg) was injected intraperitoneally 30 min before intra-nigral injection of 6-OHDA to avoid degeneration of noradrenergic neurons.[22] Then 6-OHDA (8 μg/ per rat in 2 μl saline with 0.02 % ascorbic acid) was infused by infusion pump at the flow rate of 0.2 μl/mine into the left substantia nigra. At the end of injection, guide cannula was kept for an additional 2 min and then slowly was withdrawed. All of these procedures were repeated in Sham-operated animals but they were received only 2 μl vehicle of 6-OHDA (0.9% saline containing 0.2% (w/v) ascorbic acid). After three weeks as a recovery period, only the rats that showed marked immobilization in bare test and motor imbalance in rotarod test were subjected to further experimentation. Then parkisonian rats were randomly allocated to equal groups and were treated with L-DOPA (15 mg/kg, i.p.) twice daily (9 AM, 9 PM) for 20 days. Peripheral metabolism of L-DOPA was inhibited by concomitant administration of carbidopa (1.5 mg/kg, i.p.).

Motor impairment study

Catalepsy was assessed by using of standard wooden bar test mean. Anterior limbs of rat gently extended on 9 cm high bar (0.9 cm in diameter). Elapsed time for each rat in this imposed posture was considered as a bar test time. The end point of catalepsy was designated to occur when both front paws were removed from the bar or if the animal moved its head in an exploratory manner. The cut-off time of the test was 720 seconds.

Assessement of motor imbalance was done by a rotarod apparatus. Rat was placed on the rotarod (18 RPM) and the latency to fall off the rotarod was recorded. Animals staying during 720 s were taken from the rotarod and their retention time on rotarod considered 720 s. All observations were made between 9 AM and 4 PM by an observer who was blind to the entity of treatments.

Statistical analysis

Statistical analysis of each data set was calculated by use of SigmaStat software. Data were expressed as the mean + SEM, and were analyzed by one-way ANOVA in each experiment. In the case of significant variation ($p<0.05$), the values were compared by Tukey test.

Results

The effect of intra-SNc-injection of 6-OHDA on motor-balance

The effect of intra-SNc injection of 6-OHDA on motor-balance was evaluated by rotarod test. The duration of time to fall from rotating rod was evaluated in three groups of rats: normal, sham-operated and 6-OHDA (8 μg/2 μl/rat)-lesioned groups. 6-OHDA (8 μg/2 μl/rat) induced motor imbalance ($P < 0.001$) in comparison with normal and sham operated groups (Figure 1). The results of intra-SNc injection of 6-OHDA on bar test (as a standard catalepsy test) have been shown in our previous studies (12, 22) in which it induced marked catalepsy ($P < 0.001$) when compared with normal and sham operated groups. Therefore, the results have not been shown in this paper.

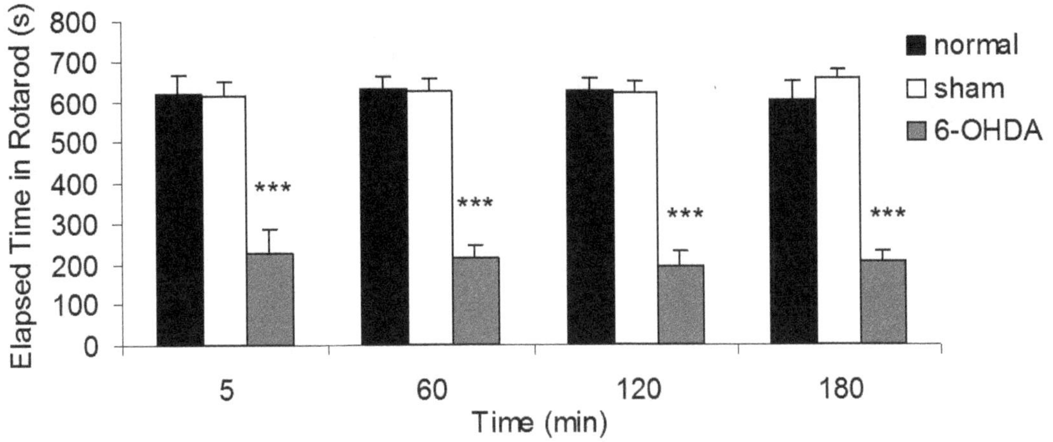

Figure 1. The results of rotarod test in control, Sham-operated and 6-OHDA (8μg/2μl/rat)- lesioned rats. Each bar presents the mean±SEM of elapsed time (s), n = 8 rats for each group; *** $p<0.001$ when compared with normal and sham operated groups.

The effect of chronic administration of L-DOPA on motor-balance

The effect of chronic injection of L-DOPA (15 mg/kg, i.p.) and its vehicle on motor- balance was investigated in 6-OHDA- lesioned rats for 20 consecutive days (Figure 2). In these groups, motor-balance was assessed by rotarod on days 5, 10, 15 and 20. L-DOPA significantly increased retention time on rotarod ($p < 0.001$, $p<0.01$ and $p<0.05$) at days 5, 10 and 15, whereas it's motor-balance improving effect was decreased at day 20. The results of same treatments on bar test are accessible in our previous paper.[12,22]. In that study we showed that L-DOPA could induce anti-cataleptic effect only until day 15.

The effect of fluoxetine on anti-cataleptic and motor-balance improving effect of L-DOPA

Three groups of animals that were pre-treated with L-DOPA (15 mg/kg twice daily, i.p.), received three different doses of fluoxetine (0.1, 0.5 and 1 mg/kg, i.p.) on day 21. The results showed that fluoxetine improved the anti-cataleptic effect of L-DOPA at the doses of 0.5 and 1 mg/kg ($p < 0.05$ and 0.01) (Figure 3, panel A), while it did not improve the effect of L-DOPA in rotarod test (Figure 3, panel B).

The effect of NAN-190 co-treatment with fluoxetine on anti-cataleptic effect of L-DOPA

On day 21, the effect co-administartion of NAN-190 (1mg/kg, i.p.) with fluoxetine (0.5 mg/kg, i.p.) was investigated in rats pre-treated with L-DOPA (15 mg/kg twice daily, i.p.). As it has been shown in Figure 4, the catalepsy-improving effect of fluoxetine was halted ($p<0.05$ and 0. 01) in the presence of NAN-190.

Discussion

According to the obtained results the acute administration of fluoxetine improved anti-parkinsonian effects of L-DOPA in 6-OHDA- lesioned rats. The 6-OHDA- lesioned rats are generally used in the study for PD and L-DOPA related adverse motor complications.[6] In this study intra-SNc injection of 6-OHDA caused marked catalepsy and motor imbalance when assessed by bar test and rotarod test, respectively. In rodents catalepsy is considered as a test for akinisia[23] and can be reproduced by 6-OHDA and neuroleptic drugs.[6,13,19] Bar test is a standard test which is used commonly to assess catalepsy in rodents.[6,19] Furthermore, unilateral injection of 6-OHDA induces motor imbalance that can be measured by rotarod as a standard motor-balance test.[6,20] Indeed unilateral lesion of substantia nigra forces a rat to change its weight abnormally for movement and equilibrium; hence this results in motor disorders.[24] Our results showed that 6-OHDA- lesioned rats fail to maintain their balances on rotarod and a significant reduction in retention time on rotarod was observed in these animals. We observed that L-DOPA abolished catalepsy in 6-OHDA- lesioned rats only on days 5, 10 and 15. The anti-cataleptic and motor imbalance improving effects of L-DOPA were attenuated markedly on day 20. It seems that long-term administration of L-DOPA causes some plastic alterations in the striatum,[14] which these neuronal changes result in L-DOPA- induced motor disorders.[25]

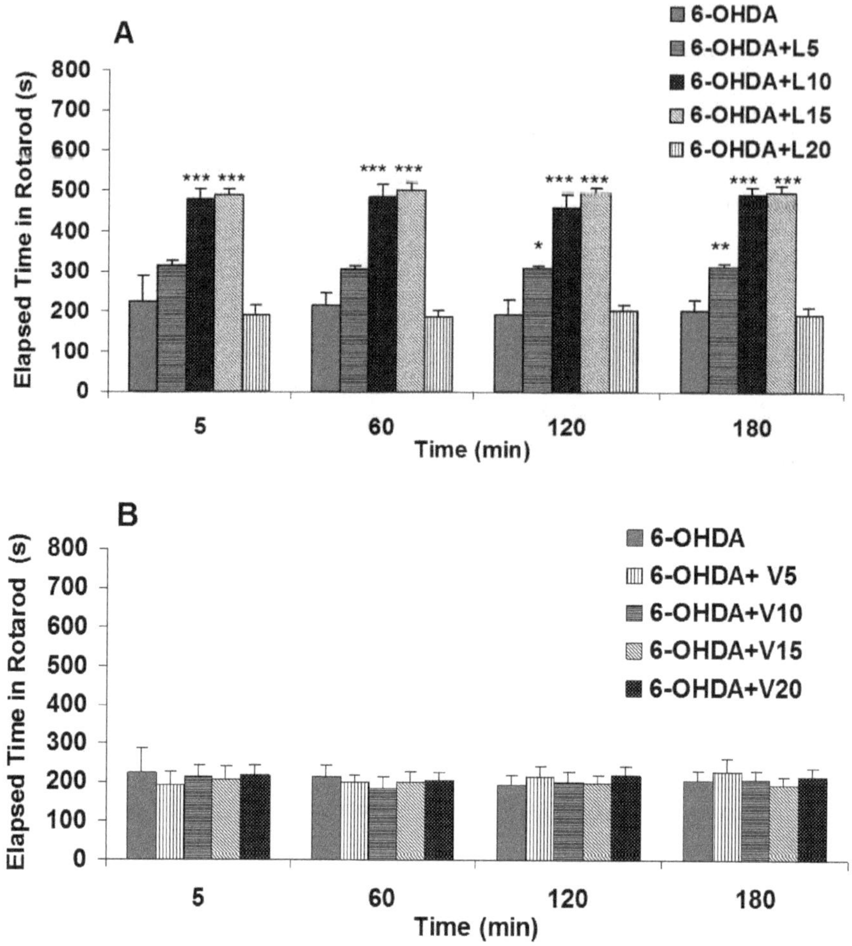

Figure 2. The results of rotarod test in 6-OHDA (8μg/2μl/rat)-lesioned rats injected with L-DOPA (15mg/kg) (Panel A) and L-DOPA's vehicle (Panel B) twice daily on the days 5, 10, 15 and 20. Each bar shows the mean±SEM of elapsed time (s), n = 8 rats for each group; *$p<0.05$, **$p<0.01$ and *** $p<0.001$ when compared with 6-OHDA lesioned rats. (L=L-DOPA on days 5, 10, 15, 20)- (V=Vehicle on days 5, 10, 15, 20).

According to the obtained results, co-administration of fluoxetine and L-DOPA enhanced anti-cataleptic effect of L-DOPA on day 21. This result confirms our study showing an anti-cataleptic effect for fluoxetine in 6-OHDA-lesioned[20] or haloperidol-treated animals.[26] Fluoxetine was not able to improve the effect of L-DOPA in rotarod on day 21. This may be due to sedative effect of fluoxetine.[27] Fluoxetine increases effect of GABA on $GABA_A$ receptors resulting in induction of sedative state.[27,28] This is in accordance to the results of other study showing that fluoxetine dose not increase rotarod elapsed time in parkinsonian rats.[29]
Under normal conditions, dopaminergic neurons regulate dopamine levels through D2 autoreceptors and dopamine transporters.[16] However serotonergic neurons have not these regulatory systems. Thus activation of these neurons impacts on L-DOPA derived dopamine and results in fluctuations in extracellular dopamine levels.[14,16] This pulsatile release of dopamine may cause intermittent dopamine receptor stimulation that eventually causes subsequent motor problems like wearing off and LID.[25] It has been suggested that in 6-OHDA-induced PD, serotonergic neurons are involved in LID.[14,16]

All components of basal ganglia receive serotonergic projection from dorsal raphe nuclei[6] which modulates nigrostriatal dopaminergic transmission.[26] It seems this system plays essential role in the modulation of motor behaviors. This effect is mediated via 5-HT_{1A} receptors within the basal ganglia circuits.[18] 5-HT_{1A} receptors are also located on dorsal raphe neurons that alter their own activity.[30] Activation of 5-HT_{1A} receptors prolongs dopamine effect in parkinsonian animals.[12] Therefore it seems that 5-HT_{1A} activators might have promising anti-parkinsonian and antidyskinetic properties. Our previous studies have shown that activation of 5-HT_{1A} receptors exert anti-cataleptic effect in parkinsonian rats.[10,19] Stimulation of this receptor could improve anti- cataleptic effect of 6-OHDA in rats.[12] It is supposed that specific serotonin reuptake inhibitors

(SSRIs) which increase serotonin levels in synaptic cleft[26] may have similar effect through affecting on 5-HT_{1A} receptors. In this study, NAN-190 (5-HT_{1A} receptor antagonist) reversed the catalepsy-improving effect of fluoxetine in L-DOPA-treated rats. Thus, we can say that fluoxetine improves anti-cataleptic effect of L-DOPA by affecting on 5-HT_{1A} receptors.

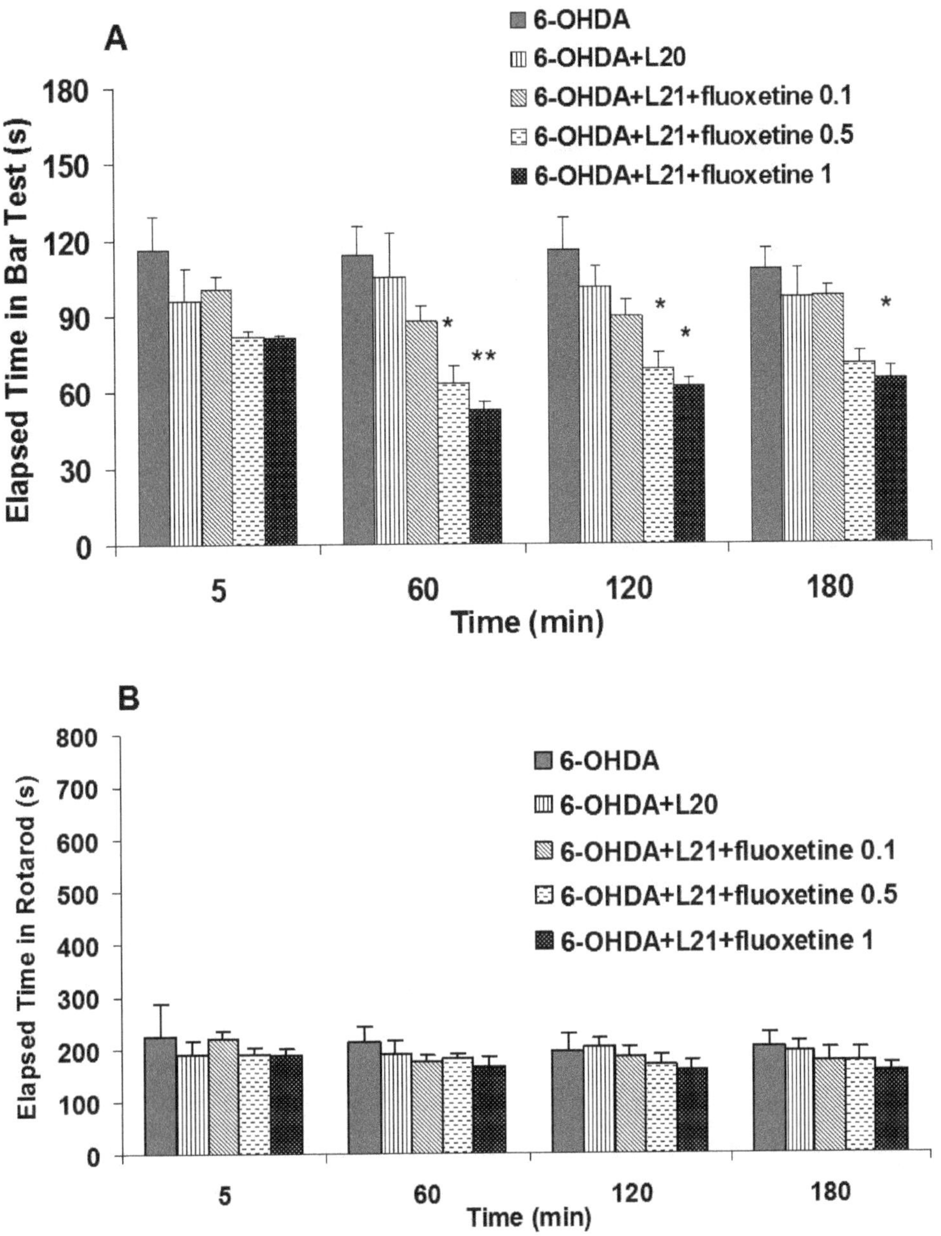

Figure 3. The bar test (panel A) and rotarod (panel B) from the co-administration of fluoxetine (0.1, 0. 5 and 1 mg/kg) with L-DOPA (15 mg/kg) on day 21 in 6-OHDA-lesioned rats and 6-OHDA lesioned rats treated with L-DOPA (15 mg/kg) on day 20. Each bar represents the mean±SEM of elapsed time (s), n = 8 rats for each group; *$p<0.05$ and ** $p<0.01$ when compared with 6-OHDA lesioned rats. (L=L-DOPA on days 20 and 21).

Aside from motor impairments, depression is other comorbid clinical problem of PD that reduces quality of life. Approximately 40% of patients with PD experience depressive syndrome.[31] SSRIs are widely used to treat depressive conditions in patients with PD.[26] Regarding to the results of this study, fluoxetine is able to improve anti-parkinsonian effect of L-DOPA. Then, it can be used as an adjuvant therapy in PD.

We conclude that fluoxetine improves anti-cataleptic effect of L-DOPA in 6-OHDA-lesioned rats. This effect is mediated by the stimulation of 5-HT_{1A} receptors. In addition, we suggest that investigation of a possible clinical application for fluoxetine should be carried out to test its usefulness in diminishing LID. Further investigations must be done for explaining exact mechanism of the interactions between serotonergic and dopaminergic neurons.

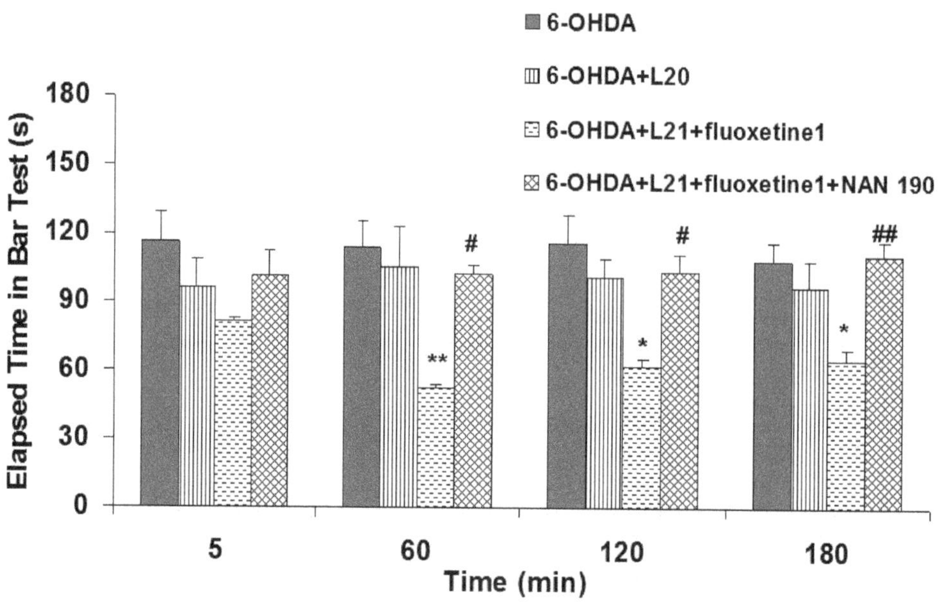

Figure 4. The bar test results from the co-administration of NAN-190 (0.5 mg/kg) with L-DOPA (15 mg/kg) and fluoxetine (0.5 mg/kg) on day 21 in 6-OHDA lesioned rats treated with L-DOPA (15 mg/kg) on day 21. Each bar represents the mean ± SEM of elapsed time (s); n = 8 rats for each group; * $p < 0.05$ and ** $p < 0.01$ when compared with 6-OHDA-lesioned rats; $^{\#}p < 0.05$ and $^{\#\#}p < 0.01$ when compared with 6-OHDA-lesioned rats co-treated with L-DOPA (15 mg/kg) and fluoxetine (0.5 mg/kg) on day 21. (L=L-DOPA on days 20 and 21).

Acknowledgment
We wish to thank Dean of Faculty of Pharmacy, Director of Drug Applied Research Center, and Research Vice-Chancellor of Tabriz University of Medical Sciences for supporting this work.

Conflict of Interest
There is no conflict of interest in this study.

References
1. Chen Q, He Y, Yang K. Gene Therapy for Parkinson's disease: Progress and Challenges. Curr Gene Ther 2005;5:71-80.
2. Nayebi AM. Hypothesis: A promising effect of 5-HT_{1A} receptor agonists in alleviating motor symptoms of Parkinson's disease. Afr J Pharm Pharmacol 2010;4:4289–90.
3. Orth M, Tabrizi SJ. Models of Parkinson's disease. Mov Disord 2003;18:729-37.
4. Carta M, Carlsson T, Munoz A, Kirik D, Bjorklund A. Involvement of the serotonin system in L-dopa-induced dyskinesias. Parkinsonism Relat Disord 2008;14:154–8.
5. Iancu R, Mohapel P, Brundin P, Paul G. Behavioral characterization of a unilateral 6-OHDA-lesion model of Parkinson's disease in mice. Behav Brain Res 2005;162:1-10.
6. Nayebi AM, Rad SR, Saberian M, Azimzadeh S, Smini M. Buspirone improves 6-hydroxydopamine-induced Buspirone improves the anti-cataleptic effect of L-DOPA catalepsy through stimulation of 5-HT_{1A} receptors in rats. Pharmacol Rep 2010;62:258–64.
7. Kalda A, Herm L, Rinken A, Zharkovsky A, Chen JF. Co-administration of the partial dopamine D2 agonist terguride with L-dopa attenuates L-dopa-induced locomotor sensitization in hemiparkinsonian mice. Behav Brain Res 2009;202:232-7.
8. Padovan-Neto FE, Echeverry MB, Tumas V, Del-Bel EA. Nitric oxide synthase inhibition attenuatesL-DOPA-induced dyskinesias in a rodent model of Parkinson's disease. Neuroscience 2009;159:927-35.
9. Carta M, Carlsson T, Munoz A, Kirik D, Bjorklund A. Serotonin-dopamine interaction in induction and maintenance of L-DOPA-induced dyskinesias. In: Progress in brain research. Di Giovanni G, Di matteo V, Esposito E, editors. Elsevier BV; 2008. 465-78.
10. Maeda T, Kannari K, Huo S, Arai A, Tomiyama M, Matsunaga M, et al. Increase of the striatal serotonergic fibers after nigrostriatal dopaminergic denervation in adult rats. Int Congr Ser 2003;1251:211–5.
11. Cenci MA, Lundblad M. Post- versus presynaptic plasticity in L-DOPA-induced dyskinesia. J Neurochem 2006;99:381-92.
12. Mahmoudi J, Nayebi AM, Samini M, Reyhani-Rad S, Babapour V. Buspirone improves the anti-cataleptic effect of levodopa in 6-hydroxydopamine-lesioned rats. Pharm rep 2011;63:908-14.
13. Munoz A, Li Q, Gardoni F, Marcello E, Qin C, Carlsson T, et al. Combined 5-HT_{1A} and 5-HT_{1B}

receptor the treatment of L-DOPA-induced dyskinesia. Brain 2008;131:3380-94.
14. Ulusoy A, Sahin G, Kirik D. Presynaptic dopaminergic compartment determines the susceptibility to L-DOPA-induced dyskinesia in rats. Proc Natl Acad Sci USA 2010;107:13159-64.
15. Carta M, Carlsson T, Kirik D, Bjorklund A. Dopamine released from 5-HT terminals is the cause of L-DOPA-induced dyskinesia in parkinsonian rats. Brain 2007;130:1819-33.
16. Carlsson T, Carta M, Winkler C, Bjorklund A, Kirik D. Serotonin neuron transplants exacerbate L-DOPA-induced dyskinesia in a rat model of Parkinson's disease. J Neurosci 2007;27:8011-22.
17. Ba M, Kong M, Ma G, Yang H, Lu G, Chen S, et al. Cellular and behavioral effects of 5-HT_{1A} receptor agonist 8-OH-DAPT in a rat model of levodopa-induced motor complication. Brain Res 2007;1127:177-84.
18. Matteo VD, Pierucci M, Esposito E, Crescimanno G, Benigno A, Giovanni GD. Serotonin modulation of the basal ganglia circuitry: therapeutic implication for parkinsons disease and other motor disorders. Prog brain Res 2008;172:423-63.
19. Mohajjel Nayebi A, Sheidaei H. Buspirone improves haloperidol-induced Parkinson disease in mice through 5-HT_{1A} receptors. DARU 2010;18:41-5.
20. Mohajjel Nayebi A, Reyhani-Rad S, Mahmoudi J, Samini M. Effect of fluoxteine on motor disorders induced by intranigral injection of 6-hydroxydopamine in rats. Pharm Sci 2010;16:45-54.
21. Paxinos G, Watson C. The rat brain in stereotaxic coordinates. Sydney: Academic press; 1982.
22. Mahmoudi J, Mohhajel Nayebi A, Samini M, Reyhani-Rad S, Babapour V. 5-HT_{1A} receptor activation improves anti-cataleptic effect of levodopa in 6-hydroxydopamine-lesioned rats. Daru 2011;19:338-43.
23. Sharma N, Rana AC, Bafan P. Effect of aqueous extract of cynodondactylon on reserpine induced catalepsy. Int J Pharm Pharm Sci 2011;3:424-6.
24. Meredith GE, Sonsalla PK, Chesselet MF. Animal models of Parkinson disease progression. Acta Neuropathol 2008;115:385-98.
25. Tomiyama M, Kimura T, Maeda Y, Kannari K, Matsunaga M, Baba M. A serotonin 5HT_{1A} receptor agonist prevents behavioral sensitization to L-DOPA in rodent model of Parkinson's disease. Neurosci Res 2005;52:185-94.
26. Pires JG, Bonikovski V, Futuro-Neto HA. Acute effects of selective serotonin reuptake inhibitors on neuroleptic-induced catalepsy in mice. Braz J Med Biol Res 2005;38:1867-72.
27. Pinna G, Costa E, Guidotti A. Fluoxetine and norfluoxetine stereospecifically facilitate pentobarbital sedation by increasing neurosteroids. Proc Natl Acad Sci USA 2004;101:6222–5.
28. Pinna G, Costa E, Guidotti A. Fluoxetine and norfluoxetine stereo specifically and selectively increase brain neurosteroid content at doses that are inactive on 5-HT reuptake. Psychopharmacology (Berl). 2006;186:362-72.
29. Dekundy A, Lundblad M, Danysz W, Cenci MA. Modulation of L-DOPA-induced abnormal involuntary movements by clinically tested compounds: further validation of the rat dyskinesia model. Behav Brain Res 2007;179:76-89.
30. Eskow KL, Gupta V, Alam S, Park JY, Bishop C. The partial 5-HT_{1A} agonist buspirone reduces the expression and development of L-DOPA-induced dyskinesia in rats and improves L-DOPA efficacy. Pharmacol Biochem Behav 2007;87:306-14.
31. Schrag A, Barone P, Brown RG, Leentjens AF, McDonald WM, Starkstein S, et al. Depression rating scales in Parkinson's disease: critique and recommendations. Mov Disord 2007;22:1077-92.

Derivative Spectrophotometric Method for Estimation of Antiretroviral Drugs in Fixed Dose Combinations

Mohite P.B. [1*], **Pandhare R.B.** [1], **Khanage S.G.** [1]

[1] *Department of Pharmaceutical Chemistry, MES's College of Pharmacy, Sonai, Ahmednagar, Maharashtra, India.*

ARTICLE INFO

Keywords:
Lamivudine
Zidovudine

ABSTRACT

Purpose: Lamivudine is cytosine and zidovudine is cytidine and is used as an antiretroviral agents. Both drugs are available in tablet dosage forms with a dose of 150 mg for LAM and 300 mg ZID respectively. ***Method:*** The method employed is based on first order derivative spectroscopy. Wavelengths 279 nm and 300 nm were selected for the estimation of the Lamovudine and Zidovudine respectively by taking the first order derivative spectra. The conc. of both drugs was determined by proposed method. The results of analysis have been validated statistically and by recovery studies as per ICH guidelines. ***Result:*** Both the drugs obey Beer's law in the concentration range 10-50 μg mL^{-1},for LAM and ZID; with regression 0.9998 and 0.9999, intercept – 0.0677 and – 0.0043 and slope 0.0457 and 0.0391 for LAM and ZID, respectively.The accuracy and reproducibility results are close to 100% with 2% RSD. ***Conclusion:*** A simple, accurate, precise, sensitive and economical procedures for simultaneous estimation of Lamovudine and Zidovudine in tablet dosage form have been developed.

Introduction

Lamivudine is chemically, 1[(2R, 5S)-2-(Hydroxy methyl)-1-3 oxathiolan-5yl] cytosine and used as an antiretroviral activity.[1] Lamivudine is an analogue of cytidine. It can inhibit both types (I and II) of HIV reverse transcriptase and also the reverse transcriptase of hepatitis B. It needs to be phosphorylated to its triphosphate form before it is active. 3TC triphosphate also inhibits cellular DNA polymerase. The chemical structure of Lamivudine is shown in Figure 1.

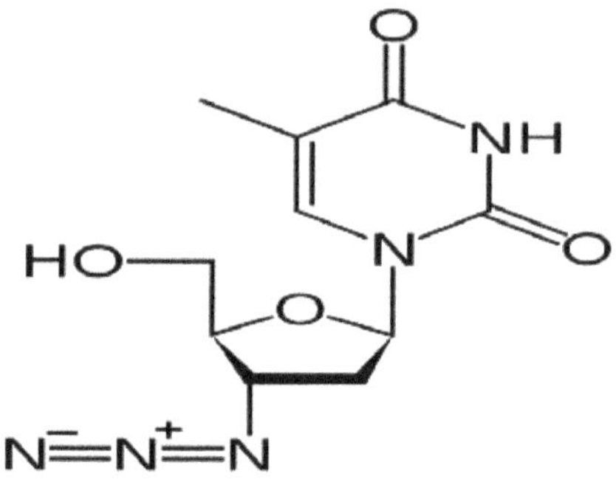

Figure 1. Structure of Lamivudine

Zidovudine is chemically, 1-[(2R, 4S, 5S) -4azido -5-(hydroxy methyl) tetrahydrofuran-2-yl]-5-methylprimidine-2,4(1H,3H)-dione and used as an antiretroviral activity.[2] The chemical structure of Lamivudine is shown in Figure 2 .

Literature survey revealed that several analytical methods including spectrophotometric[1-8], HPLC (High-performance liquid chromatography) [9-11,] ,HPTLC (High-performance thin layer chromatography) [12,13] ,RP-HPLC (Reverse phase-high performance liquid chromatography) [14,15] and LC/MS (Liquid chromatography-mass spectrophotometry)[16,17] methods have been reported for its estimation of Lamivudine and Zidovudine in various dosage forms alone or in fixed dose combination with other drugs. Like LAM, ZID is also a Nucleoside Analog. Both the drugs are available in combined dosage form with a dose of 150 mg for LAM and 300 mg for ZID respectively.

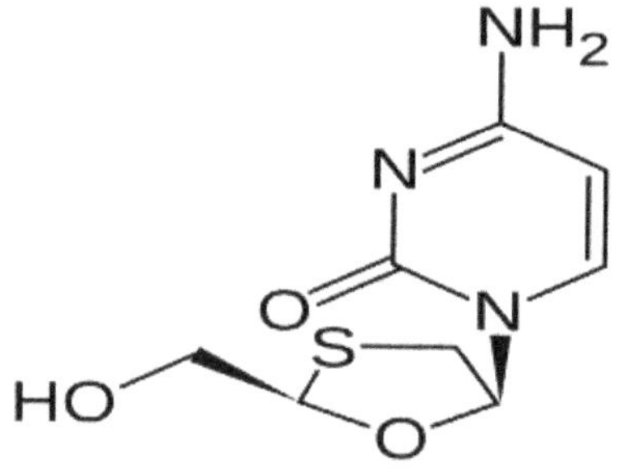

Figure 2. Structure of Zidovudine

Both these drugs are not official in Indian Pharmacopoeia, United States Pharmacopoeia.

Extensive literature survey reveals that derivative spectrophotometric method is yet not reported for simultaneous determination of LAM and ZID in tablet dosage form. In present work an attempt is being made to develop simple, precise, accurate and economical

***Corresponding author:** Mohite P.B . Department of Pharmaceutical Chemistry,MES's College of Pharmacy, Sonai, University of Pune, Pune, Maharashtra, India. E-mail:mohitepb@gmail.com

derivative spectrophotometric methods for simultaneous determination of binary drug formulation.

Materials and methods

The instrument used in the present study was JASCO double beam UV/Visible Spectrophotometer (Model V-630) with spectral bandwidth of 1 nm and 10 mm a matched quartz cell was used. All weighing was done on electronic balance (Model Shimadzu BL 320-H).

Reagents and chemicals

Analytically pure sample of LAM and ZID was kindly supplied by Cipla Pharmaceuticals Ltd. (Daund, India) and used as such without further purification. The pharmaceutical dosage form used in this study was a Combivir tablets manufactured by Glenmark Pharmaceuticals Ltd. (Sinnar, India) labeled to contain 150 mg of LAM and 300 mg of ZID. All chemicals are of AR grade and were purchased from Qualigens fine Chemicals, Mumbai, India.

First Order Derivative Spectroscopic Method [18,19]

The method is based on first order derivative spectroscopy to overcome spectral interference from other drug. First order derivative spectra of both the drugs were recorded in Figure 3. It was observed that LAM showed dA/dλ zero at 279 nm in contrast to ZID that has considerable dA/dλ at this wavelength. Further, ZID has zero dA/dλ at 300 nm while at this wavelength LAM has significant dA/dλ. Therefore these two wavelengths were employed for the estimation of LAM and ZID without any interference. The calibration curves were plotted at these two wavelengths of concentrations against dA/dλ within the above mentioned range. The equations of line obtained to determine concentrations LAM and ZID are

$$C_{LAM} = DA/D\lambda_{300} - 0.0150 / 0.0168$$

$$C_{ZID} = DA/D\lambda_{279} - 0.0124 / 0.0176$$

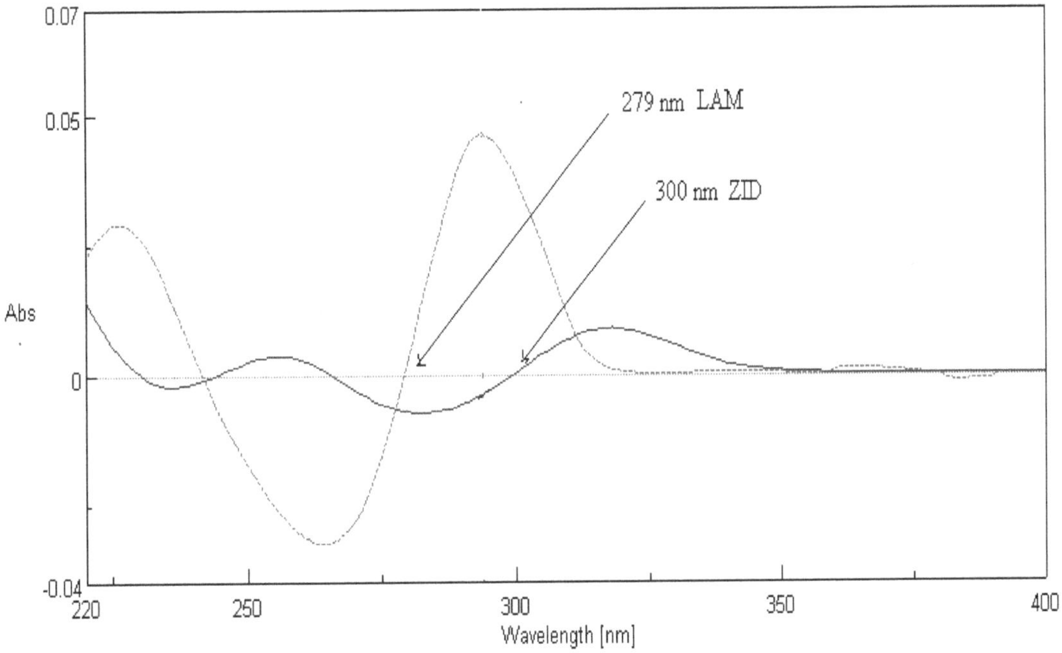

Figure 3. First order derivative overlain spectra of LAM (10 μg mL^{-1}) and ZID (10 μg mL^{-1}) in 0.1M HCl

Preparation of Standard Stock Solutions

Standard stock solutions were prepared by dissolving separately 10 mg of each drug in 100 mL of 0.1 N HCl to get concentration of 0.1 mg mL^{-1}. 1 mL of the stock solution was further diluted to 10 mL with 0.1 N HCl to get a working standard solution of concentration 10 μg mL^{-1} of both LAM and ZID and scanned in the wavelength range of 200-400 nm.

Preparation of Sample Stock Solution

Contents of twenty tablets were weighed accurately and powdered. Powder equivalent to 100 mg of ZID and 50 mg of LAM was weighed and dissolved in 50 mL of 0.1 N HCl with the aid of ultrasonication for 5 min. The solution was filtered through Whatman filter paper no. 41 to a 100 mL volumetric flask. Filter paper was washed with 0.1 N HCl, adding washings to the volumetric flask and volume was made up to the mark with 0.1 N HCl to get sample stock solution which was further diluted with 0.1 N HCl to get final concentration of solution (LAM 10 μg mL^{-1} and ZID 20 μg mL^{-1}) in the linearity range.

Results and Discussions

Linearity and range

A standard stock solution was prepared for both Lamivudine and Zidovudine; they were serially diluted to yield five standard solutions.For UV spectrophotometric method, linearity was obtained in concentration range of 10 –50 μg .mL^{-1}, for LAM and ZID; with regression 0.9998 and 0.9999, intercept – 0.0677 and – 0.0043 and slope 0.0457 and 0.0391 for LAM and ZID , respectively.The results are depicted in table1.

Accuracy and precision

The accuracy of the proposed methods was checked by recovery studies, by addition of standard drug solution to preanalysed sample solution at three different concentration levels within the range of linearity for both the drugs.Results of recovery studies are shown in Table 2. The accuracy and reproducibility is evident from the data as results are close to 100 % and the value of standard deviation and % R.S.D. were found to be < 2 %; shows the high precision of the method. The proposed method is simple, economical, rapid, precise and accurate. Hence it can be used for routine analysis of LAM and ZID in tablet formulation.

Specificity

The proposed method was found to be specific as there is no interference from other excipients.

Results of analysis of tablet formulation

Analysis of tablet formulation combivir was carried out and the amount recovered were expressed as percentage amount of tablet claim.The percentage recovery for LAM is 99.98±0.645 and ZID is 98.56±0.542 respectively.The proposed methods was evaluated by the assay (n = 6) of commercially available tablets containing LAM and ZID. The results of assay are presented in Table3.

The proposed method has an advantage two advantage over earlier developed methds. One is the of use of 0.1N HCl as solvent which is easily available and less costlier as compared to methanol and second is good recovery results. Also the derivative spectrophotometry provides greater selectivity and offers a solution in resolving a overlapping spectra.

Table 1. Linearity Results

Components	Concentration range(μg mL^{-1})	Equation for regression line	r^2
LAM	10-50	Y=0.0457x - 0.0677	0.9998
ZID	10-50	Y=0.0391 x - 0.0043	0.9999

**Mean of six determinations,R.S.D. is relative standard deviation.*

Table 2. Recovery studies of LAM and ZID

Drug	Conc of drug added		%Recovery ±S.D.*	Intra day Precision	%Recovery ±S.D.*	Inter day Precision
	μg mL^{-1}	%Level				
LAM	5	50	100.43±0.54	0.45	99.74±0.34	0.35
	10	100	100.21±0.08	0.54	99,28±0.38	0.44
	15	150	99.85±0.28	0.51	99.55±0.28	0.4
ZID	10	50	98.76±0.34	0.35	99.06±0.54	0.39
	20	100	98.98±0.29	0.46	98.88±0.69	0.43
	30	150	98.65±0.42	0.45	99.65±0.42	0.58

** Mean of three determinations*

Table 3: Results of commercial formulation analysis

Method	Formulation	Label claim (mg/Tablet)	%label claim estimated* (Mean±S.D.)	% R.S.D.
Derivative spectroscopy	Combivir	LAM	99.98±0.645	0.345
		ZID	98.56±0.542	0.412

**Mean of six determinations,R.S.D. is relative standard deviation*

Conclusion

The developed and validated spectrophotometric method employed here proved to be simple, economical, rapid, precise and accurate. Thus it can be used for routine simultaneous determination of LAM and ZID in tablet dosage form instead of processing and analyzing each drug separately.

Acknowledgement

The authors are thankful to Cipla Pharmaceuticals Ltd. (Daund, India), for providing drug samples and Principal MES College of Pharmacy, Sonai and Mula Education Society for providing facilities to carry out this work.

Conflict of interest

The authors report no conflicts of interest.

References

1. Djurdjevic P, Laban A, Markovic S, Jelikic-Stankov M. Chemometric Optimization of a RP-HPLC Method for the Simultaneous Analysis of Abacavir, Lamivudine, and Zidovudine in Tablets. *Anal Lett* 2004;37(13):2649-67.
2. Shankar DG, Reddy MVVN, Kumar JMR, Rajendra, Murthy TK.UV spectrophotometric determination of some antiHIV drugs. *Asian J Chem* 2002;14(1):433-6.
3. Garikapati DR. Development and validation of spectrophotometric method for the determination of anti-HIV drug. *Asian J Chem* 2004;16(2):1217-9.
4. Erk N. Derivative and difference UV spectrophotometric and compensation technique for the simultaneous determination of Zidovudine and Lamivudine in human serum. *Pharmazie* 2004;59:106.
5. Shankar DG, Reddy MVVN, Kumar JMR, Rajendra, Murthy TK.Spectrophotometric determination of Lamivudine and Stavudine. *Indian Jour Pharm Sci* 2002;64:504.
6. Sarma CSN, Sastri CK, Sastri CSP. Simple oxidative method for determination of Stavudine and Lamivudine. *Asian J Chem* 2002;14(2): 683-690.
7. Appalaraju S, Karadi Arvind B, Kamalapurkar OS, Sarasambi Prakash S. Spectrophotometric Determination of Lamivudine. *Asian J Chem* 2022;14(1):475-478.
8. Sarma CSN, Sastry CK, Sastry CSP. Determination of stavudine and lamivudine by visible spectrophotometry. *Acta Ciencia Indica Chem* 2002; 28: 221-225.
9. Ozkan SA, Uslu B. Rapid HPLC assay for lamivudine in pharmaceuticals and human serum. *J Liq Chromatogr Relat Technol* 2002;25(9):1447-1456.
10. Nerurkar KK, Dhorda UJ, Bhoir SI, Sudarshan M. Concurrent assay of Lamivudine and Zidovudine from combination tablets by HPLC. *Indian Jour Pharm Sci* 2003;65:412.
11. Wagh PJ, Pai N. Development and validation of HPLC method for simultaneous determination of Lamivudine and Zidovudine from pharmaceutical preparation. *Indian Drugs* 2002;39:654.
12. Wankhede SB, Gupta KR, Wadodkar SG. Simultaneous HPTLC estimation of Lamivudine and Stavudine in tablet dosage form. *Indian J Pharm Sci* 2005; 67:96.
13. Anbazhagan S, Indumathy N, Pitchaimuthu S, Krishnan S. Simultaneous quantification of stavudine, Lamivudine and Nevirapine by UV spectroscopy, reverse phase HPLC and HPTLC in tablets. *J Chromatogr* 2007; 859: 234.
14. Pai N, Desai AD. Simultaneous RP-HPLC estimation of some antiretroviral drugs fromTablets. *Indian Jour Pharm Sci* 2007; 69:118.
15. Pallad MS, Rajesh PMN, Chatter M, Bhatt AR. RP-HPLC determination of Zidovudine and Lamivudine in tab dosage form. Indian J Pharm Sci 2005;67: 110.
16. Mistri HN, Jangid AG, Pudage A, Gomes N, Sanyal M, Shrivastav P. High throughput LC–MS/MS method for simultaneous quantification of lamivudine, stavudine and nevirapine in human plasma. *J Chromatogr* 2007; 853:320.
17. Robbins B, Poston PA, Neal EF, Slaughter C, Rodman JH. Simultaneous measurement of intracellular triphosphate metabolites of zidovudine, lamivudine and abacavir (carbovir) in human peripheral blood mononuclear cells by combined anion exchange solidphase extraction and LC–MS/MS. *Jour Chromatogr* 2007; 850:310.
18. Skoog DA, Holler FJ, Nieman TA. Principles of instrumental analysis. 5th ed. Philadelphia: Harcourt Brace College Publishers; 1998.
19. Beckett AH, Stenlake JB. Practical Pharmaceutical chemistry. 4th ed. London: Athlone Press; 1988.

Esmolol: A Unique Beta-Blocker in Maintaining Cardiovascular Stability Following Neurosurgical Procedures

Hamzeh Hosseinzadeh [1], Mahmood Eydi [1], Mehdi Ghaffarlou [1], Kamyar Ghabili [2], Samad EJ Golzari [3,4*]

[1] Department of Anesthesiology, Tabriz University of Medical Sciences, Tabriz, Iran.

[2] Physical Medicine and Rehabilitation Research Center, Tabriz University of Medical Sciences, Tabriz, Iran.

[3] Medical Philosophy and History Research Center, Tabriz University of Medical Sciences, Tabriz, Iran.

[4] Students' Research Committee, Tabriz University of Medical Sciences, Tabriz, Iran.

ARTICLE INFO

Keywords:
Esmolol
Neurosurgery
Cardiovascular Stability

ABSTRACT

Purpose: Patients with increased intracranial pressure (ICP) are prone to severe cardiac and or cerebral complications following emergence from general anesthesia and especially post-extubation phase. Administering beta blockers including esmolol is believed to be helpful in providing a stable hemodynamic at the end of the surgery and recovery stages and reducing recovery phase length. ***Methods:*** In a double-blind prospective randomized clinical trial, 60 adult patients with ASA (American Society of Anesthesiologist) class of I-II scheduled to undergo elective neurosurgery operations were randomly divided into two groups receiving esmolol (n=30) and placebo (n=30) as IV infusion within four minutes prior to extubation continued by an IV infusion for 10 minutes after extubation. ***Results:*** There was a significant difference between two groups regarding the changes of systolic blood pressure and heart rate at all studied stages after extubation ($P \leq 0.05$). However, no significant difference existed between esmolol and control groups regarding recovery and extubation times emphasizing the fact that esmolol is of excellent early recovery and extubation profiles. ***Conclusion:*** Esmolol is advised to be used in preventing hyperdynamic status throughout extubation phase without extending recovery phase length.

Introduction

Patients with increased intracranial pressure (ICP) are prone to severe cardiac and or cerebral complications following emergence from general anesthesia and especially post-extubation phase which may lead to increase in oxygen consumption, and catecholamine release. This phase lasting 15 to 5 minutes could frequently be accompanied by tachycardia and hypertension.[1] This temporary encountered situation could however be endured appropriately by most patients.[2] Patients with preoperative hypertension and cardiovascular and cerebrovascular diseases and patients with increased ICP could be prone to severe cardiac and or cerebral complications.[3] Therefore, preventing postoperative and post-intubation sympathetic excitations in high-risk patients to maintain stability in the dynamic status is of great importance which may reduce the mortality and morbidity rates in these patients.[1] Esmolol, a selective beta-adrenergic receptor antagonist, is water-soluble, short acting (9 minutes) and of a rapid effect commencement. Administering esmolol throughout anesthesia reduces hyperdynamic cardiovascular responses however very few studies have been carried out to prove its efficacy at extubation and post-extubation stages. Considering the fact that pain is one of the major factors contributing to sympathetic excitement at the end of the surgery and recovery stages, we aimed to evaluate the efficacy of pre-extubation administration of esmolol on maintaining the hemodynamic stability at the end of the surgery and recovery stages and its effects on recovery phase length.

Materials and Methods

This study is a double-blind prospective placebo-control randomized clinical trial which was carried out after obtaining approval of the ethics committee of Tabriz University of Medical Sciences and informed written consents from the patients. Sixty adult patients with ASA (American Society of Anesthesiologist) class of I-II which were scheduled to undergo elective neurosurgery operations were randomly divided into two groups of 30 people. Exclusion criteria from the study included pregnant females, patients with heart rate (HR) less than 60, systolic blood pressure less than 100 mmHg, considerable hepatic, renal or

*Corresponding author: Samad EJ Golzari (MD), Medical Philosophy and History Research Center, Tabriz University of Medical Sciences, Tabriz, Iran. E-mail: dr.golzari@hotmail.com

cardiovascular complications, atrioventricular block, sick sinus syndrome, history of intolerance to beta-blockers, bronchospasm and asthma, and chronic obstructive pulmonary disease. All patients were premedicated with fentanyl (2 μg/kg IV) and lidocaine (1.5 mg/kg IV) and intubated using Sodium Thiopental (7-5 mg/kg) and Cis-atracurium (0.15 mg/kg). Anesthesia was maintained using Isoflurane (1-1.5%) and a mixture of O_2 (50%) and N_2O (50%).[4] Mechanical ventilation was maintained with a tidal volume of 10 mL/kg and at a rate to keep End-tidal CO_2 at the range of 35-30 mmHg. Repeated doses of Cis-atracurium (0.05 mg/kg) were used to provide intraoperative muscle relaxation.[5] Administration of anesthetics was terminated when suturing the skin and muscle relaxation was antagonized with neostigmine (0.05 mg/kg) and atropine (0.02 mg/kg) after reestablishment of spontaneous breathing.[6]

Esmolol group (n=30): in this group IV infusion of Esmolol (0.5 mg/kg) was administered within four minutes prior to extubation continued by an IV infusion of Esmolol at the rate of 0.15 mg/kg/min for 10 minutes after extubation.

Control group (n=30): in this group IV infusion of normal saline (0.5 ml/kg) was administered within four minutes prior to extubation continued by an IV infusion of normal saline at the rate of 0.15 ml/kg/min for 10 minutes after extubation.

Medications were prepared and coded previously by a colleague so that the coworker performing the records was unaware of the contents of the syringes. All patients were given IV lidocaine (1.5 mg/kg) 90 seconds prior to extubation. Systolic and diastolic blood pressure, mean arterial pressure and HR were recorded before and after medication administration and extubation. Vital signs were recorded every five minutes at recovery phase until the patient was discharged from the recovery unit. Time required for performing eye opening to verbal commands, spontaneous eye opening and a recognition of the location and people at the recovery unit were recorded for both groups.

All studied data were analyzed using statistical software SPSS16. To evaluate the statistics, descriptive statistical approaches (frequency, percentage, mean and standard deviation) were used. To compare qualitative variables, chi-square statistical test and to compare quantitative variables in paired groups, independent t-test was used. The changes in quantitative findings throughout the study in groups were evaluated using repeated measure of ANOVA. $P < 0.05$ was considered significant in this study.

Results

Table 1 presents the demographic findings between two groups. As it can be seen, demographic findings are equal in two groups and no statistically significant difference is observed.

Esmolol group was associated with significantly lower levels of systolic blood pressure (SBP) compared with the control group at all studied stages after extubation (All $P<0.05$) (Table 2).

Table 1. Demographic findings between two groups

	Control group	Esmolol group	P value
Age (Year)	49±17	46±16	0.42
Sex (M/F)	9.21	15.15	0.14
Weight (Kg)	71±12	73±10	0.49
Operation duration (Minutes)	186±62	184±42	0.76
ASA (II/I)	16.14	15.15	0.39

The study of the changes in diastolic blood pressure (DBP) in both groups revealed a statistically significant difference after extubation and 10 minutes after extubation ($P< 0.05$) (Table 2).

A significant difference was observed comparing the changes in HR in both groups at all HR values after extubation ($P< 0.001$ in all cases) indicating the fact that esmolol is of unique characteristic of blunting cardiovascular responses caused by catecholamine release following extubation (Table 2).

The mean of recovery phase and extubation duration for both groups have been presented in Table 3. As surprisingly observed, no significant difference regarding extubation phase length or recovery phase exists between esmolol and control groups.

Discussion

Patients with hypertension and cardiovascular or cerebrovascular diseases and patients with increased ICP could accompany severe cardiac and or cerebral complications at extubation phase.[3,7] Therefore, managing hemodynamic responses such as HR and blood pressure while disconnecting from mechanical ventilation would be of great importance.

Numerous strategies have been introduced to prevent hemodynamic responses caused by emergence from anesthesia including extubation under deep anesthesia, administration of local anesthetics, vasodilators and short acting opioids.[8]

Administering vasodilators such as sodium nitropruside, nitroglycerine and hydralazine could be associated with complications like reflexive tachycardia and increase in the plasma rennin activity.[2]

Beta-adrenergic blockers are also frequently used to suppress adrenergic activity caused by extubation especially throughout neurosurgery operations.[9,10] In the present study, esmolol, a selective short-acting beta-blocker, was administered and its preventive characteristics against cardiovascular responses caused by extubation in the surgeries involving cerebral masses were evaluated. The results obtained from the present study revealed that esmolol could be administered to prevent hemodynamic instability caused by extubation. It has previously been proven that hyperdynamic cardiovascular status caused by sympathetic excitation followed by extubation could endure for 5 to 10 minutes.[1] Considering the fact that esmolol is of very short half-life, in addition to administration of a bolus does before extubation, we used IV infusion of esmolol within 10 minutes after extubation which was associated with desirable results. In the study of Unal et al., it was stated that esmolol had the characteristic of preventing hyperdynamic status which was in line with the findings of our study.[2]

Table 2. Changes in Vital signs [Systolic Blood Pressure (SBP), Diastolic Blood Pressure (DBP) and Heart Rate (HR)] between two groups at different stages (prior to extubation until 15 minutes post-extubation)

	Stage	Control group	Esmolol group	P value
SBP	Before extubation	115 ± 14	109±17	0.16
	After extubation (immediate)	137 ± 21	115±17	<0.001
	After extubation (5 minutes)	134 ± 21	116±16	0.001
	After extubation (10 minutes)	132 ± 24	112±17	0.001
	After extubation (15 minutes)	125± 17	113±17	0.01
DBP	Before extubation	71± 13	69 ± 13	0.53
	After extubation (immediate)	85± 15	76 ± 14	0.02
	After extubation (5 minutes)	85 ± 18	77 ± 13	0.06
	After extubation (10 minutes)	84± 23	72± 14	0.01
	After extubation (15 minutes)	76± 12	74 ± 13	0.58
HR	Before extubation	77±12	73±13	0.28
	After extubation (immediate)	91±12	75±12	<0.001
	After extubation (5 minutes)	89±15	73±10	<0.001
	After extubation (10 minutes)	83±12	73±11	0.001
	After extubation (15 minutes)	81±10	71±9	<0.001

Table 3. The mean of extubation and recovery phase length (tested using three different criteria) between two groups (minutes)

	Control group	Esmolol group	P value
Extubation	4±1	4±1	0.16
Eye opening with verbal commands	12±3	11±3	0.93
Spontaneous eye opening	16±4	15±4	0.50
Orientation	21±6	20±6	0.73

Similar to our study, in the study of Dyson et al., hemodynamic changes were also less in esmolol group compared with the control group.[11] Wang et al. reported that esmolol, especially in higher doses, can reduce BP and HR increase followed by extubation which is in accordance with the results obtained from our study especially the post-extubation stage of their study.[12]

An appropriate anesthetic for neurosurgery should provide the possibility of early evaluation of the neurologic status of the patients and early diagnosis of the potential postoperative complications (for instance; hematoma and major cerebral edema) by a rapid and short recovery phase.[13] In the present study, there was no significant difference between studied groups regarding the time of eye opening (to verbal commands and spontaneous) and the recovery phase length. However in the study of Unal et al., the time of eye opening (to verbal commands and spontaneous) was recorded to be shorter in esmolol group compared with the control group.[2]

Conclusion

Sympathetic excitation followed by extubation would lead to increase in blood pressure and heart rate and therefore the patients at risk of cardiovascular and cerebral complications should be prevented from these excitations. Esmolol could safely be used in preventing hyperdynamic status throughout extubation phase without extending recovery phase length. Based on the results obtained from the present study, it could be advised to administer esmolol as one of the effective medication in cases in which control of hemodynamic status is required in high-risk patients undergoing intracranial surgeries. However, further studies with larger sample sizes to achieve more accurate results are required.

Conflict of interest

The authors report no conflicts of interest in this work.

References

1. Miller KA, Harkin CP, Bailey PL. Postoperative tracheal extubation. Anesth Analg 1995; 80: 149-72.
2. Unal Y, Ozsoylar O, Sariguney D, Arsalan M, Yardim RS. The efficacy of esmolol to blunt the hemodynamic response to endotracheal extubation in lumbar disc surgery. Res J Med Sci 2008;2: 99-104.
3. Bilotta F, Lam AM, Doronzio A, Cuzzone V, Delfini R, Rosa G. Esmolol blunts postoperative hemodynamic changes after propofol-remifentanil total intravenous fast-track neuroanesthesia for intracranial surgery. J Clin Anesth 2008;20: 426-30.
4. Agamohamdi D, Hosseinzadeh H, Golzari S, Alizadeh A, Peirovyfar A, Movassaghi R. Preincisional ipsilateral stellate ganglion block for acute post operative pain control in unilateral mastectomy. Pak J Med Sci 2011;27(4): 879-83.
5. Abdellatif AA, Ali MA. Comparison of streamlined liner of the pharynx airway (SLIPA™) with the laryngeal mask airway Proseal™ for lower abdominal laparoscopic surgeries in paralyzed, anesthetized patients. Saudi J Anaesth 2011;5: 270-6.
6. Tripathi M, Kaushik S, Dubey P. The effect of use of pyridostigmine and requirement of vecuronium in patients with myasthenia gravis. J Postgrad Med 2003;49: 311-4.
7. Guy J, Hindman BJ, Baker KZ, Borel CO, Maktabi B, Ostapkovich N, et al. Comparison of remifentanil and fentanyl in patients undergoing craniotomy for supratentorial space-occupying lesions. Anesthesiology 1997;86: 514-24.
8. Hohlrieder M, Tiefenthaler W, Klaus H, Gabl M, Kavakebi P, Keller C, et al. Effect of total intravenous anaesthesia and balanced anaesthesia on the frequency of coughing during emergence from the anaesthesia. Br J Anaesth 2007;99: 587-91.
9. O'Dwyer JP, Yorukoglu D, Harris MN. The use of esmolol to attenuate the haemodynamic response when extubating patients following cardiac surgery--a double-blind controlled study. Eur Heart J 1993;14: 701-4.
10. Blake DW. Dexmedetomidine and hemodynamic responses to simulated hemorrhage in experimental heart failure. Anesth Analg 2000;91: 1112-7.
11. Dyson A, Isaac PA, Pennant JH, Giesecke AH, Lipton JM. Esmolol attenuates cardiovascular responses to extubation. Anesth Analg 1990;71: 675-8.
12. Wang YQ, Guo QL, Xie D. Effects of different doses of esmolol on cardiovascular responses to tracheal extubation. Hunan Yi Ke Da Xue Xue Bao 2003;28: 259-62.
13. Palmer JD, Sparrow OC, Iannotti F. Postoperative hematoma: a 5-year survey and identification of avoidable risk Factors. Neurosurgery 1994;35: 1061-4.

Development of a Dispersive Liquid–Liquid Microextraction Technique for the Extraction and Spectrofluorimetric Determination of Fluoxetine in Pharmaceutical Formulations and Human Urine

Ahad Bavili Tabrizi [1]*, **Ahmad Rezazadeh** [2]

[1] *Department of Medicinal Chemistry, Faculty of Pharmacy and Biotechnology Research Center, Tabriz University of Medical Sciences, Tabriz, Iran.*

[2] *Student Research Committee, Tabriz University of Medical Sciences, Tabriz, Iran.*

ARTICLE INFO

Keywords:
Dispersive liquid-liquid-microextraction
Fluoxetine
Injectable formulation
Spectrofluorimetry
Urine

ABSTRACT

Purpose: Fluoxetine is the most prescribed antidepressant drug worldwide. In this work, a new dispersive liquid–liquid microextraction (DLLME) method combined with spectrofluorimetry has been developed for the extraction and determination of FLX in pharmaceutical formulations and human urine. ***Methods:*** For FLX determination, the pH of a 10 mL of sample solution containing FLX, was adjusted to 11.0. Then, 800 μL of ethanol containing 100 μL of chloroform was injected rapidly into the sample solution. A cloudy solution was formed and FLX extracted into the fine droplets of chloroform. After centrifugation, the extraction solvent was sedimented and supernatant aqueous phase was readily decanted. The remained organic phase was diluted with ethanol and its fluorescence was measured at 292±3 nm after excitation at 234±3 nm. ***Results:*** Some important parameters influencing microextraction efficiency were investigated. Under the optimum extraction conditions, a linear calibration curve in the range of 10 to 800 ng/mL with a correlation coefficient of r^2 = 0.9993 was obtained. Limit of detection (LOD) and limit of quantification (LOQ) were found to be 2.78 and 9.28 ng/mL, respectively. The relative standard deviations (RSDs) were less than 4%. Average recoveries for spiked samples were 93–104%. ***Conclusion:*** The proposed method gives a very rapid, simple, sensitive, wide dynamic range and low–cost procedure for the determination of FLX.

Introduction

Fluoxetine, (±)–N–methyl–Y–[4–(trifluoromethyl) phenoxy] benzene propanamine) (FLX), is a selective serotonin reuptake inhibitor in presynaptic neurons. It was introduced in 1980s, and since then, it is the most prescribed antidepressant drug worldwide. It is used to treat mental depression, obsessive–compulsive disorder, nervous bulimia, and premenstrual dysphoric disorder.[1,2]

Absolute bioavailability of oral FLX in dogs is about 72% of the intravenous dose. In humans, following a single oral dose of 40 mg, peak plasma concentrations of FLX were from 15 to 55 ng/mL and observed after 6 to 8 hours. FLX predominantly undergoes N–demethylation to norfluoxetine (NFLX), which has similar activity to FLX.[3] Both FLX and NFLX have long elimination half–lives, ranging from 1 to 6 days and from 5 to 6 days, respectively. About 11% of the dose is excreted as unchanged FLX and about 7% as NFLX. The therapeutic dose can vary from 20 to 60 mg per day depending on the treatment and the urine levels excreted are usually at mg/L levels.[3,4]

FLX has been determined in its pharmaceutical formulations by spectrophotometry,[5–9] spectrofluorimetry,[9–11] high performance liquid chromatography (HPLC),[8,12] gas chromatography (GC),[13] capillary electrophoresis (CE),[11,14] nuclear magnetic resonance spectrometry[15] and voltammetry.[16] The spectrophotometric methods are associated with some major drawbacks such as the lack of sensitivity, selectivity, tedious extraction procedures and time–

***Corresponding author:** Dr. Ahad Bavili Tabrizi (PhD), Department of Medicinal Chemistry, Faculty of Pharmacy & Biotechnology Research Center, Tabriz University of Medical Sciences, Tabriz, Iran. E–mail: a.bavili@tbzmed.ac.ir

consuming.[5-7] Other methods were time consuming, tedious and/or dedicated to sophisticated and expensive analytical instruments.[5,9]

On the other hand, several methods have been described for the determination of FLX in biological fluids. The most widely used methods involve HPLC with ultraviolet,[3,4,12,17] fluorescence,[18-20] mass spectrometry (MS)[20,21] or diode array detection.[22,23] FLX levels can also be measured in biological samples using GC,[24] GC–MS[25] and CE.[2] Liquid–liquid extraction (LLE),[3,4,18,20,21,25] solid phase extraction (SPE),[2,22,25] and solid phase microextraction (SPME)[23] are the most common sample preparation techniques to analyze FLX and NFLX in biological fluids. LLE is considered a tedious, time–consuming procedure, which can produce emulsions and requires large amounts of high purity organic solvents for analyte extraction. SPE techniques often introduce artifacts into the sample extracts and can require lengthy processing (i.e., washing, conditioning, eluting and drying).[19] Thus, there is a need for developing new and efficient methods to overcome these drawbacks.

Recently miniaturized techniques, such as DLLME has been developed for sample preparation.[26] It is based on a ternary component solvent system like homogeneous LLE and cloud point extraction (CPE). In this method, the appropriate mixture of extraction and disperser solvent is injected into aqueous sample rapidly by syringe, and a cloudy solution is formed. The analyte in the sample is extracted into the fine droplets of extraction solvent. After extraction, phase separation is performed by centrifugation and the enriched analyte in the sedimented phase is determined by proper instrumental method. The ease of the operation, speed, lower sample volume, low cost, high recovery and high enhancement factor are some advantages of DLLME.[27] With the development of DLLME, the principles and the applications of this new technique have been reviewed recently[28,29] and its application extended to separation, preconcentration and determination of organic[26,30-33] and inorganic[27,34-37] compounds in different samples. However, to the best of our knowledge, this is the first report concerning FLX extraction using the DLLME method and second one concerning liquid–phase microextraction techniques.

In this study, DLLME followed by spectrofluorimetry has been investigated and optimized for the extraction and determination of FLX in pharmaceutical formulations and human urine. The effects of various experimental parameters, such as the kind and volume of extraction and dispersive solvent, extraction time, sample solution pH, salt effect, sample volume, centrifugation time and speed were studied and optimized systematically. Using the developed method FLX can be analyzed in pharmaceutical formulations and human urine in a simpler, cheaper and more rapid manner.

Materials and Methods

Apparatus

All fluorescence measurements were made using a Shimadzu RF–5301 PC spectrofluorophotometer equipped with a 150 W Xenon lamp and quartz micro–cell with a path length of 10 mm and a volume of 700 µL. Instrument excitation and emission slits both were adjusted to 5 nm. A centrifuge from Hettich (EBA 20 model/ Andreas Hettich GmbH & Co. KG, Föhrenstr. 12, D–78532 Tuttlingen, Germany) with 15 mL calibrated centrifuge tubes (Hirschmann, EM techcolor, Germany) was used to accelerate the phase separation process. The pH–meter model M120 (Halstead, Essex, England CO9 2DX) supplied with a glass combined electrode was used for the pH measurements.

Reagents

All solvents containing chloroform, dichloromethane, carbon tetrachloride, acetone, acetonitrile, ethanol and methanol were obtained from Merck (Darmstadt, Germany).

A stock solution of 1000 µg/mL of FLX was prepared by dissolving appropriate amount of FLX hydrochloride (obtained from Dr. Abidi Pharm. Co., Tehran, Iran) in ultrapure water and stored away from the light at 4°C. This solution was stable for at least 2 weeks. Working standard solutions were prepared daily by appropriate dilution of this stock standard solution.

The ammonia buffer (1.0 mol/L, pH 11.0) was prepared from ammonium chloride (Merck) and ammonia (Merck). All chemicals used were of analytical–reagent grade or higher. Ultrapure water (Milli–Q Advantage A 10 system, Millipore) was used throughout the work.

Recommended procedures

Procedure for DLLME

The pH of a 10 mL of sample solution, containing FLX in the range 10–800 ng/mL, was adjusted to 11.0 with 1.0 mol/L ammonia buffer and the solution was placed in a 10 mL glass test tube with conical bottom. Then, 800 µL of ethanol (as disperser solvent) containing 100 µL of chloroform (as extraction solvent) was injected rapidly into the sample solution by using a 2.00–mL syringe. A cloudy solution (water, ethanol, and chloroform) was formed in the test tube. In this step, the FLX was extracted into the very fine droplets of chloroform in a few seconds. After centrifugation for 5 min at 3500 rpm, the extraction solvent was sedimented in the bottom of the conical test tube. The supernatant aqueous phase was readily decanted with a Pasteur pipette. The remained organic phase was diluted to 1 mL with ethanol and its fluorescence was measured at 292±3 nm with the excitation wavelength set at 234 ± 3 nm.

Procedure for pharmaceutical formulation

Capsule: Contents of twenty capsules (Dr. Abidi. Pharm. Co., Tehran, Iran), each containing 10 mg FLX hydrochloride, were accurately weighed individually and finely powdered. Powdered sample containing 10 mg FLX was weighed, dissolved in 50–mL ultrapure water and vigorously shaken on a vortex mixer for 30 sec. The solution was then filtered and transferred into a 100–mL volumetric flask. The residue was washed in enough ultrapure water and the solution was finally made up to the mark with water. Thus, a 100 μg/mL solution of FLX was obtained.

Syrup: 2.5 mL of syrup containing 20 mg FLX/5mL was transferred into a 100–mL volumetric flask and made up to the mark with ultrapure water. Thus, a 100 μg/mL solution of FLX was obtained. There isn't any need for filtration. These solutions were diluted quantitatively to yield concentrations in the range of working standard solution and then the FLX content was analyzed by the procedure proposed above.

Procedure for urine sample

Urine samples were obtained from healthy male volunteer who took single oral dose of 20 mg FLX capsule. The samples were collected between 0–48 h, after administration and frozen at –20 °C until analysis. The frozen urine samples were thawed at room temperature, centrifuged for 10 min at 4000 rpm and then the 0.2 mL of the supernatant solutions were subjected to the above mentioned procedure.

Results and Discussion

In this work, DLLME combined with spectrofluorimetry was developed and optimized for the extraction and determination of FLX in pharmaceutical formulations and urine samples. To obtain high extraction efficiency, the influence of different factors affecting extraction conditions, such as kind of extraction and disperser solvents and their volumes, pH of sample solution, salt effect, sample volume, extraction time, centrifugation time and speed were studied and optimized. Figures 1 and 2 show excitation and emission spectra of FLX extracted from pharmaceutical formulation and urine sample by DLLME, respectively, using the optimized conditions established for this analysis. The excitation and emission maxima were positioned at 234 ± 3 and 292 ± 3 nm, respectively.

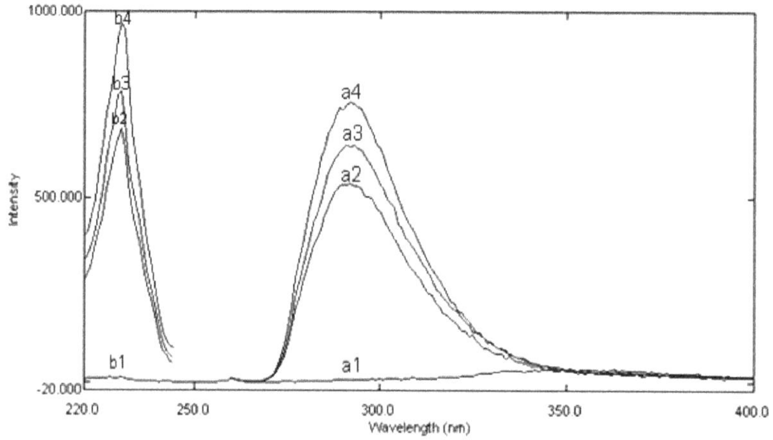

Figure 1. Excitation (b) and emission spectra (a) after DLLME: a1 & b1: reagent's blank; a2 & b2: FLX solution prepared from pharmaceutical formulation (500 ng/mL); a3 & b3: sample '2' spiked with FLX (100 ng/mL); a4 & b4: standard solution of FLX (750 ng/mL). Other conditions have been mentioned in the text.

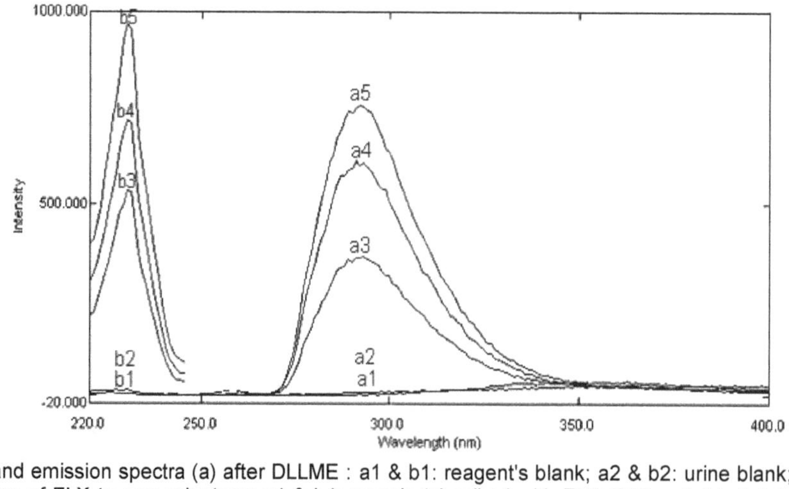

Figure 2. Excitation (b) and emission spectra (a) after DLLME : a1 & b1: reagent's blank; a2 & b2: urine blank; a3 & b3: collected urine sample after administration of FLX to one volunteer; a4 & b4: sample 'c' spiked with FLX (250 ng/mL); (a5 & b5) standard solution of FLX (750 ng/mL). Other conditions have been mentioned in the text.

Effect of pH

Obviously, pH was the key parameter for sample solution, affecting the states of analytes and the extraction efficiency. The effect of sample pH was tested in the pH range from 1 and 13. As shown in Figure 3, the signal intensity of FLX improved with the increasing of pH from 1.0 to 10.0, and then remained approximately constant in pH from 10.0–13.0. According to the literature,[19] the pK_a value of FLX is 10.05. Hence, when the pH of the aqueous sample was higher than the pK_a value of the FLX, the analyte is neutral form in aqueous solution which has a greater tendency to be extracted into the extraction solvent. Accordingly, the pH of samples was adjusted at 11.0 with 1.0 mol/L ammonia buffer.

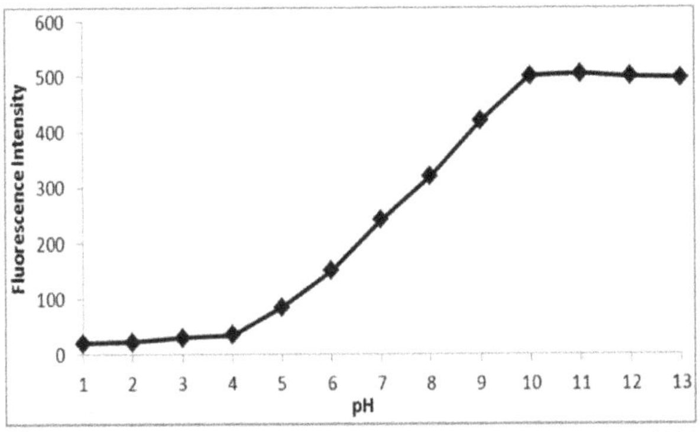

Figure 3. Effect of pH on the analytical responses; FLX (500 ng/mL), extraction with 800 µL of ethanol containing 100 µL of chloroform.

Effect of the extraction and disperser solvent type

Recovery of analytes in DLLME depends on several factors. Among these factors the main role can be ascribed to the proper choice of the pair of two solvents: the extraction one and the disperser one. Both these solvents have to meet several requirements. The extraction solvent should be denser than water. Moreover it should demonstrate low solubility in water and potential for extracting analytes. Thus, chloroform, dichloromethane and carbon tetrachloride were studied as extraction solvents. The disperser solvent has to be miscible with both the water sample and the extraction solvent. It also has to enable formation of dispersion of the extracting solvent in the water sample. Among different disperser solvents used in DLLME, methanol, ethanol, acetonitrile and acetone were studied.

In this study, all combinations of dichloromethane, chloroform and carbon tetrachloride as extraction solvents (60 µL) and methanol, ethanol, acetonitrile and acetone as dispersive solvents (500 µL) were tested and the results are shown in Figure 4. In the case of dichloromethane as extraction solvent, a two–phase system was not observed with any studied disperser solvents. This is probably due to that the density of dichloromethane is smaller than those of chloroform and carbon tetrachloride, and the miscibility of dichloromethane in the organic solvents are higher than those of chloroform and carbon tetrachloride. Thus it is not easy that dichloromethane deposited in the bottom of the test tube after spraying. The results revealed that with carbon tetrachloride and chloroform, a two–phase system was formed with all four dispersive solvents, but in the case of chloroform with ethanol more stable two–phase systems and higher signals were observed. It is probably due to higher solubility of FLX in chloroform in comparison with carbon tetrachloride. Thus chloroform and ethanol was selected as extraction and disperser solvents, respectively, in subsequent experiments.

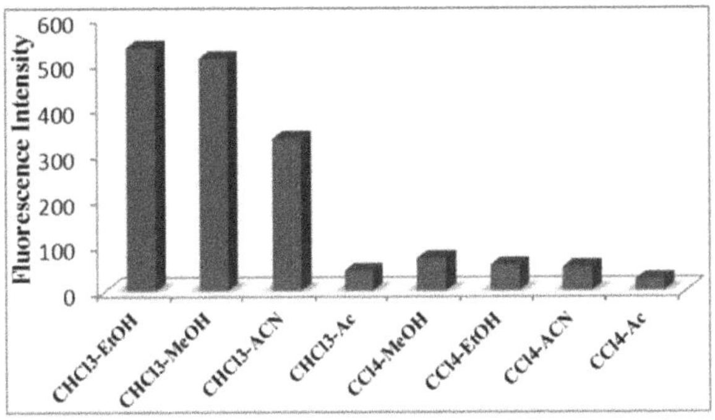

Figure 4. Effect of the type of extraction and disperser solvent on the analytical responses, EtOH: ethanol, MeOH: methanol, Ac: acetone, ACN: Acetonitrile, FLX (500 ng/mL); other conditions: 0.5 mL of 1.0 mol/L ammonia buffer; extraction with 800 µL of disperser solvent containing 100 µL of extraction solvent.

Effect of the extraction and disperser solvent volume

The effect of the volume of the extraction solvent on the analytical signals was investigated. Experiments were performed with different volumes of chloroform (in the range of 10–100 µL) as the extraction solvent by fixing the volume of the ethanol at 500 µL. Figure 5 indicates that the fluorescence intensity increased by increasing the volume of the chloroform to 80 µL and then remained approximately constant by further increasing of its volume to 100 µL. At higher volumes of extraction solvent, the ratio between the dispersive and extraction solvent decreased which probably lowered the number of formed droplets and thereby decreased the efficiency of extraction. Based on these observations, a volume of 100 µL was used for further experiments.

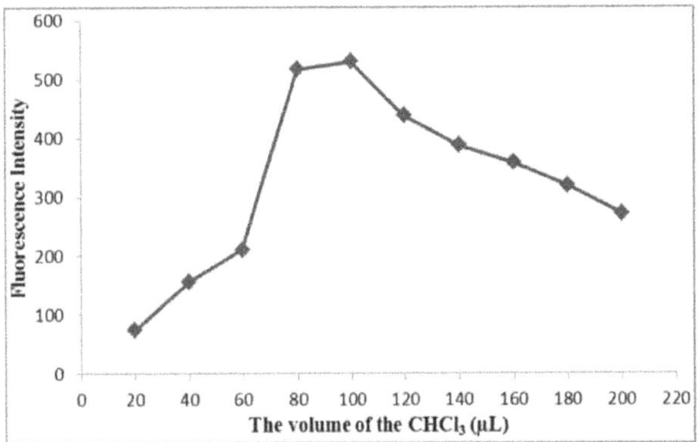

Figure 5. Effect of the extraction solvent volume on the analytical signals; other conditions have been mentioned in Figure 4.

In order to examine the effect of the disperser solvent volume, solutions containing different volumes of ethanol (in the range of 400–1800 μL) containing 100 μL of chloroform were subjected to the same DLLME procedure. As shown in Figure 6, analytical responses reached to its maximum value at 800 μL of the ethanol. At lower volumes of the disperser, tiny droplet formation may not be effective thereby lowering the extraction efficiency. At higher volumes of the dispersive solvent, the solubility of FLX in aqueous solution increases, thus lowering the partition of FLX into chloroform leading to a decrease in efficiency. Thus this volume was used in other experiments.

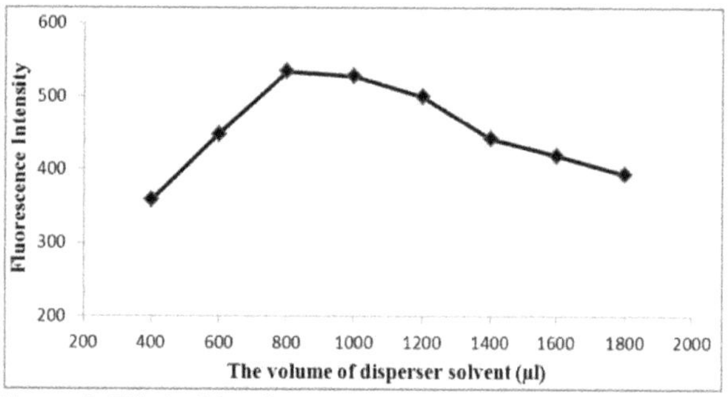

Figure 6. Effect of the disperser solvent volume on the analytical signals; other conditions have been mentioned in Figure 4.

Effect of salt addition

The effect of salt in this experiment was performed by adding different amounts of NaCl, from 0% to 20% (w/v), and other experimental conditions were kept constant. With the increase of the ionic strength, the signals were constant at first but decreased gradually by further increase of the salt concentration. Therefore, no addition of salt was employed in all subsequent experiments.

Effect of sample volume

For this purpose 2.5, 5.0, 7.5 , 10.0 and 12.5 mL aqueous solutions (containing 500 ng/mL of FLX) were selected as sample size and the DLLME procedure using ethanol as disperser solvent and chloroform as extraction solvent (200, 400, 600, 800 and 1000 μL, respectively) was performed. Results showed that by increasing sample volume up to 10 mL, the fluorescence intensity increased. This is evident from the fact that by holding sample volume/dispersive solvent volume ratio at a constant value (12.5:1), the volume of sedimented phase also remains almost constant. Therefore, by increasing sample volume and performing DLLME the concentration of analyte in the sedimented phase and consequently, the enhancement factor (EF) are also increased.

Effect of extraction time

In DLLME, extraction time is defined as interval time between injecting the mixture of disperser solvent and extraction solvent, and before starting to centrifuge. The effect of extraction time was examined in the range 0.25–20 min with constant experimental conditions. Results (not shown) revealed that the extraction time had no effect on the response of the target analyte. This could be explained by the fact that the surface area between the extraction solvent and the aqueous donor phase in DLLME is extremely large, thus the transfer of the target analyte from the aqueous phase to the extraction solvent phase is fast, achieving the equilibrium state quickly. This is the most important advantage of DLLME technique. In this method, the most time–consuming step is the centrifuging of sample solution in the extraction procedure, which is about 5 min.

Effect of other parameters

The effect of centrifugation time and speed, and the type of final diluent solvent on the analytical responses were also investigated. Based on the obtained results, 5 min, 3500 rpm and ethanol were selected as optimum centrifugation time and speed and final diluent solvent, respectively.

Validation of the method

Under the optimum experimental conditions, calibration graphs were obtained by DLLME of 10.0 mL of standard solutions containing known amount of the FLX and under the experimental conditions specified in the procedure. The calibration curve for the detection of FLX was linear over the concentration range of 10 to 800 ng/mL. The corresponding fitted equation was FI = 1.2281C–3.8067 with r^2 = 0.9993, where FI is the fluorescence intensity and C is the FLX concentration in ng/mL. The LOD and the LOQ were determined by using the criterions LOD = $3S_b/m$ and LOQ = $10S_b/m$, and found to be 2.78 and 9.28 ng/mL, respectively, where S_b is the standard deviation of the blank measurements and m is the calibration slope. These values are below the usual urinary levels in patients under daily treatment.[23] The RSD obtained for the repetitive determinations of 60, 300 and 600 ng/mL of FLX were less than 3.0% (n = 6). The inter–day repeatability was determined by analyzing five replicates of 500 ng/mL of FLX and found to be 4.02%. A comparison of the main analytical characteristics of the proposed method with those of some of the best previously reported methods are showed in Table 1. As can be seen, proposed method provides a wider dynamic range and a lower LOD, and other analytical characteristics are comparable with reported techniques.

The application of the method

The method accuracy

To investigate the accuracy of the proposed method, the solutions prepared from FLX formulations as well as drug–free urine samples were spiked at three concentration levels of 200, 400 and 600 ng/mL and extracted under the optimized conditions. Each treatment was in triplicate and the results are shown in Table 2. The recoveries for the commercial formulations and urine samples were in the range 96–104 and 93–97%, respectively.

Table 1. Analytical characteristics of reported methods (including extraction techniques) for FLX determination

Ex. & determination Method	Sample	Concentration range (μg/mL) (×10²)	Slope	r	RSD%	LOD (ng/mL)	Mean recovery (%)	Ref.
MNPs–SPE/ fluorimetry	B.S	0.500–10.0	–	0.9983	1.40	20.0	80.0–104	1
SPE–CE	B.S	0.100–20.0	6.55	0.9983	<3.10	10.0	89.0–99.0	2
LLE–HPLC	B.S	0.500–5.00	2.25	0.9992	6.20–14.1	30.0	99.8–110	4
LLE–Spectrophotometry	P.F	70.0–1000	0.020	0.9986	1.76	–	–	7
Spectrophotometry & Spectrofluorimetry	P.F ≈	3.00–60.0 0.350–5.00	0.135 0.579	0.9997 0.9992	1.52 3.37	1.00×10^2 10.0	98.0–102 97.5–100	9 ≈
Spectrofluorimetry	P.F,B.S	0.400–10.0	0.776	0.9994	<1.00	9.60	98.0–104	10
CZE	P.F	5.00–50.0	0.169	0.9998	1.50–2.20	1.00×10^2	99.3–102	11
HPLC	P.F	0.100–1.20	0.006	0.9986	<0.800	3.00	98.0	12
LPMEx.–HPLC	B.S	0.050–5.00	0.004	0.9999	5.40	LOQ=5.00	70.9	19
SPME–HPLC	B.S	0.500–20.0	31.1	0.9990	<9.00	10.0	90.0–110	23
SPE &LLE /GC–MS	B.S	0.050–75.0 & 0.100–0.800	0.920	–	<5.00	1.00 &10.0	91.0–103	25
DLLME–Spectrofluorimetry	P.F,B.S	0.100–8.00	0.228	0.9996	<3.00	2.78	93.0–104	This work

CZE= Capillary zone electrophoresis; MEKC= Micellar electrokinetic capillary chromatography; Ex.=extraction; MNPs–SPE= Magnetic nanoparticles SPE; LPMEx.=Liquid phase microextraction; P.F= Pharmaceutical formulation; B.S= Biological sample.

Table 2. Results of recoveries of spiked samples

Sample	FLX added (ng/mL)	†FLX found (ng/mL)	Recovery (%)
Capsule	200	194 ± 5.28	97
	400	384 ± 9.93	96
	600	594 ± 11.8	99
Syrup	200	204 ± 4.36	102
	400	416 ± 8.62	104
	600	588 ± 12.3	98
Human urine*	200	186 ± 3.86	93
	400	384 ± 7.32	96
	600	582 ± 9.86	97

* A 0.2 mL portion of urine sample was used for recovery experiments.
† Average of three determinations ± standard deviation.

Typical extraction and emission spectra from standard solution of FLX, real solutions prepared from commercial formulations or collected urine from one volunteer after administration of FLX and the latters spiked with FLX are shown in Figures 1 and 2, respectively. As can be seen from these figures, no additional picks due to interferences were observed at the analytical emission wavelength. Thus the coincidence of emission spectra along with reasonable recoveries demonstrates that the commercial formulations and urine matrixes had little effect on DLLME efficiency.

On the other hand, a calibration curve using spiked urine sample was made. The comparison of the slopes of standard addition and routine calibration graphs showed that there was no significant difference between these two slopes and thus there were no significant matrix effect.[2,37] Thus, the determination of FLX in urine could be made by direct comparison with aqueous standard solution, at the same instrumental conditions.

Application to the commercial formulation

The proposed method was successfully applied to the analysis of FLX in its pharmaceutical dosage form (10 mg per capsule and 20 mg/5mL syrup) and the results are summarized in Table 3. A comparison using *t*–test at 95% confidence interval demonstrates that there isn't any significant difference between achieved and labeled amounts.[38]

Table 3. Determination of FLX in pharmaceutical formulations

Sample	*FLX etermined (mg)	†Calculated t value
20 mg capsule	9.62 ± 0.23	2.86
20 mg/5mL syrup	19.7 ± 0.61	0.852

* Average of three determinations ± standard deviation.
† The tabulated t values at p = 0.05 is 4.3.[38]

Application to the human urine

A unique pharmacokinetic study was performed during two days by analyzing urine samples of a volunteer receiving a single oral dose of 20 mg FLX capsule. Urine samples were collected for 0–48 h in 6 h intervals after administration and these collections were monitored for FLX. A 0.2 mL portion of treated samples, as section of "*Procedure for urine sample*", was used for FLX determination. The commutative FLX amount found using the proposed method at different interval times, are shown in Figure 7. The found concentrations were in the range of 51 to 106 ng/mL witch were in accordance with values reported in the literature.[2] On the other hand, it must be mentioned that the proposed method can probably determine the total excreted FLX, since according to the literature,[19,20] the FLX and its NFLX metabolite have same excitation and emission wavelengths.

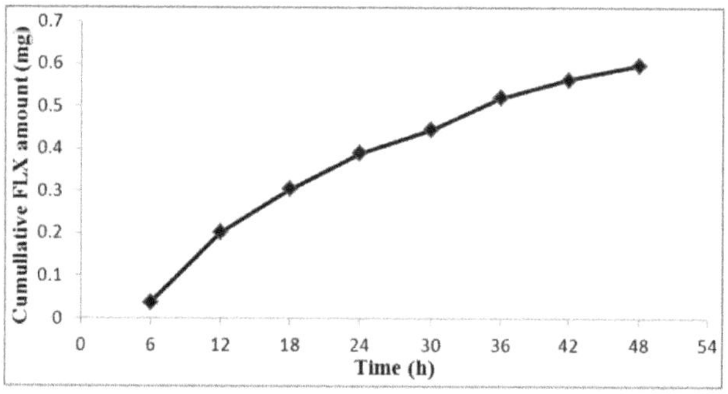

Figure 7. Time course of excreted FLX levels through urine.

Conclusion

A new DLLME method combined with spectrofluorimetry has been presented for the extraction and determination of FLX in pharmaceutical formulations and urine samples. In this method, sample preparation time as well as consumption of toxic organic solvents was minimized without affecting the sensitivity of the method. In addition, it is avoided the need of employing a high performance separation instrument for the treatment of urine samples. The proposed method gives a very rapid, simple, sensitive, wide dynamic range and low–cost procedure for the determination of FLX. The method can be further developed by combining DLLME with proper HPLC or GC method for the separation and determination of FLX and its major metabolite.

Acknowledgements

The author is grateful to the Research Office of Tabriz University of Medical Sciences for Financial support. This article was written based on a dataset of PharmD. thesis, registered in Tabriz University of Medical Sciences.

Conflict of Interest

There is no conflict of interest in this study.

References

1. Bagheri H, Zandi O, Aghakhani A. Extraction of fluoxetine from aquatic and urine samples using sodium dodecyl sulfate coated iron oxide magnetic nanoparticles followed by spectrofluorimetric determination. Anal Chim Acta 2011;716:61–5.
2. Rodriguez Flores J, Berzas Nevado JJ, Castaneda Penalvo G, Mora Diez N. Development and validation method for determination of fluoxetine and its main metabolite norfluoxetine by nonaqueous capillary electrophoresis in human urine. Talanta 2005;65:163-71.
3. Pan R–N, Chen T–H, Huang Christine SH, Hsiong CH. Pharmacokinetics and bioequivalent study of generic fluoxetine capsules preparation. J Food Drug Anal 2002;10:13-7.
4. Gao R, Higashi Y, Fujii Y. Simple determination of fluoxetine and norfluoxetine in human serum and urine by dabsylation followed by HPLC with visible light detection. J Liq Chromatogr R T 2010;33:1405-15.
5. Darwish IA. Development and validation of spectrophotometric methods for determination of fluoxetine, sertraline, and paroxetine in pharmaceutical dosage forms. J AOAC Int 2005;88:1-8.
6. Prabhakar AH, Patel VB, Giridha R. Spectrophotometric determination of fluoxetine hydrochloride in bulk and in pharmaceutical formulations. J Pharm Biomed Anal 1999;20:427-32.
7. Starczewska B, Puzanowska–Tarasiewicz H, Baranowska K. Investigation and analytical application of the reactions of eriochrome cyanine R with fluvoxamine and fluoxetine. J Pharm Biomed Anal 2000;23:477-81.
8. Raggi MA, Bugamelli F, Casamenti G, Mandrioli R, De Ronchi D, Volterra V. Analytical methods for the quality control of Prozac capsules. J Pharm Biomed Anal 1998;18:699-706.
9. Darwish IA, Amer SM, Abdine HH, Al–Rayes LI. New spectrophotometric and fluorimetric methods for determination of fluoxetine in pharmaceutical formulations. Int J Anal Chem 2009;2009:257306.
10. Berzas JJ, Alanon A, Lazaro JA. Cyclodextrin enhanced spectrofluorimetric determination of fluoxetine in pharmaceuticals and biological fluids. Talanta 2002;58:301-9.
11. Mandrioli R, Pucci V, Visini D, Varani G, Raggi M A. Rapid methods for determination of fluoxetine in pharmaceutical formulations. J Pharm Biomed Anal 2002;29:1127-34.
12. El–dawy MA, Mabrouk MM, El–Barbary FA. Liquid chromatographic determination of fluoxetine. J Pharm Biomed Anal 2002;30:561-71.
13. Berzas Nevado JJ, Villasenor Lerena MJ, Contento Salcedo AM, Aguas Nuevo E. Assay validation for three antidepressants in pharmaceutical formulations: Practical approach using capillary gas chromatography. J Pharm Biomed Anal 2005;38:52-9.
14. Berzas Nevado JJ, Contento Salcedo AM, Villasenor Llerena MJ, Aguas Nuevo E. Method development and validation for the simultaneous determination of fluoxetine and fluvoxamine in pharmaceutical preparations by capillary electrophoresis. Anal Chim Acta 2000;417:169–76.
15. Trefi S, Gilard V, Balayssac S, Malet–Martino M, Martino R. Quality assessment of fluoxetine and fluvoxamine pharmaceutical formulations purchased in different countries or via the Internet by 19F and

2D DOSY 1H NMR. J Pharm Biomed Anal 2008; 46:707-22.
16. Lencaster RP, Matos CD, Garrido J, Borges F, Garrido EM. Voltammetric quantification of fluoxetine: application to quality control and quality. J Food Drug Anal 2006;14:242–6.
17. Floriddia ML, Castorina M, Drago F. Comparative bioavailability of a new formulation of fluoxetine drops. Eur Rev Med Pharmacol Sci 2000;4:9-13.
18. Higashi Y, Gao R, Fujii Y. Determination of Fluoxetine and enantiomers in human serum and urine by isocratic HPLC and pre–column fluorescence drivatization with (R)–(+)–4–Nitro–7–(2–chloroformylpyrrolidin–1–yl)–2,1,3–benzoxadiazole. J Liq Chromatogr R T 2010;33:481-90.
19. De Freitas DF, Dobrovolskin Porto CE, Pizzamiglio Vieira E, Bastos de Siqueira MEP. Three–phase, liquid–phase microextraction combined with high performance liquid chromatography–fluorescence detection for the simultaneous determination of fluoxetine and norfluoxetine in human plasma. J Pharm Biomed Anal 2010;51:170-7.
20. Kovacevic I, Pokrajac M, Miljkovic B, Jovanovic D, Prostran M. Comparison of liquid chromatography with fluorescence detection to liquid chromatography–mass spectrometry for the determination of fluoxetine and norfluoxetine in human plasma. J Chromatogr B Analyt Technol Biomed Life Sci 2006;830:372-6.
21. Djordjevic S, Kovacevic I, Miljkovic B, Vuksanovic J, Pokrajac M. Liquid chromatographic–mass spectrometric method for the determination of fluoxetine and norfluoxetine in human plasma: application to clinical study. Il Farmaco 2005;60:345-9.
22. Sabbioni C, Bugamelli F, Varani G, Mercolini L, Musenga A, Saracino MA, et al. A rapid HPLC–DAD method for the analysis of fluoxetine and norfluoxetine in plasma from overdose patients. J Pharm Biomed Anal 2004;36:351-6.
23. Unceta N, Gomez–Caballero A, Sanchez A, Millan S. Simultaneous determination of citalopram, fluoxetine and their main metabolites in human urine samples by solid–phase microextraction coupled with high–performance liquid chromatography. J Pharm Biomed Anal 2008;46:763-70.
24. Fontanille P, Jourdil N, Villier C, Bessard G. Direct analysis of fluoxetine and norfluoxetine in plasma by gas chromatography with nitrogen–phosphorus detection. J Chromatogr B Analyt Technol Biomed Life Sci Appl 1997;692:337-43.
25. Acikkol M, Salkım D. GCMS analysis of fluoxetine and its active metabolite norfluoxetine in human urine. Marmara Pharm J 2010;14:98-103.
26. Rezaee M, Assadi Y, Milani Hosseini MR, Aghaee E, Ahmadi F, Berijani S. Determination of organic compounds in water using dispersive liquid–liquid microextraction. J Chromatogr A 2006;1116:1-9.
27. Tabrizi AB. Development of a dispersive liquid–liquid microextraction method for iron speciation and determination in different water samples. J Hazard Mater 2010;183:688-93.
28. Zgola–Grzeskowiak A, Grzeskowiak T. Dispersive liquid–liquid microextraction. Trac-Trend Anal Chem 2011;30:1382-99.
29. Nuhu AA, Basheer C, Saad B. Liquid–phase and dispersive liquid–liquid microextraction techniques with derivatization: Recent applications in bioanalysis. J Chromatogr B Analyt Technol Biomed Life Sci 2011;879:1180-8.
30. Mashayekhi HA, Abroomand–Azar P, Saber–Tehrani M, Husain SW. Rapid determination of carbamazepine in human urine, plasma samples and water using DLLME followed by RP–LC. Chromatographia 2010;71:517-21.
31. Moradi M, Yamini Y, Baheri T. Analysis of abuse drugs in urine using surfactant–assisted dispersive liquid–liquid microextraction. J Sep Sci 2011;34: 1722-9.
32. Saraji M, Hajialiakbari Bidgoli AA. Dispersive liquid–liquid microextraction using a surfactant as disperser agent. Anal Bioanal Chem 2010;397:3107-15.
33. Zeeb M, Ganjali MR, Norouzi P. Dispersive liquid–liquid microextraction followed by spectrofluorimetry as a simple and accurate technique for determination of thiamine (vitamin B_1). Microchim Acta 2010;168:317-24.
34. Yousefi SR, Shemirani F. Development of a robust ionic liquid–based dispersive liquid–liquid microextraction against high concentration of salt for preconcentration of trace metals in saline aqueous samples: application to the determination of Pb and Cd. Anal Chim Acta 2010;669:25-31.
35. Jafarvand S, Shemirani F. Supramolecular–based dispersive liquid–liquid microextraction: A novel sample preparation technique for determination of inorganic species. Microchim Acta 2011;173:353-9.
36. Abdolmohammad–Zadeh H, Sadeghi GH. Combination of ionic liquid–based dispersive liquid–liquid microextraction with stopped–flow spectrofluorometry for the preconcentration and determination of aluminum in natural waters, fruit juice and food samples. Talanta 2010;81:778-85.
37. Hashemi P, Hosseini SM, Kakanejadifard A. Dispersive liquid–liquid microextraction of Cu(II) using a novel dioxime for its highly sensitive determination by graphite furnace atomic absorption spectrometry. J Chin Chem Soc 2010;57:111-7.
38. Miller JC, Miller JN. Statistics for Analytical Chemistry. New York: Wiley;1984.

The Effect of Chronic Administration of Buspirone on 6-Hydroxydopamine-Induced Catalepsy in Rats

Hamdolah Sharifi[1], **Alireza Mohajjel Nayebi**[1,2]*, **Safar Farajnia**[1]

[1] *Drug Applied Research Center, Tabriz University of Medical Sceinces, Tabriz, Iran.*

[2] *Department of Pharmacology and Toxicology, Faculty of Pharmacy, Tabriz University of Medical Sceinces, Tabriz, Iran.*

ARTICLE INFO

Keywords:
Buspirone
Chronic
6-Hydroxydopamine
Catalepsy
Rat

ABSTRACT

Purpose: Several evidences show that serotonergic neurons play a role in the regulation of movements executed by the basal ganglia. Recently we have reported that single dose of buspirone improved 6-hydroxydopamine (6-OHDA) and haloperidol-induced catalepsy. This study is aimed to investigate effect of chronic intraperitoneal (i.p.) administration of buspirone on 6-OHDA-induced catalepsy in male Wistar rats. ***Methods:*** Catalepsy was induced by unilateral infusion of 6-OHDA (8 μg/2 μl/rat) into the central region of the SNc and was assayed by the bar-test method 5, 60, 120 and 180 min after drugs administration in 10th day. The effect of buspirone (0.5, 1 and 2 mg/kg, i.p. for 10 days) was assessed in 6-OHDA-lesioned rats. ***Results:*** The results showed that chronic injection of buspirone (0.5, 1 and 2 mg/kg, i.p. for 10 days) decreased catalepsy when compared with the control group. The best anticataleptic effect was observed at the dose of 1 mg/kg. The catalepsy-improving effect of buspirone was reversed by 1-(2-methoxyphenyl)- 4-[4-(2-phthalimido) butyl]piperazine hydrobromide (NAN-190), 0.5 mg/kg, i.p.,as a 5-HT_{1A} receptor antagonist. ***Conclusion:*** Our study indicates that chronic administration of buspirone improves catalepsy in a 6-OHDA-induced animal model of parkinson's disease (PD). We also suggest that buspirone may be used as an adjuvant therapy to increase effectiveness of antiparkinsonian drugs. In order to prove this hypothesis, further clinical studies should be done.

Introduction

PD is a neurodegenerative disease that leads to motor impairments such as tremor, rigidity, slowed body movements (bradykinesia), unstable posture and difficulty in walking .[1] This disease is characterized by the loss of dopamine (DA)-producing neurons in the ventral midbrain with cell bodies in the substantia nigra pars compacta (SNc) that project to the striatum .[2,3]
It's motor symptoms can be treated with dopaminergic drugs, however, their effectiveness diminishes as the severity of the clinical symptoms increases due to progression of the underlying neurodegeneration .[4]
It has been suggested that non-dopaminergic regions including the serotonergic neurons of dorsal raphe nucleus (DRN*)* are involved in pathology of PD .[5,6] 5-HT projections from the DRN innervate all components of the basal ganglia circuitry. The striatum and output regions of the basal ganglia (SNr and GPm) receive a dense serotonergic (5-HT) input.[5]
In addition to dopamine, 5-HT also modulates the actions of other neurotransmitters, including GABA and glutamate, as well as providing feedback mechanisms on 5-HT neurotransmission itself via an action in the DRN .[7,8] It is therefore plausible that serotonin plays a role in the regulation of movements executed by the basal ganglia .[2]
Among the subtypes of 5-HT receptors, 5-HT_{1A} receptors play a particularly significant role in the regulation of motor activity. For example, 5-HT_{1A} receptor agonists attenuate the catalepsy induced by raclopride and anti-psychotics such as haloperidol and risperidone.[9]For this reason, there has been a substantial attention on 5-HT_{1A} receptors and their involvement in motor control .[10] In an experiment by Gerber and colleagues it was found that 5-HT_{1A} receptor stimulation represented antiparkinsonian effects in 6-OHDA-lesioned rats (Gerber et al., 1988). We have shown previously that single dose of buspirone decreases haloperidol [11] and 6-hydroxydopamine-induced catalepsy .[2] This effect is most likely caused by the increase in 5-HT_{1A} receptor activation resulting in an inhibition of 5-HT release .[12]
Buspirone acts as 5-HT_{1A} receptor partial agonist and is used in chronic treatment of anxiety disorders .[13,14]
Since drugs may have completely different effects in

***Corresponding author:** Alireza Mohajjel Nayebi (PhD), Drug Applied Research Center, Tabriz University of Medical Sceinces, Tabriz, Iran.
E-mail: nayebia@tbzmed.ac.ir

acute and chronic use, thus in this study we tried to evaluate effect of chronic administration of buspirone on catalepsy induced by 6-OHDA. Furtheremore, the possible involvement of 5-HT_{1A} receptor in mediating of observed effects was investigated.

Materials and Methods

Chemicals

All chemicals were obtained from Sigma Chemical Co. (USA) except for buspirone, which was purchased from Heumann Co. (Germany). Solutions were prepared freshly on the day of experimentation. Buspirone, and 1-(2-methoxyphenyl)-4-[4-(2-phthalimido) butyl] piperazine hydrobromide (NAN-190) were dissolved in physiological saline (0.9% NaCl), and 6-OHDA was dissolved in 0.9% saline containing 0.2% (w/v) ascorbic acid. 6-OHDA was injected into the central region of the substantia nigra pars compacta (SNc) in a total volume of 8 µl /rat with a constant injection rate of 0.2 µl /min.

Animals

The experiments were carried out on male Wistar rats weighing 260-300 g. Animals were housed in standard polypropylene cages, four per cage, under a 12:12 h light/dark schedule at an ambient temperature of 25 ± 2°C and were allowed food and water ad libitum. Animals were acclimated to the testing conditions for 2 days before the behavioral experiment was conducted. All of the procedures were carried out under the ethical guidelines of the Tabriz University of Medical Sciences.

6-OHDA-induced SNc lesion

Animals were anesthetized with an *ip* injection of ketamine (50 mg/kg) and xylazine (5 mg/kg). After they were deeply anesthetized (loss of corneal and toe pad reflexes), rats were mounted in a stoelting stereotaxic frame in the flat skull position. The scalp was shaved, swabbed with povidone iodine 10% and a central incision made to expose the skull. 6-OHDA was injected thorough a guide cannula (23 gauge stainless steel) implanted in the SNc. The coordinates for this site were based on the rat brain atlas [30]: anteroposterior (AP): –5.0 mm from the bregma; mediolateral (ML): –2.1 mm from the midline and dorsoventral (DV): –7.7 from the skull.

Desipramine (25 mg/kg, *ip*) was injected 30 min before the intranigral injection of 6-OHDA to avoid the destruction of noradrenergic neurons. Then, 6-OHDA (8 µg/per rat in 2 µl saline with 0.2% ascorbic acid) was infused with an infusion pump at a constant flow rate of 0.2 µl/min into the left SNc. At the end of infusion, the injection tube was kept implanted for an additional 2 min and then was slowly retracted. Sham-operated animals were submitted to the same procedure but 2 µl vehicle (0.9% saline containing 0.2% (w/v) ascorbic acid) of 6-OHDA was infused into the SNc.

Catalepsy test

Catalepsy was measured by using a standard bar test. In this method, forepaws of rats were placed over a 9-cm-high standard wooden bar, and the duration of retention of rats in this imposed posture was considered as the bar test elapsed time. The end point of catalepsy was considered to occur when both front paws were removed from the bar or when the animal moved its head in an exploratory manner. The cut-off time of the test was 720 s. This test was carried out 5, 60, 120 and 180 min after drug administration. All observations were made between 9 a.m. and 4 p.m.

After a three-week recovery period, only the rats that were markedly immobilized in the bar test were subjected to further experimentation. Then, parkinsonian rats were divided randomly into equal groups and received once daily (9 a.m.) injections of buspirone, a 5-HT_{1A} receptor partial agonist (0.5,1 and2 mg/kg, *ip*) for 10 days. NAN-190, as a 5-HT_{1A} receptor antagonist, was injected (0.5 mg/kg, *ip*) concomitantly with the effective dose of buspirone.

Statistical analysis

Statistical analysis of each data set was calculated by use of SPSS software (version 16.0). Data were expressed as the mean+SEM, and were analyzed by one-way ANOVA in each experiment. In the case of significant variation ($p<0.05$), the values were compared by Tukey test.

Results

Catalepsy induced by 6-OHDA

Rats were divided into three groups: normal, sham operated (receiving 2 µl vehicle) and 6-OHDA (8 µg/2µl/rat)-injected rats. Drugs and vehicle were injected into the SNc through the implanted guide cannula. As shown in Figure 1, 6-OHDA was able to induce significant ($p < 0.05$ and 0.01) catalepsy in comparison with both normal and sham-operated rats (Figure 1).

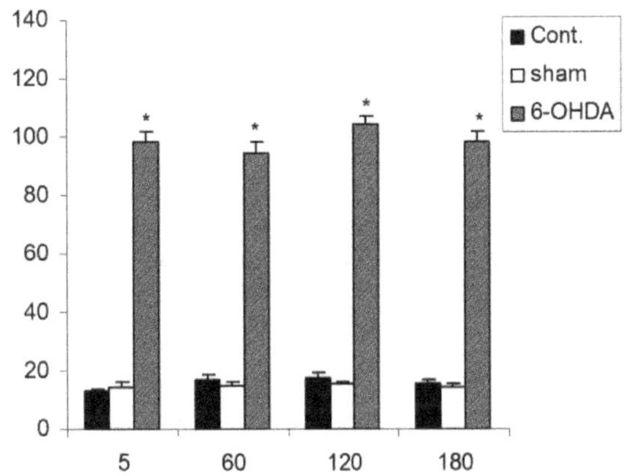

Figure 1. The bar test results of control, sham-operated and 6-OHDA (8 µg/2 µl/rat)- lesioned rats. Each bar represents the mean ± SEM of elapsed time (s); n = 8 rats for each group; * p <0.001 when compared with normal and sham-operated groups.(Cont.=control)

Effect of buspirone on 6-OHDA induced catalepsy

Four groups of 6-OHDA-lesioned rats received saline or one of three different doses of buspirone (0.5, 1 and 2mg/kg, *ip*), respectively for 10 days. The results indicated that buspirone attenuated the severity of 6-OHDA induced catalepsy ($p < 0.05$) (Figure 2).

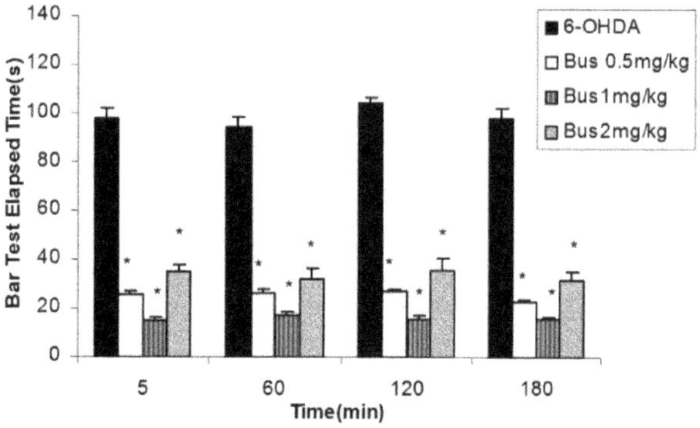

Figure 2. The bar test results of 6-OHDA (8 μg/2 μl/rat)-lesioned rats treated with Buspirone (0.5,1 and 2mg/kg,ip for 10 days). Each bar represents the mean ± SEM of catalepsy time (s); n = 8 rats for each group; * $p < 0.001$ when compared with 6-OHDA-lesioned rats. (Bus=Buspirone)

Effect of NAN-190 co-injection with buspirone on 6-OHDA-induced catalepsy

Three groups of 6-OHDA-lesioned animals respectively received saline, buspirone (1 mg/kg, *ip*) or buspirone (1 mg/kg, *ip*) with NAN-190 (0.5μmg/rat, ip). The results showed that the catalepsy-ameliorating effect of buspirone was abolished ($p < 0.05$) by NAN-190 (Figure 3).

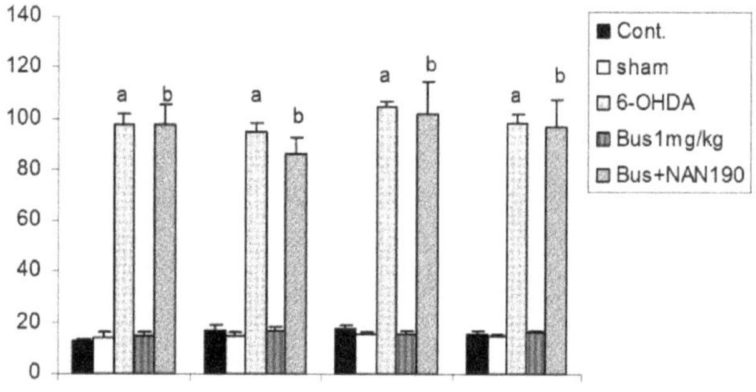

Figure 3. The bar test results from the co-administration of NAN-190 (0.5 mg/kg, ip) with buspirone (1mg/kg, ip for 10 days) in 6-OHDA-lesioned rats. Each bar represents the mean ± SEM of catalepsy time (s); n = 8 rats for each group,a, $p < 0.001$ when compared with 6-OHDA-lesioned rats; b, $p < 0.001$ when compared with 6-OHDA-lesioned rats co-treated with NAN-190(0.5mg/kg,ip) and buspirone (1 mg/kg,ip) .Cont.=control, Bus.=buspirone

Discussion

In our previous study the potential anticataleptic effects of $5\text{-}HT_{1A}$ agonists in 6-OHDA-lesioned rats were investigated in single dose administrations .[2] Since in clinic drugs are used chronically, therefore in this study we studied the potential anticataleptic effects of chronic administration of buspirone in 6-OHDA-lesioned rats. Our results showed intra-SNc injection of 6-OHDA induced catalepsy when assessed by the bar test. This is a standard test frequently used for evaluating catalepsy induced by 6-OHDA and neuroleptic drugs in rodents .[2,11,15] According to the results, buspirone, a partial agonist of $5\text{-}HT_{1A}$ receptors, improved catalepsy in 6-OHDA-lesioned rats. This confirms our previous study reporting a promising role for $5\text{-}HT_{1A}$ agonists in decreasing the motor disorders associated with PD.[2,11]

5-Hydroxytryptamine 1A ($5\text{-}HT_{1A}$) receptors are widely distributed throughout the basal ganglia. They are located on dorsal raphe neurons with efferents to the striatum and on cortical neurons that send glutamatergic projections to the basal ganglia .[12] Stimulation of $5\text{-}HT_{1A}$ receptors in these regions leads to dopamine release [16] via the inhibition of adenyl cyclase and the opening of potassium channels .[17] It seems that $5\text{-}HT_{1A}$ receptor agonists can reduce serotonin synthesis and release by activation of presynaptic, somatodendritic autoreceptors on raphe serotonergic cell bodies .[10] A potential role of $5\text{-}HT_{1A}$ agonists in the enhancement of motor activity was suggested because stimulation of somatodendritic $5\text{-}HT_{1A}$ receptors by a selective agonist such as 8-hydroxy-2-(di-n-propylamino) tetralin (8-OH-DPAT) inhibited synthesis of 5-HT to decrease its release from the nerve endings .[18]

The mechanism by which buspirone exerts an anticataleptic effect in 6-OHDA-lesioned rats was studied by using $5\text{-}HT_{1A}$ receptor antagonists. In addition to $5\text{-}HT_{1A}$ receptors, buspirone has D_2 and α_2-adrenoceptor blocking effects .[14,19] Thus, it seems that D_2 and α_2 receptors may be involved in the observed effects of buspirone. In this study the catalepsy-improving effect of buspirone was reversed by NAN-190, a $5\text{-}HT_{1A}$ receptor antagonist. This confirms the involvement of $5\text{-}HT_{1A}$ receptors in the observed effect of buspirone. According to the obtained results, we suggest that chronic administration of buspirone alleviates catalepsy in 6-OHDA-lesioned rats by acting on $5\text{-}HT_{1A}$ receptors in the SNc, and may it be used as a potential adjuvant drug together with routinely used antiparkinsonian drugs.

We investigated anticataleptic effect of different chronic doses of buspirone. The results showed that anticataleptic effect of buspirone at dose of 1 mg/kg was more than doses of 0.5 and 2. On the other hand, the anticataleptic effect of buspirone was attenuated by increasing the dose. Studies show that buspirone exerts dose-dependent opposite effects on the function of the nigrostriatal dopaminergic neurons so that at high doses, it acts as an antagonist on D_2 receptors .[13] Furthermore, the affinity of buspirone on $5\text{-}HT_{1A}$ receprots is higher than D_2 receptors .[20,21,22] Thus the possible involvement of D_2 receptors should not be neglected at it's high doses.

In conclusion our data suggest that chronic administration of buspirone improves catalepsy in 6-OHDA-lesioned rats. Inaddition we suggest that it may be used as an adjuvant therapy for improving effects of antiparkinson drugs. However, further clinical investigations should be carried out to prove it.

Acknowledgment
We wish to thank the Director of Drug Applied Research Center of the Tabriz University of Medical Sciences for supporting this study.

Conflict of Interest
There is no conflict of interest in this study.

References

1. Neha Singh, Viness Pillay, Yahya E. Choonara Advances in the treatment of Parkinson's disease. Progress in Neurobiology 2007; 81:29-44.
2. Alireza M. Nayebi, Siyamak R. Rad, Mehdi Saberian, Saeid Azimzadeh, Morteza Samini. Buspirone improves 6-hydroxydopamine-induced catalepsy through stimulation of nigral 5-HT1A receptors in rats. Pharmacological reports 2010; 62:258-264.
3. Malú G, Tansey Melissa K. McCoy, Tamy C, Frank-Cannon. Neuroinflammatory mechanisms in Parkinson's disease: Potential environmental triggers, pathways, and targets for early therapeutic intervention.Experimental Neurology 2007; 208:1-25.
4. Malú G, Tansey Matthew S. Goldberg .Neuroinflammation in Parkinson's disease: Its role in neuronal death and implications for therapeutic intervention. Neurobiology of Disease 2010; 37:510–518.
5. Susan H. Fox Rosalind Chuang , Jonathan M. Brotchie JM.Parkinson's disease – opportunities for novel therapeutics to reduce the problems of levodopa therapy. Progress in Brain Research 2008;172: 479-494.
6. Schapira AH, Bezard E, Brotchie J, Calon F, Collingridge GL, Ferger B, et al. Novel pharmacological targets for the treatment of Parkinson's disease. Nature reviews Drug discovery. 2006;5(10):845-54.
7. Di Matteo V, Pierucci M, Esposito E, Crescimanno G, Benigno A, Di Giovanni G.Serotonin modulation of the basal ganglia circuitry: therapeutic implication for Parkinson's disease and other motor disorders. Prog Brain Res 2008; 172:423-463.
8. Fox SH, Chuang R, Brotchie JM. Serotonin and Parkinson's disease: On movement, mood, and madness. Movement disorders : official journal of the Movement Disorder Society. 2009;24(9):1255-66.
9. Nobuaki Egashira, Tomomi Matsuda, Emi Koushi, Kenichi Mishima, Katsunori Iwasaki, Yukihiro Shoyama, Michihiro Fujiwara. Involvement of 5-hydroxytryptamine1A receptors in Δ9-tetrahydrocannabinol-induced catalepsy-like immobilization in mice. European Journal of Pharmacology 2006;550:117-122.
10. Laurence Mignon , William A Wolf. Postsynaptic 5-HT1A receptor stimulation increases motor activity in the 6-hydroxydopamine-lesioned rat: implications for treating Parkinson's disease. Psychopharmacology 2007; 192: 49-59.
11. Mohajjel Nayebi A, Sheidaei H. Buspirone improves haloperidol-induced Parkinson disease in mice through 5-HT1A receptors. DARU 2010; 18:41-45.
12. B Scholtissen, F R J Verhey, H W M Steinbusch, A F G Leentjens.Serotonergic mechanisms in Parkinson's disease: opposing results from preclinical and clinical data. J Neural Transm 2006;113: 59–73.
13. A G Dhavalshankh, S A Jadhav, R V Gaikwad, R K Gaonkar, V M Thorat, J J Balsara.Effects of buspirone on dopamine dependent behaviours in rats.Indian J Physiol Pharmacol 2007; 51 (4): 375–386.
14. S A Jadhav,R V Gaikwad, R K Gaonkar, V M Thorat, S C Gursale ,J J Balsara.Dose-Dependent response of central dopaminergic systems to buspirone in mice..Indian Journal of Experimental Biology 2008;46 :704-714.
15. Arturo Zazpe, Ine´s Artaiz, Ana Innera´rity, Elena del Olmo, Elena Castro, Luis Labeaga, Angel Pazos, Aurelio Orjales. In vitro and in vivo characterization of F-97013-GD, a partial 5-HT1A agonist with antipsychotic- and antiparkinsonian-like properties. Neuropharmacology 2006;51: 129-140.
16. Ichikawa J, Meltzer HY. R(+)-8-OH-DPAT, a serotonin 1A receptor agonist, potentiated S(–)-sulpirideinduced dopamine release in rat medial prefrontal cortex and nucleus accumbens but not striatum. J Pharmacol Exp Ther1999; 291:1227–1232.
17. Harrington MA, Oksenberg D, Peroutka SJ. 5-Hydroxytryptamine 1Areceptors are linked to a Gi-adenylate cyclase complex in rat hippocampus. Eur. J Pharmacol 1988; 154:95–98.
18. Darakhshan Jabeen Haleema, Erum Shireena, M.A. Haleem. Somatodendritic and postsynaptic serotonin-1A receptors in the attenuation of haloperidol-induced catalepsy. Progress in Neuro-Psychopharmacology & Biological Psychiatry 2004;28:1323-1329.
19. Gower AJ, Tricklebank MD. Alpha 2-adrenoceptor antagonist activity may account for the effects of buspirone in an anticonfilict test in the rat. Eur J Pharmacol 1988; 155:129–137.
20. Kazuo Matsubaraa, , Keiko Shimizub, Manabu Sunoa, Kento Ogawab, Toshio Awayaa, Takehiro Yamadaa, Toshihiro Nodaa, Machiko Satomia, Ko-ichi Ohtakia, Kaoru Chibaa, Yoshikazu Tasakia, Hiroshi Shionob. Tandospirone, a 5-HT1A agonist, ameliorates movement disorder via non-dopaminergic systems in rats with unilateral 6-

hydroxydopamine-generated lesions. Brain Research 2006; 1112:126-133.

21. Kristin B Dupre, Karen L Eskow, Christopher J Barnum, Christopher Bishop.Striatal 5-HT1A receptor stimulation reduces D1 receptor-induced dyskinesia and improves movement in the hemiparkinsonian rat. Neuropharmacology 2008; 55: 1321–1328.

22. Kristin B. Dupre Karen L Eskow, Giselle Negron, Christopher Bishop. The differential effects of 5-HT1A receptor stimulation on dopamine receptor-mediated abnormal involuntary movements and rotations in the primed hemiparkinsonian rat. Brain Research. 2007; 1158:135-143.

31

Antimicrobial and Cytotoxic Activity of Three Bitter Plants-*Enhydra fluctuans, Andrographis Peniculata* and *Clerodendrum Viscosum.*

M. Ruhul Amin, Ripon Mondol, M. Rowshanul Habib, M. Tofazzal Hossain*

Department of Biochemistry and Molecular Biology, Rajshahi University, Rajshahi-6205, Bangladesh.

ARTICLE INFO

Keywords:
Antimicrobial
Cytotoxic
Enhydra fluctuans
Clerodendrum viscosum
Andrographi speniculata

ABSTRACT

Purpose: In this study, three important medicinal plants (*Enhydra fluctuans* Lour, *Clerodendrum viscosum* Vent and *Andrographis peniculata* Wall) of Bangladesh were investigated to analyze their antimicrobial and cytotoxic activities against some pathogenic microorganisms and *Artemia salina* (brine shrimp nauplii). ***Methods:*** The coarse powder material of leaves of each plant was extracted separately with methanol and acetone to yield methanol extracts of leaves of *Enhydra fluctuans* (MLE), *Clerodendrum viscosum* (MLC) and *Andrographis peniculata* (MLA), and acetone extracts of leaves of *Enhydra fluctuans* (ALE), *Clerodendrum viscosum* (ALC) and *Andrographis peniculata* (ALA). The disc diffusion method and the method described by Meyer were used to determine the antimicrobial and cytotoxic activities of each plant extract. ***Results:*** Among the test samples, MLE and ALE showed comparatively better antimicrobial activity against a number of bacteria and fungi with inhibition zones in the range of 06-15 mm and according to the intensity of activity, the efficacy against microorganisms were found in the order of *Enhydra fluctuans*> *Andrographi speniculata*> *Clerodendrum viscosum.* In cytotoxicity assay, all samples were found to be active against brine shrimp nauplii (*Artemia salina*) and ALA produced lowest LC_{50} value (7.03 μg/ml). ***Conclusion:*** *Enhydra fluctuans* and *Andrographi speniculata* possesses significant antimicrobial and cytotoxic activities.

Introduction

Bacterial infection is one of the serious global health issues in 21st century.[1] There are several reports of antibiotic resistance of human pathogens to available antibiotics.[2,3] The multiple drug resistance and associated adverse effects of antibiotics on the host including hypersensitivity, immune suppression and allergic reaction are growing and because of this outlook the use of antimicrobial drugs in the future is still uncertain.[4] So there is a need of an alternative source for new antibiotics in the drug development pipeline. Natural products, either as pure compounds or as standardized plant extract provide unlimited opportunities for new drug development because of the unmatched availability of chemical diversity.[5] It is reported that Bangladesh has over 5,000 medicinal plants and uses of these plants for medicinal purposes are remarkable.[6] *Enhydra fluctuans* Lour (Traditional name: Helencha; Family: Compositae), *Clerodendrum viscosum* Vent (Traditional name: Ghetu; Family: Verbenaceae) and *Andrographis peniculata* Wall (Traditional name: Kalomegh; Family: Acanthaceae) are three such medicinally important plants bitter in taste that widely grow in Bangladesh. *Enhydra fluctuans* is nutritious and used in ascites, dropsy, anasarca and snakebite.[7] This plant has been reported to have antioxidative and analgesic activities.[8,9] *Andrographis peniculata* exhibits antihepatotoxic, antimalarial, antihepatitic, antithrombogenic, antiinflammatory, anti-snake venom and antipyretic properties[10-12] and itis also used in the treatment of upper respiratory tract infections.[13] *Clerodendrum viscosum* with antioxidative property is used in the treatment of fever, cough, bronchitis and also applied for herpetic eruptions and as vermifuge and bitter tonic.[14,15] Since there are no reports on antimicrobial and cytotoxic effects of *Enhydra fluctuans, Clerodendrum viscosum* and *Andrographis peniculata,* in this study attempts were made to evaluate the antimicrobial and cytotoxic activities of leaves of the above three important species against some pathogenic microorganisms and *Artemia salina* (brine shrimp nauplii).

***Corresponding author:** Dr. M. Tofazzal Hossain (PhD), Department of Biochemistry and Molecular Biology, Rajshahi University, Rajshahi-6205, Bangladesh. E-mail: thossainbd@yahoo.com

Materials and Methods

Plant materials

Leaves of *Enhydra fluctuans*, *Clerodendrum viscosum* and *Andrographis peniculata* were collected in the month of October, 2011 from Rajshahi district of Bangladesh and the plant material was taxonomically identified by Professor A.T.M Naderuzzaman, Department of Botany, University of Rajshahi. Voucher specimens were deposited under the accession numbers DACB-21401 for *Enhydra fluctuans*, DACB-20710 for *Clerodendrum viscosum* and DACB-18612 for *Andrographis peniculata* at the Bangladesh National Herbarium.

Extraction

The collected leaves of each plant were cleaned and shade-dried. The dried leaves were pulverized into a coarse powder by a grinding machine (FFC-15, China). Then half of each plant material was extracted with methanol and remaining part was extracted with acetone at room temperature. Each extract was filtered through filter papers and filtrate was evaporated under reduced pressure at 40°C using a rotary evaporator to have 0.87, 2.2 and 2.4 g methanol extracts of leaves of *Enhydra fluctuans* (MLE), *Clerodendrum viscosum* (MLC) and *Andrographis peniculata* (MLA), respectively whereas 3.5, 2.7 and 4.8g acetone extracts of leaves of *Enhydra fluctuans* (ALE), *Clerodendrum viscosum* (ALC) and *Andrographis peniculata* (ALA), respectively were also obtained.

Antimicrobial assay

Four Gram positive (*Bacillus subtilis* BTCC19, *Bacillus megaterium* BTCC18, *Bacillus cereus* ATCC27853 and *Sarcina lutea* ATCC28106), four Gram negative (*Escherichia coli* ATCC25922, *Shigella sonnei* ATTC8992, *Shigella shiga* ATCC27853 and *Shigella dysenteriae* ATCC14228) pathogenic bacterial strains and five fugal strains (*Aspergillus niger* ATTC235561, *Aspergillus fumigatus* ATTC10231, *Candida albicans* ATTC25889, *Human-3* sp ACCT10558 and *Fusarium sp* ACCT56390) were collected from the Institute of Biological Science (IBSC), University of Rajshahi, Bangladesh. The methanol and acetone extracts of leaves of each plant were tested separately for antibacterial activity by disc diffusion assay method.[16] *Kanamycin* disc (30 μg/disc) and *Nystatin* disc (100 μg/disc) were used as positive antibacterial and antifungal control, respectively. Blank disc impregnated with the respective solvent was used as negative control. The antibacterial activity of each extract was tested against each bacterium at concentrations of 200 μg/disc and 400 μg/disc. For antifungal screening, each extract was tested at concentration of 300 μg/disc and 500 μg/disc. Antibacterial assay plates were incubated at 37±1°C for 24 hrs, whereas antifungal assay plates were incubated at 37±1°C for 48 hrs. Each experiment was carried out in triplicates, and diameter of the zone of inhibition surrounding each disc was recorded.

Cytotoxic assay

The experiment was carried out using the method described by Meyer *et al.*[17] In brief, *Artemia salina* Leach (brine shrimp eggs) was allowed to hatch and mature as nauplii (Larvae) in seawater for 48 hrs at 25°C. Serially diluted test solutions (80 μL in DMSO from a stock solution of 5 mg/mL DMSO) were added to the seawater (5 mL), containing 10 nauplii. After incubation for 24 h at 25°C, the number of survivors was counted. The LC_{50} (50% lethal concentration, μg/ml) was determined from triplicate experiments. Ampicillin trihydrate was used as positive control.

Statistical analysis

The mortality data from cytotoxic experiment were then subjected to probit analysis for the determination of LC_{50} values using the computer software SPSS of 14 version.

Results

Results of antimicrobial test

In antibacterial study, the efficacy of MLE, MLC, MLA, ALE, ALC and ALA to inhibit the growth of four gram (+) positive bacteria and four gram (–) negative bacteria is shown in table 1 and table 2. As shown in table 1 and table 2, MLE and ALE moderately inhibited the growth of *Bacillus cereus*, *Escherchia coli*, *Shigella shiga* and *Shigella sonnei* with the zone of inhibition in the range 06 to 14 mm. ALA and MLA showed activity against *Sarcina lutea*, *Escherichia coli* and *Shigella sonnei* and produced zone of inhibition between 06 to 11 mm (Table 2). MLC and ALC were found inactive against the tested bacteria at concentration of 200 μg/disc, whereas at concentration of 400 μg/disc, it showed mild activity against *Sarcina lutea*, *Escherichia coli* and *Shigella sonnei* exhibiting their zones of inhibition of 06 to 08 mm in diameter (Table 2).

In antifungal activity test, ALE produced zone of inhibition between 07 to 15 mm against *Aspergillus niger*, *Fusarium* sp and *Aspergillus fumigatus* whereas MLE exhibited activity against *Aspergillus niger* and *Fusarium sp* (Table 3). Both MLA and ALA showed moderate activity only against *Human-3* sp and produced inhibition zone ranging from 08 to 14 mm (Table 4). MLC and ALC had no antifungal activity.

Results of cytotoxic assay

All test sample (i.e., MLE, MLC, MLA, ALE, ALC and ALA) showed potent cytotoxicity against brine shrimp nauplii (*Artemia salina*) in comparison with ampicillin trihydrate (LC_{50}: 21.38 μg/ml) (Table 5). Among the samples, ALA (LC_{50}: 7.03 μg/ml) showed the highest toxicity and the mortality was not shown in the negative control experiment.

Discussion

In the continuation of new antimicrobial drug discovery, methanol and acetone extracts of leaves of *Enhydra fluctuans*, *Clerodendrum viscosum* and

Andrographis peniculata (MLE, MLC, MLA, ALE,ALC and ALA)were investigated, which are being used as a successive medicinal plant in different diseases by folk practitioner in our locality.[7]

Table 1. *In vitro* antibacterial activity of leaves of *Enhydra fluctualns*

Name of microorganism	Zone of inhibition				
	MLE		ALE		Kanamycin
	Dose (µg/disc)				
	200	400	200	400	30
Bacillus subtilis	R	R	R	R	32 ± 1.0
Bacillus megaterium	R	R	R	R	34 ± 1.5
Bacillus cereus	06 ± 0.3	10 ± 1.0	06 ± 0.6	10 ± 1.0	28 ± 1.8
Sarcina lutea	R	R	R	R	35 ± 1.4
Escherichia coli	06 ± 0.6	08 ± 0.3	06 ± 0.3	10 ± 0.6	31 ± 2.1
Shigella sonnei	06 ± 0.6	11 ± 0.5	08 ± 0.6	11 ± 0.3	26 ± 1.2
Shigella shiga	06 ± 0.3	14 ± 0.5	07 ± 0.6	12 ± 1.0	30 ± 1.8
Shigella dysenteriae	R	R	R	R	36 ± 2.0

Data are expressed as mean ± S.E.M (Standard error of mean); MLE: Methanol extract of leaves of Enhydra fluctualns; ALE: Acetone extract of leaves of Enhydra fluctualns; R: Resistance

Table 2. *In vitro* antibacterial activity of leaves of *Clerodendrum viscosum* and *Andrographis peniculata*.

Name of microorganism	Zone of inhibition								
	MLC		ALC		MLA		ALA		Kanamycin
	Dose (µg/disc)								
	200	400	200	400	400	200	400	200	30
Bacillus subtilis	R	R	R	R	R	R	R	R	34 ± 1.3
Bacillus megaterium	R	R	R	R	R	R	R	R	30 ± 1.8
Bacillus cereus	R	R	R	R	R	R	R	R	28 ± 1.5
Sarcina lutea	R	08 ± 0.6	R	07 ± 1.0	06 ± 0.3	11 ± 0.6	06 ± 0.6	09 ± 0.3	30 ± 1.1
Escherichia coli	R	06 ± 0.3	R	06 ± 0.3	06 ± 1.0	08 ± 1.0	06 ± 0.3	10 ± 0.3	32 ± 1.6
Shigella sonnei	R	08 ± 1.8	R	07 ± 1.0	R	08 ± 0.5	08 ± 1.0	11 ± 0.7	38 ± 0.9
Shigella shiga	R	R	R	R	R	R	R	R	26 ± 1.5
Shigella dysenteriae	R	R	R	R	R	R	R	R	31 ± 1.2

Data are expressed as mean ± S.E.M (Standard error of mean); **MLC**: Methanol extract of leaves of *Clerodendrum viscosum*; **ALC**: Acetone extract of leaves of *Clerodendrum viscosum*; **MLA**: Methanol extract of leaves of *Andrographis peniculata*; **ALA**: Acetone extract of leaves of *Andrographis peniculata*; **R**: Resistance

Table 3. *In vitro* antifungal activity of leaves of *Enhydra fluctualns*

Name of microorganism	Zone of inhibition				
	MLE		ALE		Nystatin
	Dose (µg/disc)				
	300	500	300	500	100
Aspergillus niger	07 ± 0.6	13 ± 0.3	07 ± 1.0	15 ± 0.6	25 ± 1.1
Aspergillus fumigatus	R	R	R	13 ± 0.5	30 ± 1.8
Human-3sp	R	R	R	R	28 ± 1.0
Fusarium sp	06 ± 0.6	09 ± 0.3	06 ± 1.0	10 ± 1.0	31 ± 1.5

Data are expressed as mean ± S.E.M (Standard error of mean); MLE: Methanol extract of leaves of Enhydra fluctualns; ALE: Acetone extract of leaves of Enhydra fluctualns; R: Resistance

Table 4. *In vitro* antifungal activity of leaves of *Clerodendrum viscosum* and *Andrographis peniculata.*

Name of microorganism	Zone of inhibition								
	MLC		ALC		MLA		ALA		Nystatin
	Dose (μg/disc)								
	300	500	300	500	300	500	300	500	100
Aspergillus niger	R	R	R	R	R	R	R	R	25 ± 1.1
Aspergillus fumigatus	R	R	R	R	R	R	R	R	30 ± 1.8
Human-3 sp	R	R	R	R	07 ± 1.8	07 ± 1.8	07 ± 1.8	07 ± 1.8	28 ± 1.0
Fusarium sp	R	R	R	R	R	R	R	R	31 ± 1.5

Data are expressed as mean ± S.E.M (Standard error of mean); **MLC**: Methanol extract of leaves of *Clerodendrum viscosum*; **ALC**: Acetone extract of leaves of *Clerodendrum viscosum*; **MLA**: Methanol extract of leaves of *Andrographis peniculata*; **ALA**: Acetone extract of leaves of *Andrographis peniculata*; **R**: Resistance

Table 5. Cytotoxicity of the leaves of Enhydra fluctuans, Clerodendrum viscosum and Andrographis peniculata against brine shrimp nauplii.

Sample	LC_{50} (μg/mL)
Amphicillin trihydrate	21.38 ± 0.29
MLE	13.33 ± 0.47
ALE	11.37 ± 0.19
MLC	10.58 ± 0.76
ALC	13.68 ± 0.30
MLA	10.81 ± 0.84
ALA	7.03 ± 0.53

Data are expressed as mean ± S.E.M (Standard error of mean)

In the present investigation, mild to moderate antimicribial activity of these crude extracts were found against the test microorganisms at the concentrations of 200 and 400 μg/disc. Among the samples, the methanol (MLE) and acetone (ALE) extracts of leaves of *Enhydra fluctuans* showed better efficacy against both gram positive (+) and gram negative (-) bacteria as well as three pathogenic fungi. In literature, it has been found that the presence of terpenoids, flavonoids, steroids and glycosides like chemicals in crude extract plays an important role for producing antimicrobial activity.[18-20] The presence of phytoconstitutents like alkaloids, steroids, flavonoids, terpenoids, glycosides etc, in the leaves of *Enhydra fluctuans*, *Clerodendrum viscosum* and *Andrographis peniculata* has been previously confirmed by several studies[7] and these phytoconstitutents possibly might have contributed to the anti-bacterial activity of the three plants.

In the Brine Shrimp lethality study, all extracts obtained from the leaves of the three plants were tested for their cytotoxicity against brine shrimp nauplii and showed positive results indicating that these are biologically active. Several studies have shown that brine shrimp bioassay has been an excellent method to screen the cytotoxic property of medicinal plants and for the isolation of a great variety of biologically active compounds.[21] Finally the overall results of this study act a scientific basis to investigate the relationship between the phytochemicals of the three plant extracts and the biological activities that may explore the actual antimicrobial and cytotoxic chemical constituents present in the crude extracts. Our future studies to isolate these active phytochemicals and determine their activities against microorganisms, are in progress.

Acknowledgement

The authors are thankful to the Institute of Biological Science (IBSc), Rajshahi University, for providing the pure cultures of the test microorganisms to carry out this research work.

Conflict of interest

The authors have declared that there is no conflict of interest.

References

1. Morris AK, Masterton RG. Antibiotic resistance surveillance: action for international studies. J Antimicrob Chemoth 2002;49:7-10.
2. Levy SB, Marshall B. Antibacterial resistance worldwide: causes, challenges and responses. Nat Med 2004;10:S122-9.
3. Taubes G. The bacteria fight back. Science 2008;321:356-61.
4. Parekh J, Chanda V. In vitro Antimicrbail activity and Phytochemical analysis of some Indial medicinal plants. Turk J Biol 2007;31:53-8.
5. Cos P, Vlietinck AJ, Berghe DV, Maes L. Anti-infective potential of natural products: How to develop a stronger in vitro 'proof-of-concept'. J Ethnopharmacol 2006;106:290-302.
6. Biswas KR, Ishika T, Rahman M, Khan T, Swarna A, Monalisa MN, et al. Medicinal Plants Used for Preventive Medicinal Purposes: a Survey in Muktipara Village, Chuadanga District, Bangladesh. American-Eurasian Journal of Sustainable Agriculture 2011;5:247-51.

7. Ghani A. Medicinal Plants of Bangladesh. 2nd ed. Dhaka: Asiatic Society of Bangladesh; 2003.
8. Sannigrahi S, Mazuder UK, Pal DK, Parida S, Jain S. Antioxidant Potential of Crude Extract and Different Fractions of Enhydra fluctuans Lour. Iran J Pharm Res 2010;9:75-82.
9. Rahman MT, Begum N, Alimuzzaman M, Khan MOF. Analgesic activity of Enhydra fluctuans. Fitoterapia 2002;73:707-9.
10. Choudhury BR, Poddar MK. Andrographolide and Kalmegh (Andrographis paniculata) extract: effect on intestinal brush-border membrane bound hydrolases. Methods Find Exp Clin Pharmacol 1985;7:617-21.
11. Choudhury BR, Poddar MK. Andrographolide and Kalmegh (Andrographis paniculata) extract: in vivo and in vitro effect on hepatic lipid peroxidation. Methods Find Exp Clin Pharmacol 1984;6:481-5.
12. Choudhury RB, Haque SJ, Poddar MK. In vitro and in vivo effects of kalmegh(andrographis paniculata) extract and andrographolide on hepatic microsomal drug metabolizing enzymes. Planta Med 1987;53:135-40.
13. Coon JT, Ernst E. Andrographis paniculata in the treatment of upper respiratory tract infections: a systematic review of safety and efficacy. Planta Med 2004;70:293-8.
14. Liza SA, Rahman MO, Uddin MZ, Hassan MA, Begum M. Reproductive Biology of Three Medicinal Plants. Bangl J Plant Taxon 2010; 17:69-78.
15. Rahman MM, Rumzhum NN, Zinna K. Evaluation of Antioxidant and Antinociceptive Properties of Methanolic Extract of Clerodendrum viscosum Vent. Stamford J Pharm Sci 2011;4:74-8.
16. Rois JJ, Reico MC, Villar A. Antimicrobial Screening of natural products. J Enthopharmocol 1988;23:127-49.
17. Meyer BN, Ferrigni NR, Putnam JE, Jacobsen LB, Nichols DE, Mclaughlin JL. Brine shrimp: a convenient general bioassay for active plant constituents. Planta Med 1982;45:31-4.
18. Mandalari G, Bennett RN, Bisignano G, Trombetta D, Saija A, Faulds CB, et al. Antimicrobial activity of flavonoids extracted from bergamot (Citrus bergamia Risso) peel, a byproduct of the essential oil industry. J Appl Microbiol 2007;103:2056-64.
19. Maiyo ZC, Ngure RM, Matasyoh JC, Chepkorir R. Phytochemical constituents and antimicrobial activity of leaf extracts of three Amaranthus plant species. African Journal of Biotechnology 2010; 9:3178-82.
20. Viji M, Murugesans S. Phytochemical analysis and antibacterial activity of medicinal plant Cardiospermum halicacabum Linn. J Phytol 2010; 2:68-77.
21. Quignard EL, Pohlit AM, Nunomura SM, Pinto AC, Santos EV, Morais SK, et al. Screening of plants found in Amazonas state for lethality towards brine shrimp. Acta Amazon 2003;33: 93-104.

Development and Validation of an HPLC Method for the Analysis of Sirolimus in Drug Products

Ziba Islambulchilar [1,2,3], Saeed Ghanbarzadeh [1,4], Shahram Emami [3], Hadi Valizadeh [1,5], Parvin Zakeri-Milani [1,6]*

[1] *Faculty of Pharmacy, Tabriz University of Medical Sciences, Tabriz, Iran.*

[2] *Faculty of Pharmacy, Zanjan University of Medical Sciences, Zanjan, Iran.*

[3] *Student Research Committee, Tabriz University of Medical Sciences, Tabriz, Iran.*

[4] *Drug Applied Research Center, Tabriz University of Medical Sciences, Tabriz, Iran.*

[5] *Research Center for Pharmaceutical Nanotechnology, Tabriz University of Medical Sciences, Tabriz, Iran.*

[6] *Liver and Gastrointestinal Diseases Research Center, Tabriz University of Medical Sciences, Tabriz, Iran.*

ARTICLE INFO

Keywords:
Sirolimus
HPLC
Method development
Validation
Ultraviolet
Chromatography

ABSTRACT

Purpose: The aim of this study was to develop a simple, rapid and sensitive reverse phase high performance liquid chromatography (RP-HPLC) method for quantification of sirolimus (SRL) in pharmaceutical dosage forms. ***Methods***: The chromatographic system employs isocratic elution using a Knauer- C18, 5 mm, 4.6 × 150 mm. Mobile phase consisting of acetonitril and ammonium acetate buffer set at flow rate 1.5 ml/min. The analyte was detected and quantified at 278nm using ultraviolet detector. The method was validated as per ICH guidelines. ***Results***: The standard curve was found to have a linear relationship ($r^2 > 0.99$) over the analytical range of 125–2000ng/ml. For all quality control (QC) standards in intraday and interday assay, accuracy and precision range were -0.96 to 6.30 and 0.86 to 13.74 respectively, demonstrating the precision and accuracy over the analytical range. Samples were stable during preparation and analysis procedure. ***Conclusion***: Therefore the rapid and sensitive developed method can be used for the routine analysis of sirolimus such as dissolution and stability assays of pre- and post-marketed dosage forms.

Introduction

Sirolimus (SRL, formerly rapamycin: $C_{51}H_{79}NO_{13}$, CAS: 53123-88-9) is a lactone-lactam macrolide antibiotic with immunosuppressant and anticancer effects. It was first identified as an antifungal agent produced by the Streptomyces hygroscopicus bacterium and was subsequently demonstrated to be a potent immunosuppressive agent that was approved by the U.S. Food and Drug Administration (FDA) to be used beside cyclosporine or tacrolimus in kidney transplantation. In contrast to tacrolimus and cyclosporine, which inhibit the production of cytokines, sirolimus binds to the FK (peptidyl-prolyl cis-trans isomerase) binding protein which modulates the activity of the mammalian Target Of Rapamycin (mTOR).The mTOR inhibits Interleukin-2-mediated signal transduction, resulting in cell cycle stop in the G1-S phase and prevents cell cycle progression and proliferation, hence blocks the response of T- and B-cell activation by cytokines. These pharmacological properties allow rapamycin not only to be a promising immunosuppressant with the absence of nephrotoxicity but also to be a possible chemotherapeutic agent against many types of solid tumor. SRL is a white to off-white powder, insoluble in water, very slightly soluble in hexane and petroleum ether, soluble in methanol, diethyl ether, and N, N-dimethylformamide (DMF) and freely soluble in benzyl alcohol, chloroform, acetone, and acetonitrile (ACN).[1-9] Validation of new analytical methods for pharmaceutical products is a requirement of Current Good Manufacturing Practice (cGMP) regulations. As stated by the current International Conference on Harmonization (ICH) guideline, accuracy, precision, linearity and stability of test methods are some of the analytical parameters which require assays validation.[3,10-13] Several types of analytical methods have been used for quantification of SRL, including immunoassay, HPLC ultraviolet, and HPLC mass spectrometric detection (HPLC-MS or HPLC/MS/MS). The immunoassay is not commercially available, and there is an acute need for an accurate, rapid, and simple chromatographic assay to determine SRL in drug development procedure and also post marketing investigations.[4,7,14,15] Considering the less complication

***Corresponding author:** Parvin Zakeri-Milani (PhD), Department of Pharmaceutics, Faculty of Pharmacy, Tabriz University of Medical Sciences, Tabriz, Iran. 51664. E-mail: pzakeri@tbzmed.ac.ir

and readily availability of HPLC-UV method in research laboratories and clinic a simple and rapid chromatographic method in the present study was developed to routine analysis of sirolimus concentration.

Materials and Methods

Chemicals

Sirolimus was obtained from Poli (Lazio, Italy). HPLC grade solvents, such as methanol and acetonitril (ACN) were purchased from Merck (Darmstadt, Germany). Double-distilled water was used during the entire HPLC procedure. Analytical grade ammonium acetate, sodium lauryl sulphate (SLS) and sodium hydroxide were obtained from Merck (Darmstadt, Germany).

HPLC conditions

The RP-HPLC (Beckman, Florida, USA) with a variable wavelength ultraviolet spectrophotometric detector (166 gold) set at 278 nm. System Gold software was used for data acquisition and system Gold nouveau software was used for data reporting and analysis.

For the preliminary analysis different columns in combination with different solvent systems were tried out. Analytical column used for analysis was Knauer ODS 5 mm, 4.6 × 150 mm. Column temperature was set at 55°C. The mobile phase was a mixture of 70% ACN and 30% ammonium acetate buffer (The buffer was prepared by dissolving 0.8 g ammonium acetate in 1000 ml water, adjusted to pH 5.8 with NaOH 1N). Injection volume was 150 µl which injected into the column using a Hamilton (Bonaduz, Switzerland) injector syringe and the isocratic flow rate was set at 1.5 ml/min. SRL was detected by UV absorption at 278 nm.

Preparation of standard solutions

The primary stock solution of sirolimus was prepared by dissolving 10 mg sirolimus in methanol in a 50 ml volumetric flask to yield a concentration of 200 µg/ml. One ml of obtained solution was diluted in 100 ml volumetric flask with sodium lauryl sulphate (0.4% in water) solution. Finally, working standard solutions were prepared by serially dilution with SLS solution to obtain sirolimus concentrations of 125, 250, 500, 1000, 1500, and 2000 ng/ml.

Method Validation

The optimized RP-HPLC method was validated according to ICH guidelines with respect to linearity range, sensitivity, accuracy, precision, and stability.

Linearity

The linearity of an analytical method indicates its ability to obtain the response directly proportional to the concentration of the analyte in the sample within a definite range. The standard curves in the range of 125-2000 ng/ml were prepared on 3 consecutive days. Each set of standards was injected into the column from lowest to highest concentration.

Limits of Detection (LOD) and Quantitation (LOQ)

LOD and LOQ settle on the sensitivity of the method. LOD is the lowest concentration of the analyte detected by the method and LOQ is the minimum measurable concentration. There are three different methods indicated in ICH guidelines for determination of LOD and LOQ. The first method relies on visual evaluation method, second, signal to noise ratio method (the signal-to-noise ratio of 3:1 and 10:1 were taken as LOD and LOQ respectively) and third is the slope method (were calculated by the equations LOD = yb + 3.3sb, and LOQ = yb + 10sb where yb is the signal of the blank and sb is its SD), which were calculated using Gold nouveau software.[7,10,12,13,16-19] In this study we used the slope method for determination of LOD and LOQ.

Accuracy and Precision

Three quality control samples with concentrations at three levels (low, medium and high) within calibration range were used in triplicates to determine the accuracy and precision of the method. The mean measured concentrations for all prepared samples were considered for intraday and interday accuracy and precision evaluation. Accuracy was assessed via calculating the percentage deviation of the calculated concentration and the theoretical concentration while the precision was determined by calculating the coefficient of variation percentage (CV %) for intra- and inter-day runs. The acceptable value for accuracy is less than ±15% deviation from the nominal values and, CV% ≤ ±15% for precision.[1,3,7,13,16,18,20]

Stability

The stability of the drug in analytical solution was checked by replicate analysis (N = 3) of the three control samples (in low, medium and high concentrations) for 6 h (considering the approximate time required for preparation of samples and analysis by HPLC method) after storage at ambient temperature. In all sample stability experiments, the results were compared with the sirolimus initial concentrations. The acceptable relative error was considered to be ±15 %.[13,14,21-23]

Results and Discussion

Linearity

Linearity of the method was confirmed by preparing sirolimus standard curves for the analytical range of 125–2000 ng/ml. Statistical analysis using least square regression indicated excellent linearity for SRL in the mentioned range. A good correlation between SRL peak heights and drug concentration was observed with $r^2 \geq 0.99$ for all standard curves (Table 1). Concentration curves for SRL had a mean slope, intercept and r^2 of 0.099, -9.82 and 0.996 respectively.

Representative chromatogram of serial concentrations of SRL in the range 125 nm to 2000 nm is shown in Figure 1. The retention time was approximately 8 min.

LOD and LOQ

The LOD and LOQ were calculated by the equations LOD = yb + 3.3sb and LOQ = yb + 10sb where yb is the signal of the blank and sb is its SD. Based on these equations, the calculated LOD and LOQ values for SRL were 22.03 and 56.2 ng/ml, respectively.

Table 1. Linearity data of SRL calibration curves on 3 consecutive days

Standard curve	Slope	Intercept	r^2
Day 1	0.078	14.34	0.996
Day 2	0.067	-79.51	0.994
Day 3	0.091	35.70	0.996
Mean	0.099	-9.82	0.996
RSD	0.15	-6.24	0.001

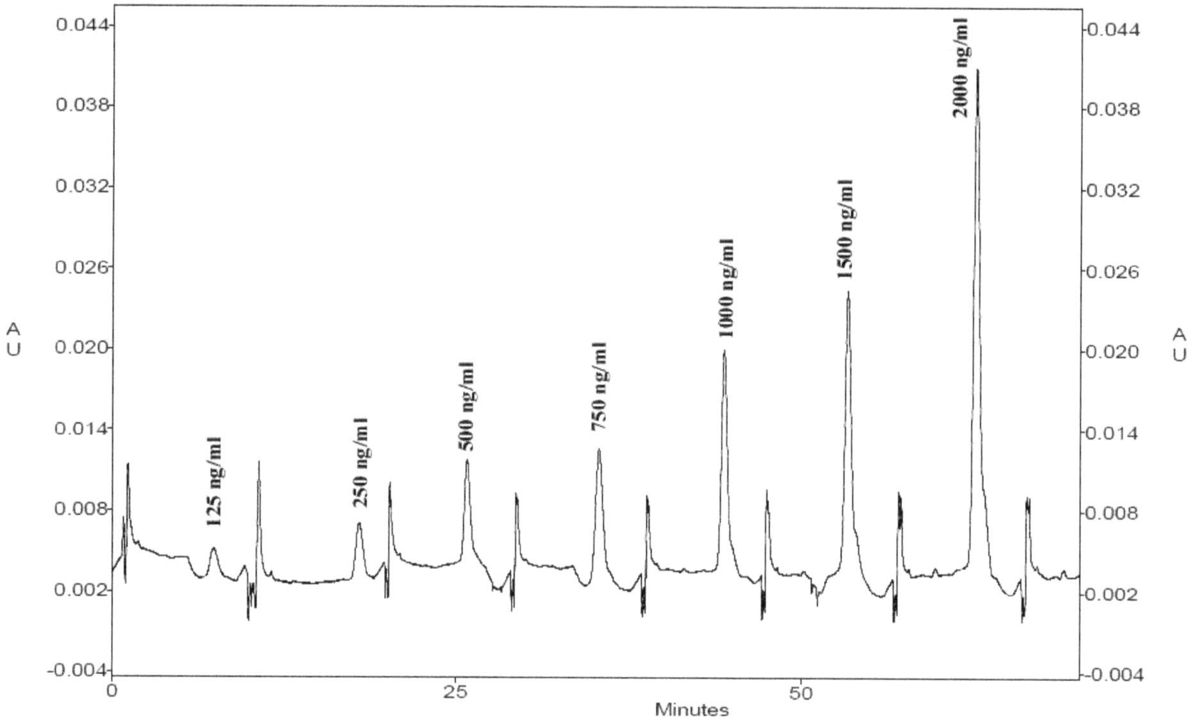

Figure 1. Chromatogram of serial concentrations of sirolimus

Accuracy and Precision

In this study intra- and inter-day precision was expressed as percent of coefficient of variation (CV %). Accuracy was expressed as the mean percentage of analyte recovered in the assay. The Intra-day precision, accuracy and relative errors range were 0.86-9.18%, 100.59-102.44% and 0.59-2.44%, respectively. Corresponding results for inter-day evaluations were 12.29-13.74%, 99.04-106.30% and 0.96-6.3%, respectively. Precision (CV %) and relative error percent acquired at each concentration should not exceed ±15%. The results of the precision and accuracy for intra- and inter-day are shown in Table 2. The results illustrate a good repeatability of response of HPLC system to different concentrations.

Stability

The stability of working standard samples was determined at ambient temperature by analyzing the solutions over a period of 6 h (Table 3). The aim was to ensure that the preparation of samples and analysis time did not contribute to the degradation and indicate that the samples will remain stable during the course of the analysis .The solutions were considered stable if the variability in the assay results was less than 15 % of initial.[14,21-23] The stability of sirolimus SRL has been investigated previously and was shown that SRL even in whole blood was stable for 30 days at 4°C.[4,24] Therefore the results that SRL was stable during sample preparation and the analysis times are confirmed.

Conclusion

The analytical method described in this paper has good accuracy, precision, linearity and is suitable for SRL assay. As the method was successfully validated based on ICH guidelines, it can be readily used in quality control laboratories for the routine pharmaceutical analysis. Also this simple and rapid method can simplify performance in developing new formulations. Further investigations are necessary to adopt this method to protein binding analysis and clinical monitoring of plasma level in therapeutic drug monitoring (TDM) studies and dose adjustment.

Table 2. Intra-day and inter-day accuracy and precision obtained from calibration curves with three levels of QC samples.

Added concentration (ng/ml)	Intra-day				Inter-day			
	Mean measured (ng/ml)	Precision (CV %)	Accuracy (%)	Relative Error %	Mean calculated (ng/ml)	Precision (CV %)	Accuracy (%)	Relative Error %
1000	1021.85 ±93.37	9.188	102.18	2.18	990.41 ±151.47	12.294	99.041	0.96
1500	1508.88 ±75.32	5.020	100.59	0.59	1534.62 ±256.92	13.742	102.308	2.30
2000	2048.92 ±17.61	0.864	102.44	2.44	2126.15 ±333.58	12.689	106.307	6.30

Table 3. SRL Stability after 6h in ambient temperature

Initial concentration (ng/ml)	Measured concentration (mean ± SD, ng/ml)	Deviation %
250	263.3±7.05	5.32
1000	925.29±10.5	-7.47
2000	1855.56±12.93	-7.25

Acknowledgments

The authors would like to thank the authorities of Faculty of Pharmacy, Tabriz University of Medical Sciences, for providing analytical facilities. This paper is based on a PhD thesis (number 42 and 54) submitted in Faculty of Pharmacy, Tabriz University of Medical Sciences.

Conflict of Interest

There is no conflict of interest in this study.

References

1. Asensi Diez R, Quesada Sanz MP, Valverde Molina E, de Ramon Garrido E, Gomez Maldonado J, Munoz Castillo I. Comparison of high-resolution liquid chromatography versus microparticle enzyme immunoassay for the measurement of sirolimus levels in renal transplantation. Farm Hosp 2006;30(3):142-8.
2. Chen KH, Tsai MK, Lai IR, Lin Wu FL, Hu RH, Lee PH. Favorable results of concomitant tacrolimus and sirolimus therapy in Taiwanese renal transplant recipients at 12 months. J Formos Med Assoc 2008;107(7):533-9.
3. Di Marco GS, de Andrade MC, Felipe CR, Alfieri F, Gooding A, Silva HT Jr, et al. Determination of sirolimus blood concentration using high-performance liquid chromatography with ultraviolet detection. Ther Drug Monit 2003;25(5):558-64.
4. Jones K, Saadat-Lajevard S, Lee T, Horwatt R, Hicks D, Johnston A, et al. An immunoassay for the measurement of sirolimus. Clin Ther 2000;22(Suppl B):B49-61.
5. Molnar-Kimber KL. Mechanism of action of rapamycin (Sirolimus, Rapamune). Transplant Proc 1996;28(2):964-9.
6. Nikitin AV. [Sirolimus: mechanism of action, use in combined chemotherapy of cancer]. Antibiot Khimioter 2007;52(1-2):39-41.
7. Salm P, Taylor PJ, Pillans PI. The quantification of sirolimus by high-performance liquid chromatography-tandem mass spectrometry and microparticle enzyme immunoassay in renal transplant recipients. Clin Ther 2000;22 Suppl B:B71-85.
8. Sehgal SN. Rapamune (Sirolimus, rapamycin): an overview and mechanism of action. Ther Drug Monit 1995;17(6):660-5.
9. Sehgal SN. Rapamune (RAPA, rapamycin, sirolimus): mechanism of action immunosuppressive effect results from blockade of signal transduction and inhibition of cell cycle progression. Clin Biochem 1998;31(5):335-40.
10. Bohnert S, Vair C, Mikler J. Development and validation of a sensitive HPLC method for the quantification of HI-6 in guinea pig plasma and evaluated in domestic swine. J Chromatogr B Analyt Technol Biomed Life Sci 2010;878(17-18):1407-13.
11. Ruzilawati AB, Wahab MS, Imran A, Ismail Z, Gan SH. Method development and validation of repaglinide in human plasma by HPLC and its application in pharmacokinetic studies. J Pharm Biomed Anal 2007;43(5):1831-5.
12. Shou M, Galinada WA, Wei YC, Tang Q, Markovich RJ, Rustum AM. Development and validation of a stability-indicating HPLC method for simultaneous determination of salicylic acid, betamethasone dipropionate and their related compounds in Diprosalic Lotion. J Pharm Biomed Anal 2009;50(3):356-61.
13. Zakeri-Milani P, Barzegar-Jalali M, Tajerzadeh H, Azarmi Y, Valizadeh H. Simultaneous determination of naproxen, ketoprofen and phenol red in samples from rat intestinal permeability studies: HPLC method development and validation. J Pharm Biomed Anal 2005;39(3-4):624-30.

14. Islambulchilar Z, Valizadeh H, Zakeri-Milani P. Rapid HPLC determination of pioglitazone in human plasma by protein precipitation and its application to pharmacokinetic studies. J AOAC Int 2010;93(3):876-81.
15. Wilson D, Johnston F, Holt D, Moreton M, Engelmayer J, Gaulier JM, et al. Multi-center evaluation of analytical performance of the microparticle enzyme immunoassay for sirolimus. Clin Biochem 2006;39(4):378-86.
16. Kuehl PJ, Angersbach BS, Stratton SP, Myrdal PB. Development of an HPLC method for the analysis of Apomine in a topical cream formulation. J Pharm Biomed Anal 2006;40(4):975-80.
17. Taylor PJ, Salm P, Lynch SV, Pillans PI. Simultaneous quantification of tacrolimus and sirolimus, in human blood, by high-performance liquid chromatography-tandem mass spectrometry. Ther Drug Monit 2000;22(5):608-12.
18. Zochowska D, Bartlomiejczyk I, Kaminska A, Senatorski G, Paczek L. High-performance liquid chromatography versus immunoassay for the measurement of sirolimus: comparison of two methods. Transplant Proc 2006;38(1):78-80.
19. Zakeri-Milani P, Valizadeh H, Islambulchilar Z. Comparative bioavailability study of two cefixime formulations administered orally in healthy male volunteers. Arzneimittelforschung 2008;58(2):97-100.
20. Zakeri-Milani P, Nemati M, Ghanbarzadeh S, Hamishehkar H, Valizadeh H. Fasted state bioavailability of two delayed release formulations of divalproex sodium in healthy Iranian volunteers. Arzneimittelforschung 2011;61(8):439-43.
21. Souri E, Jalalizadeh H, Saremi S. Development and validation of a simple and rapid HPLC method for determination of pioglitazone in human plasma and its application to a pharmacokinetic study. J Chromatogr Sci 2008;46(9):809-12.
22. Holt DW, Lee T, Johnston A. Measurement of sirolimus in whole blood using high-performance liquid chromatography with ultraviolet detection. Clin Ther 2000;22(Suppl B):B38-48.
23. Bhatt J, Jangid A, Venkatesh G, Subbaiah G, Singh S. Liquid chromatography-tandem mass spectrometry (LC-MS-MS) method for simultaneous determination of venlafaxine and its active metabolite O-desmethyl venlafaxine in human plasma. J Chromatogr B Analyt Technol Biomed Life Sci 2005;829(1-2):75-81.
24. Gomes NA, Laud A, Pudage A, Joshi SS, Vaidya VV, Tandel JA. Validated LC-MS/MS method for determination of Alverine and one of its hydroxy metabolites in human plasma along with its application to a bioequivalence study. J Chromatogr B Analyt Technol Biomed Life Sci 2009;877(3):197-206.

How spherical crystallization improves direct tableting properties

Maryam Maghsoodi*

Drug applied Research Center and Faculty of Pharmacy, Tabriz University of Medical Sciences, Tabriz, Iran.

ARTICLE INFO

Article Type:
Review Article

Keywords:
Direct tabletting
Spherical crystallization
Flowability
Compactability

ABSTRACT

Direct tableting has been renewed as a preferable process by simply mixing and compressing powder to save time and cost in comparison with granule tableting. Direct compression tableting as a technique has been successfully applied to numerous drugs on the industrial scale, although the success of any procedure, and resulting mechanical properties of tablets, is strongly affected by the quality of the crystals used. Good flowability, packability and compactability are prerequisite for drug to be prepared by direct tableting. When the mechanical properties of the drug particles are inadequate a primary granulation is necessary. The use of spherical crystallization as a technique appears to be an efficient alternative for obtaining suitable particles for direct tableting. Spherical crystallization is a particle design technique, by which crystallization and agglomeration can be carried out simultaneously in one step and which has been successfully utilized for improvement the micromeritic properties of crystalline drugs. In this review, we will discuss how the micromeritic properties of the particles such as flowability, packability and compactability can be improved by spherical crystallization technique.

Introduction

Today the tablet is the most popular dosage form, representing 50% of all oral drug delivery systems, and accounting for 70% of all pharmaceutical preparations produced. From the manufacturing point of view, the initial capital outlay is high but tablets can be produced at much higher rate than any other dosage form. The dry dosage form promotes stability, and tablets are readily portable and consumed. The formulation of a tablet is optimized to achieve several goals. The focus today in the business is better drug delivery concepts, but also to make the simple standard formulations as economical as possible to produce. One of the most economical solutions is to find direct compressible formulations and this is especially of interest for large volume products. The required number of unit operations in direct compression is lower which means less equipment and space, lower labour costs, less processing time, and lower energy consumption. However, the use of this technique, although conceptually quite simple, depends on generating appropriate: (a) particle size and particle size distribution of the materials, (b) flowability of the crystals, (c) bulk density of the powder, in order to feed the correct amount of drug into a die cavity, and (d) compactibility of the powder. Despite some drug crystals exhibiting such appropriate properties, many materials display poor flowability and compactibility.[1] Direct tableting of latter materials has been successfully industrialized by coformulating higher amounts of fillers (≥75%). However, direct compression in the production of high dose formulations is limited, since large quantities of excipients are ordinarily required to produce suitable tablets.[2] To overcome this problem, the physicomechanical properties of drug need to be modified to improve flowabiility, packability and compressibility, so that powder can be delivered stably into die cavity and produce mechanically strong tablets. It is well known that the physical properties of the pharmaceutical raw materials such as crystal size, crystal shape, degree of agglomeration, and agglomerate properties can be modified by crystallization techniques to such an extent that these materials to be suitable for particular applications. Crystallization variables such as temperature profile, solvent composition, method and rate of supersaturation generation, hydrodynamics can be used to produce crystals with specific physicmechanical properties.

One interesting crystallization technique in which synthesis, crystallization, separation and agglomeration can be carried out in one step has been defined as spherical crystallization.[3] Indeed, this technique can promote the effectiveness of mixing, filling and tabletting procedures via producing spherical agglomerates with improved physicomechanical properties like compressibility, packability and flowability.[5-7] Spherical crystallization was firstly introduced into pharmaceutical manufacturing by

***Corresponding author:** Maryam Maghsoodi (PhD), Faculty of Pharmacy, Tabriz University of Medical Sciences, Tabriz 51664, Iran.
E-mail: maghsoodim@tbzmed.ac.ir

Kawashima et al.[8,9] as a simple technique to produce spherical agglomerates appropriate for direct tabletting. Spherical crystallization may occur via two mechanisms: spherical agglomeration (SA) and emulsion solvent diffusion (ESD). In both mechanisms there are a good solvent and a poor solvent which their miscibility govern the mechanism of the spherical crystallization. In the ESD mechanism, the pure good solvent and poor solvent are miscible but as affinity between good solvent and drug is stronger than that of good solvent and poor solvent. Accordingly, emulsion droplets are first formed by mixing good solvent solution of the drug with poor solvent.[10] Then, crystallization occurs within droplets as a consequence of counter diffusion of good and poor solvents. In spite of the apparent simplicity of ESD mechanism, finding a suitable emulsifier is really time consuming and difficult.

The SA occurs in three solvent systems, in which good solvent and poor solvent are miscible.[11] The drug is precipitated immediately by mixing a good solvent solution of the drug with a poor solvent as they are freely miscible and the affinity between solvents is stronger than the affinity between good solvent and drug. The third solvent, termed "binder liquid" is usually immiscible with poor solvent but wets the dispersed crystals and collects the crystals to form agglomerates through the action of capillary forces.[12]

It was revealed from several studies spherical crystallization exhibited improved micromeritic properties of spherical agglomerated crystals over single crystals which assists in pharmaceutical processing and expedites the production of tablets by direct tabletting. In this review it has been discussed how the micromeritic properties such as flowability, packability and compactibility of particle obtained by spherical crystallization can be improved.

Flowability and packability

Improvement in flowabity and packability of the agglomerated crystals prepared by spherical crystallization in comparison with the single crystals has been shown in several investigation.[13-17] Kawashima *etal.* in 1994 produced the agglomerates of acebutolol hydrochloride by spherical crystallization. It was shown in this study that the prepared agglomerates had lower angle of repose compared to single crystals which indicated to improved flowability of the agglomerate.[13] According to their results, mean diameter and standard deviation of agglomerates was respectively larger and smaller than those of the single crystals. Therefore, better flowability of the agglomerates was attributed to their larger particle size and narrow size distribution. In other work, the effect of particle size on the angle of repose of the agglomerated and single crystals was[15] studied and it was shown that the angle of repose of agglomerates was smaller than that of original crystals over the entire studied particle size range. Therefore, it was assumable that inaddition of particle size there is another reason for improvement of flowability of agglomerated crystals. It was concluded that good flowability for agglomerates were attributed to the spherical shape and smooth surface, since the area of contacts in the powder bed for spherical shapes was smaller than that for other particle shapes. In various studies which in spherical crystallization was applied to prepare the agglomerates the packing process achieved by tapping was described by percent compressibility (Eq.1), Kawakita (Eq.2) and Kuno(Eq.3) equations as follows.[18-20]

$$\text{Compressibility\%} = {(\rho_f - \rho_o)}/{\rho_f} \times 100 \qquad \text{Eq.1}$$

$$n/C = 1/ab + n/a \quad \text{Kawakita's equation}$$

$$C = (V_o - V_n)/V_n \qquad \text{Eq.2}$$

$$\ln(\rho_f - \rho_n) = -Kn + \ln(\rho_f - \rho_o) \quad \text{Kuno's equation} \qquad \text{Eq.3}$$

Where n is the number of tapping; V_o and V_n are the initial volume of powder bed before tapping and the volume powder bed after the nth tapping, respectively; ρ_o and ρ_n are the densities of powder bed at the initial stage and at the nth tapping respectively; a, b and k are constants representing flowability and packability of powder under mechanical force. As the results of several studies showed the low value of the percent compressibility and parameter a of Kawakita equation for agglomerated crystals indicated their high packability[13,15,16,21] and the larger parameter b and k in kawakita's and of Kuno's equations respectively, for agglomerates indicated to their slower apparent packing velocity. The slow packing velocity which indicated to low proportion of the consolidation of powder per tap was attributed to high flowability and packability of the agglomerates which result in closely packing of the agglomerates even without tapping. Moreover, as reported by some works, improved packing properties of agglomerates compared to single crystals was due to their larger closest packing density.[16,21] Flowability and packability of the agglomerated Acebutolol hydrochloride crystals were comprehensively investigated by measuring interparticle frictions when sheared.[13] In this work the mechanical characteristics (e.g. friction angle, cohesive stress) of the agglomerates were determined from the yield locus, which was constructed by measuring tensile stress and shear stress of the preconsolidated powder bed. The yield locus was described by Warren Spring[22] as represented by equation 4.

$$\left(\frac{\tau}{C}\right)^n = (\sigma + \sigma_T)/\sigma_T \qquad \text{Eq.4}$$

Where τ is shear stress, C is cohesive stress, σ is vertical stress and σ_T is tensile stress. According to this study, the angle of friction, shear cohesive stress and shear index of agglomerates were lower than those of single crystals. Such a low frictional force might be due to the decrease in frictional static electric charge of agglomerates. The major principal stress required to fracture the powder compact (i.e. uniaxial compression strength), was determined by drawing the Mohr circle contacting the yield locus and passing through the origin. The lower tensile stress and uniaxial compression strength proved the reduced cohesiveness of the agglomerates. Thus decreasing friction and cohesive forces during packing, resulted in improved packability and flowability of the agglomerates. According to these studies, it is expectable that the agglomerates flow smoothly from the hopper into the die and hence tablets with appropriate uniformity in weight can be produced from the agglomerates.[15]

Compactability

In several works, it has been reported that the tablet compressed with the agglomerated crystals exhibited higher tensile strength than that of compressed single original crystals.[13-15,23-25] Superior strength characteristics of the agglomerated crystals to single crystals indicated that a stronger bonding occurred during compression of agglomerated crystals than in the case of single crystals. In Jbilou et al. study it was indicated that the improvement of compression ability of the ibuprofen agglomerated crystals compared to marketed single crystals in spite of their higher crystallinity, might be related to the isotropy of the agglomerate texture.[14] However, in several studies, increasing the contact points to bind particles as a consequence of fracturing of agglomerated crystals has been mentioned as one of the main reasons for improvement in compactibility of agglomerated crystals.[13,15,16] For example, Morishima et al.[15] indicated that the improved compactibility of agglomerated crystals was related to their structural characteristics.

During the early stage of the compression process, the agglomerates consisted of numerous small crystals fragmented and resulted in large relative volume change.

According to results of this study, the specific surface area of the agglomerates increased with increasing the compaction pressure from 0.5 to 5 MPa while no change was observed in the case of single crystals. This fact confirmed the fracturing properties of the agglomerates compared to single crystals. Furthermore, it was shown that, in the case of single crystals, there was a good linear relationship between the porosity and the logarithm of the tensile strength for each size fraction. On the other hand, compacts made from smaller crystals showed superior tensile strength compared to those made from larger crystals with the same porosity. This could be explained by considering the fact that smaller crystals could be compacted more tightly as a result of higher interparticle contact points compared to larger crystals which was in agreement with some other works.[26,27] Regarding the agglomerates, the tensile strength of the compacts was close to that of single crystal, which was similar in constitutive crystal size. Having considered this finding and the fact that a good linear relationship between porosity and the tensile strength was also observed for agglomerates, it was concludable that the tensile strength of the compacts obtained from the agglomerates was mainly determined by the size of their constitutive crystals.

Kawashima et al[13] also showed the tensile strengths of tablets from agglomerated crystals were higher than those from single crystals when compared at the same compression pressure and porosity of the tablet. However, they emphasized that the production of fresh surfaces by fracturing during the compression process is necessary to bind the particles strongly for tabletting. To confirm the effect of fresh surface, newly produced by fragmentation during compression, on interparticle bonding, tablets were prepared with ground agglomerates and single crystals in mortar. The tensile strength of tablets with ground agglomerates was drastically reduced whereas such phenomena were not found with the original single crystals. This result was attributed to this fact that if the fractured surface is exposed to air for a time after breaking, no improvement in interparticle bonding occurs because of the decrease in the free energy of the surface when adsorbed with air. In this study it was found that produced surfaces by fracturing of the agglomerates in addition of increasing contact points to bind of particle, enhances the plastic interparticle bonding.[13] In this study and some other works the compression process was analyzed by Heckel equation which showed that a surface freshly prepared by fracture increased plasticity of particles, resulting in a lower compressive force required for compressing the agglomerates under plastic deformation compared to that for single crystals.[13,16,28] On the other hand, according to several researches, it is well known that better compacts result from the compression of plastic materials.[29-31] Plastic deformation can be quantitatively measured by stress relaxation at constant strain. Greater relaxation pressure, which is measured when plastic deformation requires higher energy, indicates increasing intimate interparticle contacts and consequently formation of strong bonds.[32] According to studies which elucidated plastic deformation based on relaxation stress, agglomerated crystals showed more rapid and extensive relaxation than single crystals which indicated agglomerated crystals exhibited a greater degree of plastic deformation under compression than single crystals.[15,16,25] Moreover, in another work[23] which deformation of agglomerated crystals as a single particle was studied based on the stress- strain curve it was found that the deformation of these particles was mainly plastic. Marshall and York[33] reported that the deformation characteristics of a drug crystallized from different systems were different which might be responsible for improving plasticity of the crystals when recrystallized and agglomerated from different crystallization system. Also as mentioned previously, in some works increasing plasticity of the agglomerated crystals was attributed to structural characterstics of them which produced fresh surfaces of particle with higher plasticity as a consequence of fragmentation. In some researches lower elastic recovery of the agglomerated crystals than that of the single crystals was also reported.[25,34] For example, Kawashima et al.[25] showed the elastic recovery of the agglomerated crystals of acebutolol hydrochloride was lower than that of the single crystals because more energy was consumed for plastic deformation in the former case than in the latter. In turn, the lower elastic recovery of the agglomerated crystals resulted in lower ejection pressure for agglomerated crystals compared with that the single crystals as explained below. It is known that the ejection force is the sum of the adhesive force, the friction force and the residual force. According to results of this study, there was no significant difference in residual pressure between agglomerated crystals and single crystals. Therefore, the lower ejection pressure might be due to the lower adhesive force and the lower friction force during ejection of the tablet from the die cavity for the agglomerated crystals compared to single crystals. The elastic recovery of the compressed tablet and the interaction of the material and wall are two main factors that are determined the adhesive force of the tablet to the die wall. Furthermore, in comparison with the agglomerated crystals and those of single it is obvious that the friction force of the former is lower because of lower elastic recovery.

Therefore, the two facts of the smaller adhesive force and friction force in the tablet releasing period resulted in lowered ejection pressure for agglomerated crystals compared to their single counterparts.

In summary, according to results of various investigation it can be concluded that remarkable fragmentation, increased plastic deformation and lowered elastic recovery of the agglomerated crystals during tableting process were responsible for improving the compactibility of the agglomerated crystals compared to single crystals.

Conclusion

This study has brought forward that agglomerated crystals may receive properties that make them aimable for direct tabletting. Improvement in flowabity and packability of the agglomerated crystals obtained by spherical crystallization method in comparison with the single crystals has been shown in several investigations which were attributed to their larger particle size, spherical shape, and smooth surface. Improved flowability and packability should be of great advantage in uniform feed of the agglomerates into the die cavity and their smooth compression in the direct tabletting process. According to several studies, the compactibility improvement brought to crystals by the agglomerate form was clear. It was shown in these studies, the tablet agglomerated crystals compared to single crystals had greater tensile strength which implied the fact that a stronger bonding occurred during compression of agglomerated crystals than in the case of single crystals. The higher tensile strength of the tablets from agglomerated crystals is mainly due to the greater plastic deformation of the agglomerated crystals resulting in greater permanent inter particle contact and stronger bond force than in the case of single crystals.

Conflict of Interest

There is no conflict of interest in this study.

References

1. Tanguy D, Marchal P. Relations between the properties of particles and their process of manufacture. 13th Symposium on Industrial Crystallization: 1996; Toulouse-France: 715.
2. York P, Shekunov BYu. Crystallization processes in pharmaceutical technology and drug delivery design. J Cryst Growth 2000; 211:122-36.
3. Nocent M, Bertocchi L, Espitalier F, Baron M, Couarraze G. Definition of a solvent system for spherical crystallization of salbutamol sulfate by quasi-emulsion solvent diffusion (QESD) method. J Pharm Sci 2001; 90(10):1620-7.
4. Kawashima Y, Cui F, Takeuchi H, Niwa T, Hino T, Kiuchi K. Parameters determining the agglomeration behavior and the micrometric properties of spherically agglomerated crystals prepared by the spherical crystallization technique with miscible solvent systems. Int Natl J Pharm 1995;119: 139-47.
5. Lasagabaster A, Martin C, Goni MM. Preparation of spherically agglomerated crystals of the 3, 5-diglucoside of cyaniding (cyanin). J Chem Tech Biotechnol 1994;60(4): 397–403.
6. Farnand JR, Smith HM, Puddington IE. Spherical agglomeration of solids in liquid suspension. Can J Chem Eng 1961;39: 94–7.
7. Gordon MS, Chowhan LT. Manipulation of naproxen particle morphology via the spherical crystallization technique to achieve a directly compressible raw material. Drug Dev Ind Pharm 1990;16:1279-90.
8. Kawashima Y, Aoki S, Takenaka H. Spherical agglomeration of aminophylline crystals during reaction in liquid by the spherical crystallization technique. Chem Pharm Bull 1982;30: 1837-43.
9. Kawashima Y, Okumura M, Takenaka H. Spherical crystallization: direct spherical agglomeration of salicylic acid crystals during crystallization. Science 1982;216(4550): 1127-8.
10. Sano A, Kuriki T, Kawashima Y, Takeuchi H, Hino T, Niwa T. Particle design of tolbutamide by

spherical crystallization technique. V. Improvement of dissolution and bioavailability of direct compressed tablets prepared using tolbutamide agglomerated crystals. Chem Pharm Bull 1992;40: 3030–5.
11. Kawashima Y. New processes-application of spherical crystallization to particulate design of pharmaceuticals for direct tabletting and coating, and new drug delivery systems. In: Chulia D, Deleuil M, Pourcelot Y, editors. Powder technology and pharmaceutical processes New York: Elsevier; 1994. p. 493-512.
12. Kawashima Y, Okumura M, Takenaka H. The effects of temperature on the spherical crystallization of salicylic acid. Powder Technol 1984;39: 41–7.
13. Kawashima Y, Cui F, Takeuchi H, Niwa T, Hino T, Kiuchi K. Improvements in flowability and compressibility of pharmaceutical crystals for direct tabletting by spherical crystallization with a two solvent system. Powder Technol 1994; 78: 151-7.
14. Jbilou M, Ettabia A, Guyot-Hermann AM, Guyot JS. Ibuprofen agglomeration prepared by phase separation. Drug Dev Ind Pharm 1999;25(3): 297-305.
15. Morishima K, Kawashima Y, Takeuchi H, Niwa T, Hino T, Kawashima Y. Tabletting properties of bucillamine agglomerates prepared by the spherical crystaliization technique. Int J Pharm 1994; 105: 11-8.
16. Kawashima Y, Imai M, Takeuchi H, Yamamoto H, Kamiya K. Development of agglomerated crystals of Ascorbic acid by the spherical crystallization techniques. Powder Technol 2003; 130: 283-9.
17. Maghsoodi M. Effect of process variables on physicomechanical properties of the agglomerates obtained by spherical crystallization technique. Pharm Dev Technol 2011; 16(5): 474-82.
18. Carr RL. Evaluation flow properties of solids. Chem Eng 1965; 72: 163-8.
19. Kawakita K, Ludde KH. Some considerations on powder compression equations. Powder Technol 1971; 4: 61-8.
20. Kuno H. Chapter 5. In: Kubo T, Jimbo G, Saito E, Takahashi H, Hayakawa S. Editors. Powder Theory and Application. Maruzen; Tokyo 1979, 341-346.
21. Kawashima Y, Okumura M, Takenaka H, Kojima A. Direct preparation of spherically agglomerated salicylic acid crystals during crystallization. J Pharm Sci 1984;73(11): 1535-8.
22. Tsunakawa H, Kunii D, Takagi F, Sugita M, Tamura T, Haze H: "Comparing the Flow Properties of Bulk Solids by Tri- axial Shear, Unconfined Yield and Direct Shear Tests". J Soc Powder Technol 1986;23:678- 684.
23. Katta J, Rasmuson AC. Spherical crystallization of benzoic acid. Int J Pharm 2008; 348(1): 61-9.
24.Maghsoodi M, Barghi L. Design of agglomerated crystals of ibuprofen during crystallization: influence of surfactant. Iran J Basic Med Sci 2011; 14(1): 161-9.
25. Kawashima Y, Cui F, Takeuchi H, Niwa T, Hino T, Kiuchi K. Improved static compression behaviors and tablettabilities of spherical agglomerated crystals produced by the spherical crystallization technique with two solvent system. Pharm Res 1995; 12(7): 1040-4.
26. McKenna A, McCafferty DF. Effect of particle size on the compaction mechanism and tensile strength of tablets. J Pharm Pharmacol 1982;34: 347-51.
27. Vromans H, Bolhuis GK, Lerk CF. Magnesium stearate susceptibility of directly compressible materials as an indication of fragmentation properties. Powder Technol 1988;54: 39-44.
28. Paradkar AR, Pawar AP, Chordiya JK, Patil VB, Ketkar AR. Spherical crystallization of celecoxib. Drug Dev Ind Pharm 2002;28 (10):1213-20.
29. Schlanta S, Milosovich G. Compression of pharmaceuitical powders: I. Theory and instrumentation. J Pharm Sci 1964; 53: 562-4.
30. David S, Augsburger LL. Plastic flow during compression of directly compressible fillers and its effect on tablet strength. J Pharm Sci 1977;66: 155-9.
31. Cutt T, Fell JT, Rue PJ, Spring MS. Granulation and compaction of a model system: II. Stress relaxation. Int J Pharm 1987;39: 157-61.
32. Patel CI, Staniforth JN. Determination of the apparent failure viscosity of tablets. J Pharm Pharmacol 1987;39:647-65.
33. Marshall PV, York P. The compaction properties of nitrofurantoin samples crystallized from different solvents. Int J Pharm 1991;67: 59-65.
34. Thati J, Rasmuson AC. On the mechanisms of formation of spherical agglomerates. Eur J Pharm Sci. 2011;42: 365–79.

Phytochemical Screening and Antimicrobial Properties of a Common Brand of Black Tea (*Camellia sinensis*) Marketed in Nigerian Environment

Olosunde O. Funmilayo [1], Abu-Saeed Kamaldeen [1]*, Abu-Saeed Muhammad Buhari [2]

[1] *Research Unit, Peace Standard Pharmaceuticals, Ilorin. Nigeria.*

[2] *Department of Microbiology, University of Ilorin Teaching Hospital, Ilorin. Nigeria.*

ARTICLEINFO

Keywords:
Phytochemical screening
Antimicrobial properties
Black tea
Nigeria

ABSTRACT

Purpose: This study is aimed at determining chemical constituents and antimicrobial activities of a common brand of black tea (Lipton®) in Nigeria. ***Methods:*** Standard methods were employed for testing carbohydrates, tannins, saponins, flavonoids, alkaloids, steroids and terpenes in the tea. Antimicrobial activities of methanolic and aqueous extracts of the tea on four standard strains of organisms: *Escherichia coli*, *Pseudomonas aeruginosa*, *Staphylococcus aureus* and *Bacillus subtilis* were also determined by standard methods. ***Results:*** Results showed that the tea contains tannin and reducing sugar. Concentrations of 1%, 2%, 4%, 6%, 8% and 10% aqueous and methanolic extract of black tea were prepared and their zones of inhibition determined against the four test organisms using the cup plate method. This was compared with zones for standard disc Gentamicin (10 μg) and Erythromycin (15 μg). *Pseudomonas aeruginosa* was sensitive to 2% to 10% aqueous extracts and intermediate to 6%, 8% and 10% methanolic extracts. *E. coli* was intermediately sensitive to 6%, 8% and 10% aqueous extract and 2% to 10% methanolic extracts. *B. subtilis* was intermediately sensitive to 4%, 6% and 8% aqueous extract and 4% to 10% methanolic extract but sensitive to 10% aqueous extract. *Staph.aureus* was intermediately sensitive to 4% to 10% aqueous extracts and 2% to 10% methanolic extracts. *B. subtilis* had the lowest MIC values of both aqueous and methanolic extracts. ***Conclusion:*** In conclusion, this study has shown that Lipton® has antimicrobial properties on *E.coli*, *Staph.aureus*, *B.subtilis* and *Ps.aeruginosa* and contains tannin and reducing sugar.

Introduction

Tea is the second most commonly drunk liquid after water and the most common beverage drunk.[1] Tea, the drink, is an infusion of variously processed leaves and flowers of one of the varieties of an evergreen shrub botanically called *Camellia sinensis*. Black tea is one of a varieties of preparations made from *Camellia sinensis*. Others include green teas, white tea and oolong tea. The processes of obtaining the various types of tea are different.

The chemical compositions of *C. sinensis* is not completely known but is understood to be quite complex. Black tea is more complex than green tea partly because of the oxidation process that occurs during fermentation.[2] Chemical reactions take place when dried and finished tea is extracted into water increasing the complexity of the chemical mix in a cup of tea. When left to stand, further chemical reactions still takes place in the tea. *C. sinensis* has been used for different purposes which could be classified as edible use, medicinal use (Internal and external uses) and other uses which include dye, essential oil, food flavouring and perfumery.[3]

C. sinensis has been reported to have physiological and pharmacological effects,[4,5] strengthening capillary, slows down catabolism of catecholamine, exert anti inflammatory effects by enhancing effect of Vitamin C. It acts as an anti oxidant, also as hypocholesterolemic action. It inhibits angiotensin converting enzyme and the growth of implanted malignant cells.[6] One of the earliest reports of *C. sinensis* regarding its anti microbial activity is its recommendation by an army surgeon in soldiers' water bottles as a prophylactic against typhoid.[7]

There are several reports on the antibacterial effects of tea in vitro and in vivo mainly on intestinal pathogen.[8-10] The Japanese and others in a series of well conducted systemic studies showed that tea extract inhibit and kill various species of *Staphylococcus*, *Salmonella*, *Shigella* and *Vibrio*.[11]

The aim of this study is to determine the chemical constituents of a common brand of black tea (Lipton®) found in the Nigerian environment and to compare its

***Corresponding author:** Abu-Saeed Kamaldeen, Research Unit, Peace Standard Pharmaceuticals, Ilorin. Nigeria.
Email: kamal.abusaeed@yahoo.com

antimicrobial properties with standard antimicrobial agents using Gentamicin and Erythromycin disc.

Materials and Methods

Extraction of Black tea

Aqueous extraction was done as follows: sterile distilled water was allowed to boil, 100ml of the water was measured into a conical flask with five (5) Lipton® bags and allowed to extract (infusion) for about two minutes.

Alcoholic extraction was done using 90% Methanol. About 100ml of Methanol was measured with a measuring cylinder into a conical flask containing five Lipton® tea bags and allowed to extract for 12 hours.

The Aqueous and Methanolic extracts were poured into separate crucibles and evaporated to dryness on a water bath (Aqueous at less than 100°C and Methanolic at 60°C). Two grams (2g) of powdered dry extract was dissolved in 20ml volume each of distilled water of both Aqueous and Methanolic extract to produce 10% solutions. Serial dilution was done to obtain 8%, 6%, 4%, 2% and 1% concentrations. The different concentrations were made inside labelled, sterile bottles.

Preliminary phytochemical screening of the extracts

About 2g of the dried extract was weighed and dissolved in distilled water. The solution obtained was then subjected to various phytochemical screening to identify the chemical components present in the extract using qualitative chemical tests with the use of chemical reagents. Standard methods were employed for testing carbohydrates, tannins, saponins, flavonoids, alkaloids, steroids and terpenes.[12,13]

Antimicrobial screening of the extract

Culture of the test organisms (*Escherichia coli* ATCC 25722, *Pseudomonas aeruginosa* ATCC 27853, *Staphylococcus aureus* ATCC 25923 and *Bacillus subtilis* NCTC8325B76) were prepared by an inoculating surface scrapes on solid media into 5ml of sterile nutrient broth which was then incubated at 37°C overnight. The overnight cultures were diluted to obtain approximately 10^6 colony forming units according to standard practice (1 in 1000 dilutions for Gram positive and 1 in 5000 dilutions for Gram negative organisms). Already prepared 20ml sterile nutrient agar were melted and allowed to cool to body temperature and poured into sterile petri dish. The melted agar were allowed to solidify and then flooded with the required final dilution of the organism, the excess was discarded and the petri dishes labelled. This was allowed to diffuse into the agar for 30minutes. Wells were made on the already flooded agar using cup borer (10mm) and the wells were sealed with a drop of the melted agar. Then 0.1ml of the prepared extract concentrates to be tested was then filled into the hole and labelled. This was allowed to diffuse for at least an hour and then incubated for 24 hours at 37°C. The diameter of the zones where growth was inhibited was measured in millimetres (mm) and recorded. For the sensitivity test of standard antibiotics instead of drilling holes, the sensitivity disc (Gentamicin and Erythromycin) were placed on the agar in the petri disc and labelled. This was allowed to stand for one hour to enable antibiotics to diffuse. The plates were incubated at 37°C for 24 hours. The zones where growth was inhibited was measured (in mm) and recorded.

The Minimum Inhibitory Concentration (MIC) was determined by plotting the graph of log concentration against the diameter in mm. The MIC from the graph was the antilog of the intercept value obtained at the Y-axis (log conc.) axis.

Results

As shown on Table 1, the phytochemical screening carried out on the Lipton brand of *Camellia sinensis* extract was found to contain reducing sugar and tannins.

Generally, the observed mean zone of inhibition on Table 2 shows an increase in zone with increase in the *C. sinensis* concentrate. However, there were instances of repeated zone of inhibition like 4% and 6% aqueous concentration on *B. subtilis*. There were instances of low zone of inhibition between two high zones like 4% aqueous extract on *Ps. aeruginosa* and 2% and 4% Methanolic concentrates of *Ps. aeruginosa* and *E.coli* respectively. High zone of inhibition between two low zones were observed at 4% aqueous and 8% aqueous concentrate of *Staph.aureus* and *Ps.aeruginosa* respectively.

With the exception of 4% methanolic concentrate the zone of inhibition on *Staph.aureus* is almost the same ranging between 14.5 to 15.5mm using CLSI standard values; all the organisms were sensitive to Gentamicin while only *Ps.aeruginosa* and *B.subtilis* showed moderate or intermediate sensitivity to Erythromycin. Gentamicin gave a higher zone of inhibition as compared to erythromycin showing that it is more effective.

Figures 1 and 2 show the graphs of log concentration against diameter for methanolic and aqueous extracts on various organisms respectively. Table 3 above shows the MIC values of aqueous and methanolic extract of *C.sinensis* which indicates the minimum concentration required to inhibit the growth of an organism calculated from figures 1 and 2.

Table 1. Phytochemical screening of lipton® (*Camellia sinensis*) extract

Phytochemical compound	Result
Carbohydrate	Absent
Reducing sugar	Present
Tannin	Present
Saponin	Absent
Flavonoid	Absent
Alkaloid	Absent
Steroid and triterpenes	Absent

Table 2. Mean zone of inhibitions of various concentrations of aqueous extract, methanolic extract and standard disc (gentamicin 10µg, erythromycin 15µg) on *Escherichia coli, Pseudomonas aeruginosa, Bacillus subtilis, Staphylococcus aureus*

Mean zone of inhibition														
-	Aqueous extract (mm)						Methanolic extract (mm)						Standard disc (mm)	
Organisms	1%	2%	4%	6%	8%	10%	1%	2%	4%	6%	8%	10%	G	E
Ps. Aeruginosa	-	19	11.5	22	26.5	22	11	10.5	12.5	14	16	15.5	27	16
E. coli	-	12.5	13	15	16.5	17.5	-	14	13.5	15.5	16	16.5	24.5	6.5
B. subtilis	12.5	12	15	15	16.5	18	-	13	14.5	15	16	17	25.5	14
Staph aureus	8.5	12	15.5	14	16	16.5	-	15	9	15.5	14.5	15	28	12

Cup borer size: 1cm (10mm) ; G: Gentamicin; E: Erythromycin
Clinical and laboratory standard institute (CLSI) values:
Gentamicin (10µg): sensitivity (>18mm), intermediate (-), resistance (>13mm)
Erythromycin (15µg): sensitivity (>18mm), intermediate (14-17mm), resistance (>13mm).

Discussion

From the agar diffusion experiment carried out to determine the susceptibility of *Ps.aeruginosa, Staph.aureus, B.subtilis* and *E.coli* to different concentrations of black tea extract, almost all the organisms were sensitive at all concentration with the exception of 1% aqueous extract on *Ps.aeruginosa* and *E.coli* and 1% methanolic extract on *E.coli, B.subtilis* and *Staph.aureus*. The antimicrobial properties could be as a result of the presence of tannin which is known generally for antimicrobial activity.

The inconsistency in the zone of inhibition aside from other factors such as batch work that could affect the result could also be as a result of unavoidable variation in the time of preparation of the concentrate and its use. A cup of black tea when left to stand for a while changes colour from black to milky black colour especially when left to cool. This physical change could indicate chemical changes or reaction taking place in the black tea.

Using the Clinical and Laboratory Standard Institute (CLSI) standard value for Gentamicin and Erythromycin, *Ps.aeruginosa* gave a similar zone of inhibition to the sensitivity value of Erythromycin and Gentamicin at 4% aqueous extract and above and *B.subtilis* at 10% aqueous extract. Using the 14 to 17mm CLSI intermediate value for Erythromycin, *Ps.aeruginosa, E.coli, B.subtilis* and *Staph.aureus* gave similar zone of inhibition to the intermediate sensitivity value of Erythromycin at 6%, 2%, 4%, 6% methanolic extract and above respectively. For the aqueous extract, *E.coli, B.subtilis* and *Staph.aureus* similar zones were at 6%, 4% and 4% concentrations and above respectively. Organisms that gave zone of inhibition from 13 and below matches with the resistance value of both Gentamicin and Erythromycin at the various concentrations.

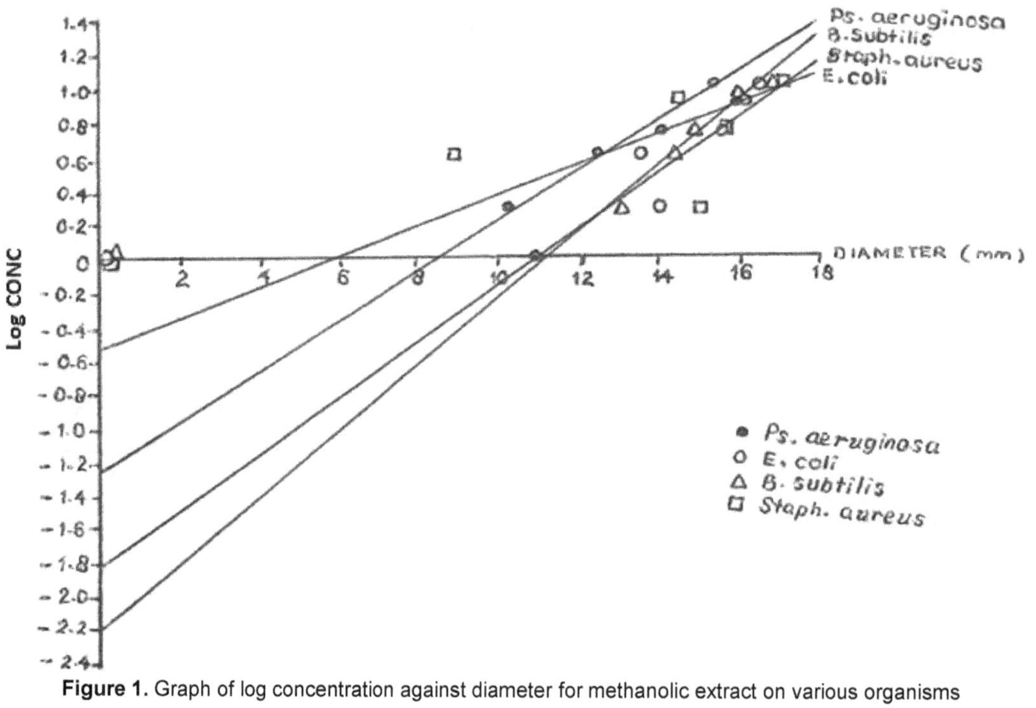

Figure 1. Graph of log concentration against diameter for methanolic extract on various organisms

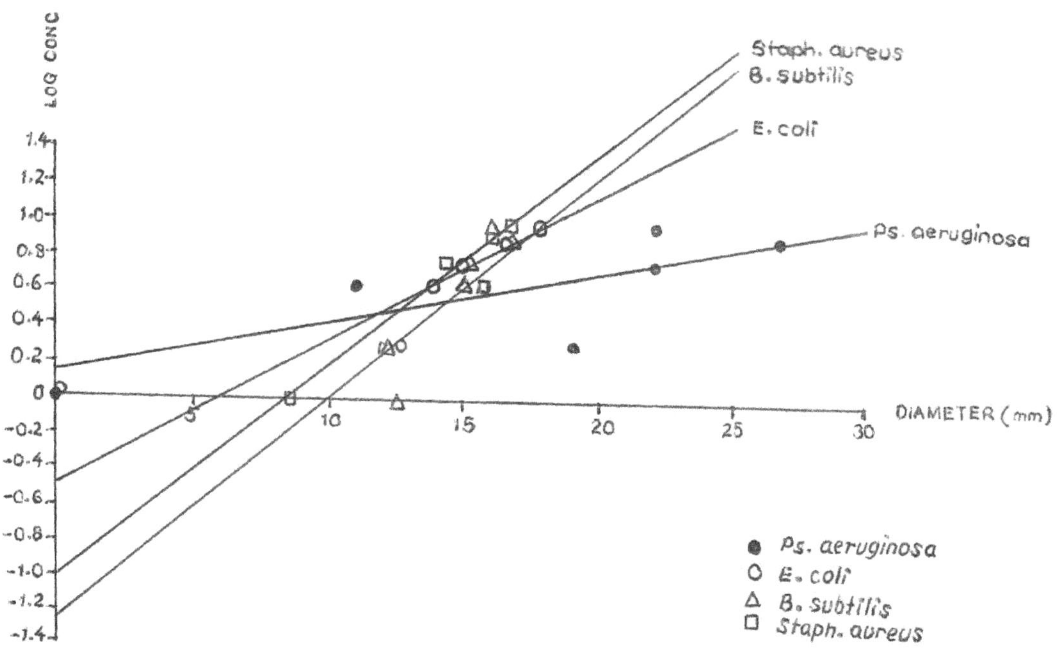

Figure 2. Graph of log concentration against diameter for aqueous extract on various organisms

Table 3. MIC value of aqueous and methanolic extract of *Camellia sinensis*

-	MIC value (x 10 μg/ml)	
Organisms	**Aqueous**	**Methanolic**
Ps.aeruginosa	1.413	0.050
Staph.aureus	0.089	0.013
E.coli	0.280	0.250
B.subtilis	0.056	0.005

The MIC value of an agent is the lowest concentration that prevents growth after overnight incubation. For quantitative estimates of antibiotics activities, dilutions of the antibiotic may be incorporated into broth or agar medium and incubated with the test organism. The MIC value obtained graphically showed that the aqueous extract has increasing MIC values on the organism in the following order: *B.subtilis*, *Staph.aureus*, *E.coli* and *Ps.aeruginosa*. The methanolic extract on the other hand has increasing MIC value on the organism in the order *B.subtilis*, *Staph.aureus*, *Ps.aeruginosa* and *E.coli*. The smaller the MIC value the more effective the extract, that is, the smaller the concentration required to inhibit the growth of the organism hence methanolic extract on *B.subtilis* is the most effective and aqueous extract on *Ps.aeruginosa* is the least effective.

Generally, the methanolic extract gave smaller MIC values on each organism than the aqueous extract. This could be as a result of the inherent antimicrobial property of the methanol itself. Considering the zone of inhibition however, once the aqueous extract starts eliciting its effect, it gives greater zone of inhibition than the methanolic extract. This can be seen in *B.subtilis* though it has a 0.05μg/ml methanolic MIC value did not inhibit at 10% concentration while *Ps.aeruginosa* with 14.13μg/ml of aqueous extract MIC value was inhibited at 2%. These differences might be as a result of the mechanism of action of the tea and also because of difference in their cell walls.

Conclusion

Within the limits of experimental errors, it was found out that Lipton brand of *Camellia sinensis* contains tannin and reducing sugar. It has also been shown to have antimicrobial properties on *E.coli, Staph.aureus, B.subtilis* and *Ps.aeruginosa*. From the MIC values obtained, *B.subtilis* requires the least concentration of either methanolic or aqueous extract to inhibit its growth.

Conflict of interest

The authors report no conflicts of interest.

References

1. Okubo S, Ikigai H, Toda M, Shimamura T. The anti-haemolysis activity of tea and coffee. Lett Appl Microbiol 1989; 9(2):65-6.
2. Hamilton-Miller JMT. Antimicrobial properties of tea (Camellia sinensis L.) Antimicrob Agents Chemother 1995;39 (11): 2375-7.
3. Samman S, Sandstrom B, Toft MB, Bukhaye K, Jensen M, Sorensen S, et al. Green tea extracts to

foods reduces non home-iron absorption. AM J Clinc Nutri 2001; 73(3):607-12.
4. Min Z, Paige X. Quantitative analysis of the active constituents in green Tea. Pyrometer Res 1991; 5:239-40.
5. Stagg GV, Millin DJ. The nutritional and therapeutic value of tea-a review. J Sci Food Agric 1975; 26: 1439-59.
6. Hattori M, Kusumoto IT, Namba T, Ishıgami T, Hara Y. Effect of tea polyphenols on glucan synthesis by glucosyltransferase from Streptococcus mutans. Chem Pharm Bull 1990;38(3):717-20.
7. Using tea to fight typhoid. Tea and Coffee Journal 1923;129.
8. Das DN. Studies on the antibiotic activity of tea. J ind Chem Soc 1962. 39:849-54.
9. Ryu E. Prophylactic effect of tea on pathogenic micro-organism infection to human and animals (1). Int J Zoonoses 1980; 7(2): 164-70.
10. Scalbert A. Antimicrobial properties tannins. Phytochemistry 1991. 30: 3875-83.
11. Toda M, Okubo S, Hiyoshi R, Shimamura T. The bactericidal activity of tea and coffee. Lelt Appli Microbial 1989; 8: 123-5.
12. Trease GE, Evans WC. Introduction and General Methods in Pharmacognosy. 14th ed. London: Alden press; 2002.
13. Sofowora EA. Traditional medicine and medicinal plant of Africa. Nigeria: Spectrum books publishers; 1982.

Permissions

 Every chapter published in this book has been scrutinized by our experts. Their significance has been extensively debated. The topics covered herein carry significant findings which will fuel the growth of the discipline. They may even be implemented as practical applications or may be referred to as a beginning point for another development.

The contributors of this book come from diverse backgrounds, making this book a truly international effort. This book will bring forth new frontiers with its revolutionizing research information and detailed analysis of the nascent developments around the world.

We would like to thank all the contributing authors for lending their expertise to make the book truly unique. They have played a crucial role in the development of this book. Without their invaluable contributions this book wouldn't have been possible. They have made vital efforts to compile up to date information on the varied aspects of this subject to make this book a valuable addition to the collection of many professionals and students.

This book was conceptualized with the vision of imparting up-to-date information and advanced data in this field. To ensure the same, a matchless editorial board was set up. Every individual on the board went through rigorous rounds of assessment to prove their worth. After which they invested a large part of their time researching and compiling the most relevant data for our readers.

The editorial board has been involved in producing this book since its inception. They have spent rigorous hours researching and exploring the diverse topics which have resulted in the successful publishing of this book. They have passed on their knowledge of decades through this book. To expedite this challenging task, the publisher supported the team at every step. A small team of assistant editors was also appointed to further simplify the editing procedure and attain best results for the readers.

Apart from the editorial board, the designing team has also invested a significant amount of their time in understanding the subject and creating the most relevant covers. They scrutinized every image to scout for the most suitable representation of the subject and create an appropriate cover for the book.

The publishing team has been an ardent support to the editorial, designing and production team. Their endless efforts to recruit the best for this project, has resulted in the accomplishment of this book. They are a veteran in the field of academics and their pool of knowledge is as vast as their experience in printing. Their expertise and guidance has proved useful at every step. Their uncompromising quality standards have made this book an exceptional effort. Their encouragement from time to time has been an inspiration for everyone.

The publisher and the editorial board hope that this book will prove to be a valuable piece of knowledge for researchers, students, practitioners and scholars across the globe.

List of Contributors

Maryam Maghsoodi
Drug applied Research Center and Faculty of Pharmacy, Tabriz University of Medical Sciences, Tabriz, Iran

Elham Hemati, Bahram Qadermazi and Zahra Yari
Student Research Committee, Tabriz University of Medical Sciences, Tabriz, Iran

Nazli Saeedi Kouzehkonani
Drug Applied Research Center, Tabriz University of Medical Sciences, Tabriz, Iran

Mohammad Ali Eghbal
Drug Applied Research Center, Tabriz University of Medical Sciences, Tabriz, Iran
Department of Pharmacology and Toxicology, Faculty of Pharmacy, Tabriz University of Medical Sciences, Tabriz, Iran

Sara Mostafalou
Drug Applied Research Center, Tabriz University of Medical Sciences, Tabriz, Iran
Department of Pharmacology and Toxicology, Faculty of Pharmacy, Tabriz University of Medical Sciences, Tabriz, Iran
Students Research Committee, Tabriz University of Medical Sciences, Tabriz, Iran

Mohammad Abdollahi
Faculty of Pharmacy, and Pharmaceutical Sciences Research Center, Tehran University of Medical Sciences, Tehran, Iran

S. Safari and M.H. Zarrintan
Department of Pharmaceutics, Faculty of Pharmacy, Tabriz University of Medical Sciences, Tabriz, Iran

M. Soleimani
Department of Hematology, Faculty of Medical Science, Tarbiat Modares University, Tehran, Iran

F. A. Dorkoosh, M. Rafiee Tehrani and H. Akbari
Department of Pharmaceutics, Faculty of Pharmacy, Tehran University of Medical Sciences, Tehran, Iran

B. Larijani
Endocrinology and Metabolism Research Center, Tehran University of Medical Sciences, Tehran, Iran

Mohite P.B.
Department of Pharmaceutical Chemistry, MES's College of Pharmacy, Sonai, Ahmednagar, Maharashtra, India
Research Scholar, Department of Pharmacy, Vinayaka Missions University, Salem, Tamilnadu, India

Bhaskar V.H.2
Department of Pharmaceutical Chemistry, MP Patel College of Pharmacy, Kapadwanj, Gujrat,India

Badir Delf Loveymi
Faculty of Pharmacy, Tabriz University of Medical Sciences, Tabriz, Iran
Biotechnology Research Center, Tabriz University of Medical Sciences, Tabriz, Iran

Mitra Jelvehgari
Faculty of Pharmacy, Tabriz University of Medical Sciences, Tabriz, Iran
Drug Applied Research Center, Tabriz University of Medical Sciences, Tabriz, Iran

Parvin Zakeri-Milani
Faculty of Pharmacy, Tabriz University of Medical Sciences, Tabriz, Iran
Liver and Gastrointestinal Diseases Research Center, Tabriz University of Medical Sciences, Tabriz, Iran

Hadi Valizadeh
Faculty of Pharmacy, Tabriz University of Medical Sciences, Tabriz, Iran
Research Center for Pharmaceutical Nanotechnology, Tabriz University of Medical Sciences, Tabriz, Iran

Mina Islambulchilar
School of Pharmacy, Zanjan University of Medical Sciences, Zanjan, Iran
Faculty of Pharmacy, Tabriz University of Medical Sciences, Tabriz, Iran
Student Research Committee, Tabriz University of Medical Sciences, Tabriz, Iran

Mohammad Reza Sattari
Faculty of Pharmacy, Tabriz University of Medical Sciences, Tabriz, Iran
Infectious & Tropical diseases research center, Tabriz University of Medical Sciences, Tabriz, Iran

Mohammad Sardashti
Faculty of Pharmacy, Tabriz University of Medical Sciences, Tabriz, Iran
Student Research Committee, Tabriz University of Medical Sciences, Tabriz, Iran

Farzaneh Lotfipour
Faculty of Pharmacy, Tabriz University of Medical Sciences, Tabriz, Iran
Hematology and Oncology Research Center, Tabriz University of Medical Sciences, Tabriz, Iran

Laleh khodaie
Drugs Applied Research Center, Tabriz University of Medical Sciences, Tabriz, Iran
Student Research Committee, Tabriz University of Medical Sciences, Tabriz, Iran
Faculty of Pharmacy, Tabriz University of Medical Sciences, Tabriz, Iran

Abbas Delazar
Drugs Applied Research Center, Tabriz University of Medical Sciences, Tabriz, Iran
Faculty of Pharmacy, Tabriz University of Medical Sciences, Tabriz, Iran

Farzaneh Lotfipour and Hossein Nazemiyeh
Faculty of Pharmacy, Tabriz University of Medical Sciences, Tabriz, Iran

Mohammad-Hosein Zarrintan
Faculty of Pharmacy, Tabriz University of Medical Sciences, Tabriz, Iran

Parvin Zakeri-Milani
Faculty of Pharmacy, Tabriz University of Medical Sciences, Tabriz, Iran
Liver and Gastrointestinal Diseases Research Center

Niaz Mousavian-Fathi
Faculty of Pharmacy, Tabriz University of Medical Sciences, Tabriz, Iran
Student Research Committee, Tabriz University of Medical Sciences, Tabriz, Iran

Saeed Ghanbarzadeh
Faculty of Pharmacy, Tabriz University of Medical Sciences, Tabriz, Iran
Drug Applied Research Center, Tabriz University of Medical Sciences, Tabriz, Iran

Hadi Valizadeh
Faculty of Pharmacy, Tabriz University of Medical Sciences, Tabriz, Iran
Research Center for Pharmaceutical Nanotechnology, Tabriz University of Medical Sciences, Tabriz, Iran

Eskandar Moghimipour and Somayeh Handali
Nanotechnology Research Center, Ahvaz Jundishapur University of Medical Sciences, Ahvaz, Iran

Morteza Azhdarzadeh
Research Center for Pharmaceutical Nanotechnology, Tabriz University of Medical Sciences, Tabriz, Iran
Students Research Committee, Tabriz University of Medical Sciences, Tabriz, Iran

Hadi Valizadeh
Research Center for Pharmaceutical Nanotechnology, Tabriz University of Medical Sciences, Tabriz, Iran
Faculty of Pharmacy, Tabriz University of Medical Sciences, Tabriz, Iran

Farzaneh Lotfipour
Faculty of Pharmacy, Tabriz University of Medical Sciences, Tabriz, Iran
Biotechnology Research Center, Tabriz University of Medical Sciences, Tabriz, Iran

Parvin Zakeri-Milani
Faculty of Pharmacy, Tabriz University of Medical Sciences, Tabriz, Iran
Liver and Gastrointestinal Diseases Research Center, Tabriz University of Medical Sciences, Tabriz, Iran

Ghobad Mohammadi
Faculty of Pharmacy, Kermanshah University of Medical Sciences, Kermanshah, Iran

Fatemeh Fathiazad
Department of Pharmacognosy, Faculty of Pharmacy, Tabriz University of Medical Sciences, Iran

Masoumeh Mazandarani
Islamic Azad University Gorgan Branch, Gorgan, Iran

Sanaz Hamedeyazdan
Department of Pharmacognosy, Faculty of Pharmacy, Tabriz University of Medical Sciences, Iran
Student Research Committee, Tabriz University of Medical Sciences, Tabriz, Iran

Fithriyatun Nisa, Adam Hermawan, Retno Murwanti and Edy Meiyanto
Cancer chemoprevention research center, Faculty of pharmacy, universitas gadjah mada, Sekip Utara II, Yogyakarta 55281, Indonesia

Maryam Maghsoodi
Drug applied Research Center and School of Pharmacy, Tabriz University of Medical Sciences, Tabriz, Iran

Katayoun Derakhshandeh and Zahra Yari
School of Pharmacy, Kermanshah University of Medical Sciences, Kermanshah, Iran

Josephine Leno Jenita
Department of Pharmaceutics, Dayananda Sagar College of Pharmacy, Kumaraswamy Layout, Bangalore - 560078, Karnataka, India

Negar Bashardoust
Department of Pharmaceutics, Dayananda Sagar College of Pharmacy, Kumaraswamy Layout, Bangalore - 560078, Karnataka, India
Student Research Committee, Tabriz University of Medical Sciences, Tabriz, Iran

Parvin Zakeri-Milani
Faculty of Pharmacy, Tabriz University of Medical Sciences, Tabriz, Iran
Drug Applied Research Center, Tabriz University of Medical Sciences, Tabriz, Iran

Sattari Mohammadreza
Neurosciences Research Centre, Tabriz University of Medical Sciences, Tabriz, Iran
Faculty of Pharmacy, Tabriz University of Medical Sciences, Tabriz, Iran

Islambulchilar Mina
Infectious and Tropical Diseases Research Centre, Tabriz, Iran
Faculty of Pharmacy, Tabriz University of Medical Sciences, Tabriz, Iran

Toluyi Mohsen
Students Research Committee, Tabriz University of Medical Sciences, Tabriz 51664-14766, Iran

Mashayekhi Siminozar
NPMC, Tabriz University of Medical Sciences, Tabriz 51664-14766, Iran
Faculty of Pharmacy, Tabriz University of Medical Sciences, Tabriz, Iran

Hadi Valizadeh
Faculty of Pharmacy, Tabriz University of Medical Sciences, Tabriz, Iran
Research Center for Pharmaceutical Nanotechnology, Tabriz University of Medical Sciences, Tabriz, Iran

Parvin Zakeri-Milani
Faculty of Pharmacy, Tabriz University of Medical Sciences, Tabriz, Iran
Liver and Gastrointestinal Diseases Research Center, Tabriz University of Medical Sciences, Tabriz, Iran

Aynoor Farajnia
Student Research Committee, Tabriz University of Medical Sciences, Tabriz, Iran
Drug Applied Research Center, Tabriz University of Medical Sciences, Tabriz, Iran

Wenqiong Mai and Xican Li
School of Chinese Herbal Medicine, Guangzhou University of Chinese Medicine, Guangzhou, China

Dongfeng Chen
School of Basic Medicine, Guangzhou University of Chinese Medicine, Guangzhou, China

Shantaram Gajanan Khanage
Research scholar, Department of Pharmacy,Vinayaka Missions University, Salem, Sankari main road, NH-47,Tamilnadu, India

S. Appala Raju
Department of Pharmaceutical chemistry, H.K.E.'S College of Pharmacy, Sedam road, Gulbarga, Karnataka, India

Popat Baban Mohite and Ramdas Bhanudas Pandhare
Department of Pharmaceutical chemistry, M.E.S. College of Pharmacy, Sonai, Tq-Newasa, Dist.-Ahmednagar, Maharashtra, India

Eskandar Moghimipour
Nanotechnology Research Center, Jundishapur University of Medical Sciences, Ahvaz, Iran

Anayatollah Salimi
Nanotechnology Research Center, Jundishapur University of Medical Sciences, Ahvaz, Iran
Department of Pharmaceutics, Faculty of Pharmacy, Jundishapur University of Medical Sciences, Ahvaz, Iran

Fatemeh Leis
Department of Pharmaceutics, Faculty of Pharmacy, Jundishapur University of Medical Sciences, Ahvaz, Iran

Daryosh Mohammadnejad and Ayda Azami
Drug Applied Research Center, Tabriz University of Medical Sciences, Tabriz, Iran

Ali Abedelahi, Jafar Soleimani-rad and Morteza Rashtbar
Department of Anatomical Sciences, Tabriz University of Medical Sciences, Tabriz, Iran

Ameneh Mohammadi-roshandeh
Department of Anatomical Sciences, Hamedan University of Medical Sciences, Hamedan, Iran

Afshin Zahedi
Faculty of Veterinary Medicine, Islamic Azad University, Rasht Branch, Rasht, Iran

Fatemeh Fathiazad
Department of Pharmacognosy, faculty of Pharmacy, Tabriz University of Medical Sciences, Tabriz, Iran

Arash Khaki
Women's Reproductive Health Research Center, Tabriz University of Medical Sciences, Tabriz, Iran

Behnam Ahmadnejad
Faculty of Veterinary Medicine, Islamic Azad University, sciences & Research campus Branch, Tehran, Iran

Leila Barghi
Faculty of Pharmacy, Tabriz University of Medical Sciences, Tabriz, Iran
Student Research Committee, Tabriz University of Medical Sciences, Tabriz, Iran

Jaleh Barar
Faculty of Pharmacy, Tabriz University of Medical Sciences, Tabriz, Iran

Davoud Asgari
Faculty of Pharmacy, Tabriz University of Medical Sciences, Tabriz, Iran
Research Center for Pharmaceutical Nanotechnology, Tabriz University of Medical Sciences, Tabriz, Iran

Hadi Valizadeh
Faculty of Pharmacy, Tabriz University of Medical Sciences, Tabriz, Iran
Drug Applied Research Center, Tabriz University of Medical Sciences, Tabriz, Iran

Ayuob Aghanejad
Research Center for Pharmaceutical Nanotechnology, Tabriz University of Medical Sciences, Tabriz, Iran
Faculty of Pharmacy, Tehran University of Medical Sciences, Tehran, Iran

Ashish Jain and Satish Nayak
Bansal College of Pharmacy, Kokta, Anand Nagar, Bhopal-462021, India

Vandana Soni
Department of Pharmaceutical Sciences, Dr H.S.Gour Vishwavidyalaya, Sagar 470003, M.P. India

Yahya Rahimpour
Biotechnology Research Center and Student Research Committee, Tabriz University of Medical Sciences, Tabriz, Iran

Hamed Hamishehkar
Pharmaceutical Technology Laboratory, Drug Applied Research Center, Tabriz University of Medical Sciences, Tabriz, Iran

Heibatullah Kalantari, Mohsen Rezaei, Masoud Mahdavinia, Mojtaba Kalantar, Zivar Amanpour and Golnaz Varnaseri
Faculty of Pharmacy, Toxicology Research Center, Ahvaz Jundishapur University of Medical Sciences, Ahvaz, Iran

Javad Mahmoudi and Morteza Samini
Department of Pharmacology, Science and Research Branch, Islamic Azad University, Tehran, Iran

Alireza Mohajjel Nayebi
Department of Pharmacology and Toxicology, Faculty of Pharmacy, Tabriz University of Medical Science, Tabriz 51664, Iran
Drug Applied Research Center, Tabriz University of Medical Sciences, Tabriz 51664, Iran

Siyamak Reyhani-Rad
Department of laboratory sciences, Marand Branch, Islamic Azad University, Marand, Iran

Mohite P.B., Pandhare R.B. and Khanage S.G.
Department of Pharmaceutical Chemistry, MES's College of Pharmacy, Sonai, Ahmednagar, Maharashtra, India

Hamzeh Hosseinzadeh, Mahmood Eydi and Mehdi Ghaffarlou
Department of Anesthesiology, Tabriz University of Medical Sciences, Tabriz, Iran

Kamyar Ghabili
Physical Medicine and Rehabilitation Research Center, Tabriz University of Medical Sciences, Tabriz, Iran

Samad EJ Golzari
Medical Philosophy and History Research Center, Tabriz University of Medical Sciences, Tabriz, Iran
Students' Research Committee, Tabriz University of Medical Sciences, Tabriz, Iran

Ahad Bavili Tabrizi
Department of Medicinal Chemistry, Faculty of Pharmacy and Biotechnology Research Center, Tabriz University of Medical Sciences, Tabriz, Iran

Ahmad Rezazadeh
Student Research Committee, Tabriz University of Medical Sciences, Tabriz, Iran

Hamdolah Sharifi and Safar Farajnia
Drug Applied Research Center, Tabriz University of Medical Sceinces, Tabriz, Iran

Alireza Mohajjel Nayebi
Department of Pharmacology and Toxicology, Faculty of Pharmacy, Tabriz University of Medical Sceinces, Tabriz, Iran

M. Ruhul Amin, Ripon Mondol, M. Rowshanul Habib and M. Tofazzal Hossain
Department of Biochemistry and Molecular Biology, Rajshahi University, Rajshahi-6205, Bangladesh

Ziba Islambulchilar
Faculty of Pharmacy, Tabriz University of Medical Sciences, Tabriz, Iran
Faculty of Pharmacy, Zanjan University of Medical Sciences, Zanjan, Iran
Student Research Committee, Tabriz University of Medical Sciences, Tabriz, Iran

Saeed Ghanbarzadeh
Faculty of Pharmacy, Tabriz University of Medical Sciences, Tabriz, Iran
Drug Applied Research Center, Tabriz University of Medical Sciences, Tabriz, Iran

Hadi Valizadeh
Faculty of Pharmacy, Tabriz University of Medical Sciences, Tabriz, Iran
Research Center for Pharmaceutical Nanotechnology, Tabriz University of Medical Sciences, Tabriz, Iran

Parvin Zakeri-Milani
Faculty of Pharmacy, Tabriz University of Medical Sciences, Tabriz, Iran
Liver and Gastrointestinal Diseases Research Center, Tabriz University of Medical Sciences, Tabriz, Iran

Shahram Emami
Student Research Committee, Tabriz University of Medical Sciences, Tabriz, Iran

Maryam Maghsoodi
Drug applied Research Center and Faculty of Pharmacy, Tabriz University of Medical Sciences, Tabriz, Iran

Olosunde O. Funmilayo and Abu-Saeed Kamaldeen
Research Unit, Peace Standard Pharmaceuticals, Ilorin. Nigeria

Abu-Saeed Muhammad Buhari
Department of Microbiology, University of Ilorin Teaching Hospital, Ilorin. Nigeria

Index

www.ingramcontent.com/pod-product-compliance
Lightning Source LLC
LaVergne TN
LVHW060600210926
848485LV00005B/1349